# Hypochondriasis:
# Modern Perspectives
# on an Ancient Malady

# HYPOCHONDRIASIS
## Modern Perspectives
## on an Ancient Malady

Edited by
### VLADAN STARCEVIC, M.D.

*University of Belgrade*
*School of Medicine and*
*Institute of Mental Health*
*Belgrade, Yugoslavia*
*and*
*Hunter Mental Health Services*
*and University of Newcastle*
*Newcastle, Australia*

### DON R. LIPSITT, M.D.

*Department of Psychiatry*
*Mount Auburn Hospital*
*Cambridge, Massachusetts*
*and*
*Harvard Medical School*
*Boston, Massachusetts*

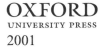

OXFORD
UNIVERSITY PRESS
2001

# OXFORD
UNIVERSITY PRESS

Oxford   New York
Athens   Auckland   Bangkok   Bogotá   Buenos Aires   Calcutta
Cape Town   Chennai   Dar es Salaam   Delhi   Florence   Hong Kong   Istanbul
Karachi   Kuala Lumpur   Madrid   Melbourne   Mexico City   Mumbai
Nairobi   Paris   São Paulo   Shanghai   Singapore   Taipei   Tokyo   Toronto   Warsaw

and associated companies in
Berlin   Ibadan

Published by Oxford University Press, Inc.,
198 Madison Avenue, New York, New York, 10016
http://www.oup-usa.org

Library of Congress Cataloging-in-Publication Data
Hypochondriasis : modern perspectives on an ancient malady/
edited by Vladan Starcevic and Don R. Lipsitt.
p. ; cm.   Includes bibliographical references and index.
ISBN 0-19-512676-9
1. Hypochondria.
I. Starcevic, Vladan,
II. Lipsitt, Don R.
[DNLM: 1. Hypochondriasis. WM 178 H998 2001]   RC552.H8 H97 2001   616.85'25—dc21   00-035956

*Cover Illustration*
   Courtesy of the Fogg Art Museum, Harvard University Art Museums,
   Gift of Carl Pickhardt, Class of 1931. Copyright © Presidents and Fellows
   of Harvard College, Harvard University.

9 8 7 6 5 4 3 2 1

Printed in the United States of America
on acid-free paper

To Katarina, for all her unwavering understanding and support, and to Andrej and Rastko, for the irretrievable time taken away from them

—V. S.

With love, to Merna, who was always there when I needed her, even when she needed me more; for her courage and encouragement, forbearance, tested patience, and support over these many months

—D. R. L.

*Acknowledgment*
Daniel Lipsitt, without whose technological wizardry and multiple rescues from computer meltdown, this book may never have made it to hard copy

—D. R. L.

# Contents

## III. Treatment Considerations

## Appendices

# Contributors

ARTHUR J. BARSKY, M.D.
*Professor of Psychiatry, Harvard Medical
School; Director of Psychosomatic
Research, Brigham and Women's
Hospital, Boston, Massachusetts, USA*

GERMAN E. BERRIOS, B.A. (Oxford),
M.D., Dr. Med. honoris causa
(Heidelberg), F.R.C Psych., F.B.Ps S.
*Consultant Neuropsychiatrist, Department
of Psychiatry, University of Cambridge;
Addenbrooke's Hospital, Cambridge,
United Kingdom*

BRIAN A. FALLON, M.D.
*Director, Somatic Disorders Research
Program, The New York State
Psychiatric Institute, Columbia
University Department of Psychiatry,
New York, New York, USA*

GIOVANNI A. FAVA, M.D.
*Associate Professor of Psychosomatic
Medicine, University of Bologna School
of Medicine, Bologna, Italy; Clinical
Professor of Psychiatry, State
University of New York at Buffalo,
Buffalo, New York, USA*

MICHAEL HOLLIFIELD, M.D.
*Assistant Professor, Departments of
Psychiatry and Family and Community
Medicine, University of New Mexico
Health Sciences Center, Albuquerque,
New Mexico, USA*

LAURENCE J. KIRMAYER, M.D.
*Professor and Director, Division of Social
and Transcultural Psychiatry,
Department of Psychiatry, McGill
University; Director, Culture and
Mental Health Research Unit, Sir
Mortimer B. Davis–Jewish General
Hospital, Montreal, Quebec, Canada*

DON R. LIPSITT, M.D.
*Clinical Professor of Psychiatry, Harvard
Medical School; Medical Director,
Institute for Behavioral Science in
Health Care, Mount Auburn Hospital,
Cambridge, Massachusetts, USA*

KARL J. LOOPER, M.D.
*Resident, Department of Psychiatry, McGill
University, Montreal, Quebec, Canada*

LARA MANGELLI, PSY.D.
*Research Fellow, Department of
Psychology, University of Bologna,
Bologna, Italy*

RUSSELL NOYES, Jr., M.D.
*Professor of Psychiatry, Department of
Psychiatry, University of Iowa College
of Medicine; Director of the Anxiety
Clinic, University of Iowa Hospitals
and Clinics, Iowa City, Iowa, USA*

ISSY PILOWSKY, M.D.
*Professor of Psychiatry, University of
Adelaide, Adelaide, Australia; Visiting
Professor, Department of Psychological
Medicine, University of Sydney, Sydney,
Australia*

PAUL M. SALKOVSKIS, PH.D.
*Professor of Cognitive Psychology,
University of Oxford Department of
Psychiatry, Warneford Hospital, Oxford,
United Kingdom; Professor of Clinical
Psychology and Applied Science,
Department of Psychology, Institute of
Psychiatry, London, United Kingdom*

ANNE E. M. SPECKENS,
M.D., PH.D.
*Psychiatrist and Cognitive-Behavioral
Therapist, Department of Psychiatry,
Leiden University Medical Center,
Leiden, The Netherlands*

VLADAN STARCEVIC, M.D., PH.D.
*Associate Professor of Psychiatry,
University of Belgrade School of
Medicine; Director, Day Clinic,
Institute of Mental Health; Belgrade,
Yugoslavia; Consultant Psychiatrist,
Hunter Mental Health Services,
University of Newcastle, Newcastle,
Australia*

HILARY M. C. WARWICK, M.D.
*Senior Lecturer in Psychiatry, Department
of Psychiatry, St. George's Hospital
Medical School, London, United
Kingdom*

# Introduction

Vladan Starcevic
Don R. Lipsitt

Can a persistent belief in a non-existent illness be an illness itself?
Appleby, 1987

L'hypocondrie: Symptome àla croisée des chemins ou chemin à la croisée des syndromes?

Is hypochondriasis a symptom standing at the crossroads or a road crossing syndromes?
Collin et al., 1989

How can an illness that has endured for more than two millennia arouse so much controversy? A full understanding of the diversity of opinion swirling about hypochondriasis entails facing, accepting, tolerating, and responding to the challenging issues that accompany hypochondriasis as a symptom, as a syndrome, as a sign, as an illness, and as social commentary. A panoply of associated dimensions is called into view, including aspects of the mind-body relationship, ambiguity and uncertainty in medicine, the imperfection of human nature, interpersonal trust and mistrust, the limitations imposed on us by our bodies, and the pervasiveness of death anxiety in our lives.

Other attributes assigned to hypochondriasis are that it is a defense mechanism; a peculiar cognitive style; a means of nonverbal communication; a pattern of reacting to stress; an abnormal illness behavior; an obsessional trait or some other enduring personality pattern; and an aspect of identity. Thus, hypochondriasis appears to be a paradigm of psychopathological complexity and interrelatedness, and, in that sense, it occupies a rather unique place. Both physicians and laypersons rise to the challenge by either passionately endorsing or totally disregarding particular attitudes toward the "condition"; where hypochondriasis is at issue, relatively few people remain neutral.

This situation is also reflected in disagreements between experts on whether hypochondriasis is a valid and independent diagnostic category and in disagreements on various definitions of hypochondriasis, including those put forward by accepted diagnostic systems. These definitions emphasize that hypochondriasis is a persistent and excessive preoccupation with fear and/or belief that the person has become seriously ill, despite all reassurance and evidence to the contrary.

Regardless of how hypochondriasis is defined, there is apparent agreement about the diversity of its manifestations. Thus, at one pole, some people who are given the label "hypochondriac" are, in fact, well-functioning individuals who seem only to pay marked attention to matters like physical exercise or healthy diets. Others become easily distressed by minor bodily symptoms or they develop transient and mild manifestations of hypochondriasis, usually in response to traumatic experiences or in the course of concurrent physical disease. A similar situation is encountered among medical students, usually by their second year. Hypochondriasis is often a part of the clinical presentation of other mental disorders, most notably panic disorder, depression, and personality disturbance, and in these cases it is referred to as *secondary hypochondriasis*.

Hypochondriasis may be a mental disorder *per se*, when it is also referred to as *primary hypochondriasis*. As such, it tends to be chronic and often co-occurs with other psychiatric conditions. It is classified among somatoform disorders, although some consider it more akin to anxiety or personality disorders. It is patients with this type of hypochondriasis who usually fit the stereotype of this condition; they examine every minor change in their bodies and subject themselves to countless medical investigations. In turn, such behavior has an adverse impact on the quality of life of these people, impairs their functioning, and overburdens the health care system. At the other pole of hypochondriacal phenomena are hypochondriacal or somatic delusions, not always easily distinguished from intense nonpsychotic hypochondriacal preoccupations.

The more complex the nature of illness, the more complex its treatment is bound to be. All treatment begins with an adequate assessment. Individuals with hypochondriacal manifestations may present special requirements because of the stigmatizing and deprecating attitudes with which they are often approached. It is common knowledge that "hypochondriacs" are not physicians' favorite patients. The risk that many patients may be rejected as "incurable" or "malingerers" hovers over the encounter with sufferers of hypochondriasis as in perhaps no other clinical situation. Persons with hypochondriasis need not only relief from morbid preoccupation with disease and a substantial decrease in health-related concerns, but also a sense of being understood. Understanding the essential underlying needs will provide a sound backdrop for the compassionate treatment of hypochondriacal patients.

Even when it is conducted adequately, the treatment of hypochondriasis can be a complex, challenging, and long-lasting process. It requires a skillful and flexible therapist who is capable of accepting the patient "as is," of deciphering the patient's somatic "idiom of distress," and of tolerating the frustrating behaviors that appear to be simultaneously seeking and rejecting help. We believe that establishing and maintaining a therapeutic relationship is the *sine qua non* of treatment regardless of whether other therapy modalities are also applied.

At the beginning of the new millennium, with increasing costs of medical care worldwide and rapid changes in modern society, hypochondriasis poses new challenges. It is timely to examine current knowledge of hypochondriasis to see how well we are equipped to respond to these challenges. In offering modern perspectives on hypochondriasis, we aim to produce a text on this ancient disorder that will provide "state-of-the-art" knowledge on hypochondriasis for years to come. More specifically, the purposes of our book are as follows:

- To demonstrate how present-day concepts of hypochondriasis are linked with its rich history (Chapters 1, 5, 8, and 11)
- To re-examine controversial conceptual issues surrounding hypochondriasis and consider ways of overcoming the corresponding obstacles (Chapters 2, 4, 5, 6, 8, 9, 10, and 11)
- To critically review diagnostic and nosological problems in hypochondriasis (Chapters 1, 2, 5, 8, and 11)
- To re-examine the heterogeneity of hypochondriasis and its relationships with other mental disorders (Chapters 2, 4, 5, 6, and 9)
- To present current views on the etiology, pathogenesis and psychopathology of hypochondriasis (Chapters 8, 9, and 10)
- To present advances in the assessment of hypochondriasis (Chapters 3 and 15)
- To present results of clinical and epidemiological research on hypochondriasis (Chapters 2, 4, 5, 6, 7, 9, 10, and 11)
- To describe principles of the therapeutic relationship in hypochondriasis and present main treatment approaches to hypochondriasis (Chapters 7, 12, 13, 14, and 15).
- To provide guidelines for treating hypochondriasis (Chapters 7, 12, 13, 14, and Epilogue)

In consideration of the different and competing views on hypochondriasis, we elected to present the subject of the book from various perspectives, representing each major "school of thought." Therefore, contributions were solicited from authors who are world experts in their respective fields. While we expect that the book will not reconcile theoretical differences between various orientations, we nonetheless hope to promote a dialogue between the "camps," in the service of achieving a well-balanced integration of different "models" of hypochondriasis.

Mainly intended for practicing clinicians, including psychiatrists, psychiatric residents, clinical psychologists, other mental health workers, primary care physicians, and other medical specialists, this book offers up-to-date information on epidemiology, clinical presentation, etiology and pathogenesis, diagnostic criteria and assessment, differential diagnosis, relationship with other mental disorders, course, prognosis, and treatment of hypochondriasis. We hope that such information will help clinicians to make appropriate diagnostic decisions and to tailor their treatment approaches to the specific needs and characteristics of their patients. Because the majority of patients with hypochondriasis are seen and treated by primary care physicians, one chapter is devoted to the primary care perspective on this disorder.

Considering that individuals with hypochondriasis and their families, as well as the general lay public, need accurate and current information, we believe this volume will also be of interest to them.

In the end, there may be more questions posed and issues raised than answers given and solutions offered. Nevertheless, our objectives will have been met if the pages that follow engage readers in a consideration of their views or their practice. With this, we may "cross the road" into an era of greater enlightenment and solace as we embark on our journey to resolve the "riddle" of hypochondriasis and to decrease confusion surrounding this condition.

### References

Appleby L. 1987. Hypochondriasis: an acceptable diagnosis? *British Medical Journal* 294:857.

Collin A., Reynaert C., Janne P., Vause M. 1989. L'hypocondrie: Symptome à la croisée des chemins ou chemin à la croisée des syndromes? *Acta Psychiatrica Belgica* 89:19–30.

# I

# Clinical and Diagnostic Considerations

# Hypochondriasis:
# History of the Concept

## GERMAN E. BERRIOS

Dans l'histoire si long-temps embrouillée de l'hypocondrie, il n'est pas moins curieux d'étudier les médecins qui ont écrit sur cette maladie que les malades qui en ont été le sujet. Les uns et les autres ont également concouru à rendre obscur ce qu'ils attachaient une si grande importance à éclairer.

In the long and confused history of hypochondriasis, the study of the doctors who wrote on it is not less interesting than the study of the patients themselves. Both have contributed to make obscure the very topic that they wanted to clarify.

Leuret, 1834

Like any other field of empirical research, psychiatric history has to confront general and specific problems. Among the latter, two are particularly salient to the "hypochondriacal disorders." One pertains to the *validity* and explanatory power of the so-called continuity hypothesis, (the "Greeks to the present" tale); the other relates to the finding of a *definition* of hypochondriasis that may survive historical translocation.

## Matters Historiographical

### The Continuity Hypothesis

The main justification for writing a historical account of hypochondriasis that starts with the Greeks and ends up in the present is the fact that it is in keeping with the official view that science is a cognitive enterprise "inching toward the truth." Whether correct or not, this type of account is handy in that it confirms the naïve belief that "latest is truest," flatters current scientists into believing that they are "closer to the truth" than anyone else before, and keeps collaborateur historians in useful employment (on the issue of the "historicity of truth," see Campbell, 1992).

The "continuity hypothesis" is beset with conceptual problems, but only one will be briefly mentioned here, namely the nature of the element from which it derives its appealing linearity (on the theme of a "history of ideas," see Lovejoy, 1936; Bevir, 1999). One can envisage such to be a word, a concept, a behavior or combinations thereof. The commonest mechanism is decontextualized words. This is the way, for example, in which dictionaries and encyclopedias manage to create the mirage of continuity and progress. Melancholia and mania are good examples of that: Nothing but the terms alone provide the glue that holds together those histories of melancholia since the Greeks to the present day.

There is much debate on whether concepts can ever provide support for continuity narratives. The issue here is whether psychiatric concepts are always theoretically (and hence historically) tethered or whether some exist *sub specie aeternitatis* ("under the aspect of eternity"). Only those who believe in the latter feel inclined to support the view that concept on occasions provides the glue for a continuity tale.

Another possibility is the most desirable to medical historians but, alas, the rarest: It takes the form of certain behaviors that are so stereotyped they resist cultural and temporal translocation. For example, tics, hallucinations, and delirium are states that the historian can find clearly described in the literature of the ages. In this case, a history of delirium from the Greeks to the present can be said to be a history of the way in which a very stable behavior has been talked about and explained for the last 25 centuries. But even here there are problems, for sponsors of the continuity tales must explain the stability of the said behavior: Medical historians feel naturally inclined to view it as the expression of some neurobiological disorder. In contrast, social constructionists might wish to explain behavioral stability in terms of social factors. This closes the conceptual loop and starts the fun. Fortunately, we do not have to resolve this problem here. Nonetheless, the usefulness of this historiographical excursus has been to throw new light on the following question: From the Greeks on, what is the history of hypochondriasis about? We can now say that it is unlikely to be about some stable behavior related to some tenebrous brain structure. It is far more likely that it is just about the avatars of a fascinating *term*.

## Defining Hypochondriasis

Defining and classifying "hypochondriasis" is not an easy matter as at least three issues must be resolved. One concerns the nature of the referent: Is it a "RRUS"—

that is, a *real*, *recognizable*, *unitary* and *stable* object of inquiry? Second, is this RRUS valid in all possible cultural universes? Third, what slot should it occupy in a nosology of "mental" disorders? For example, on what empirical evidence has it been subordinated to the "somatoform" disorders?

A good example of such difficulties running riot can be found in the current *International Classification of Diseases* (ICD-10) definitions (World Health Organization, 1992), which shows the hopelessness of pretending to construct operational definitions out of ordinary language terms. For example, by using vague words such as "preoccupation," "belief," and so on, interchangeably, the authors of F45 have caused undue confusion. Then there is the whimsical nature of the taxonomy. It would seem *de facto* (if not *de jure*) that a high-level class has been constructed: Somatoform disorders (F45). This, in turn, includes five orders: Somatization disorder (F45.0), Undifferentiated somatoform disorder (F45.1), Hypochondriacal disorder (F45.2), Somatoform autonomic dysfunction (F45.3), and Persistent somatoform pain disorder (F45.4). The order Hypochondriacal disorder, in turn, contains five species: body dysmorphic disorder, dysmorphophobia (nondelusional), hypochondriacal neurosis, hypochondriasis, and nosophobia. *Vis-à-vis* this classification, there are two options: one that it reflects a fact of nature, the other, that it does not. Because no evidential database has been made available by the ICD creators, one must assume that the classification in question is more or less a matter of opinion. If so, how can these definitions and classifications be used as the starting point for a real history of hypochondriasis?

In an attempt to deal with the two problems listed above, the historical account to be presented in this chapter will focus on the period stretching from the seventeeth century to the nineteenth century (when the core conceptual structures were worked out) and will visit the Greeks only for etymological clarification. It will not deal with the twentieth century and hence with the history of psychoanalytical hypotheses (for this, see Berrios and Mumford, 1995, or Chapter 8 of this text). It goes without saying that the history of hypochondriasis has also been written about from other perspectives (e.g., Fischer-Homberger, 1983; Kenyon, 1965; Meister, 1980; Place, 1986).

## History of the Word

The word *hypochondrium* was used by Hippocrates to refer to the regions of the abdomen lying under the rib cage. For example, he reported a woman in postpartum who "suffered in her right ὑποχόνδριόν (hypocondrion)" (Case IV, Epidemics I, Hippocrates, 1972). By the time of Celsus, the anatomical locus in question was included under the wider concept of *praecordia:* "1. The lower chest in front of the heart; 2. The region over the diaphragm, and 3. The upper abdomen below the ribs (*hypochondria*)" (Celsus, 1935, p. 100).

The Greek belief that the abdominal organs were the source of disordered emotions was still prevalent at the time of Plato (Warrington, 1965). For example, in the *Timaeus* Plato wrote: "That part of the soul which desires meats and drinks and the other things of which it has need by reason of the bodily nature, they placed between the midriff and the boundary of the navel . . . and there they bound it like a wild animal which was chained up with man" (Plato, 1973, p. 1194). Diocles Carystus (circa 350 BCE) seems to have been one of the first to report complaints of the digestive organs associated with pathology of the "hypochondria" (Ladee, 1966, p. 7). Classical writers went on to establish a firm association between the hypochondria or praecordia and, at least, two clusters of "symptoms:" one pertained to digestive symptomatology, flatulence, and so on (as in Diocles) and another to melancholia (as in Paulus de Aegina, c. A.D. 625–690). It is important to remember that during this period melancholia had little or nothing to do with depressive illness (Berrios, 1988).

The Greek view held sway up to the early seventeenth century when references to hypochondriacal or flatuous melancholia can still be found: "Besides fear and sorrow, sharp belchings, fulsome crudities, heat in the bowels, wind and rumblings in the guts, vehement gripping, pain in the belly and stomack" (Burton, 1621/1883, p. 269). Interestingly enough, Burton went on to quote Crato's prescient remark that "in this hypochondriacal or flatuous melancholy, the symptoms are so ambiguous that the most well-trained physicians cannot identify the part involved" (p. 269).

## The History of the Concept and Behaviors

Between the classical thinking of Robert Burton (1577–1640) and the views of Thomas Willis (1621–1675) and Thomas Sydenham (1624–1689) there is a conceptual abyss: This was mostly due to the fact that new definitions of medical observation, causality, disease, and treatment had developed in the interim. This is also the time when the distinction between delusional and attitudinal or personality-related hypochondriasis is made, and when it becomes a "nervous disorder" (in the sense of Willis, see below).

### The Great Dichotomy

It is during the seventeenth century that the two great descriptive and explanatory models of hypochondriasis appeared in the form of two classical narratives. They have since controlled thinking in this field. As part of his *Novelas Ejemplares,* Cervantes (1547–1616) published "El Licenciado Vidriera" (Cervantes, 1916), the tale of a successful undergraduate at the University of Salamanca who after being given a love potion developed the delusion that he was made of glass. The story of the lengths he went to protect himself from breakage constitutes a classical description of what during the nineteenth century was to be called "delusional hypochondriasis": sudden onset, identifiable causal factor, lack of interaction with a physician, perceived by others as an illness, and delusional control of behavior. Sampayo (1986) has identified an Erasmian influence in Cervantes's novel. Likewise, the glass delusion had been known in European literature ever since the late fifteenth century (Speak, 1990). By the end of the seventeenth century, John Locke (1632–1704) decided to use it as a prototypical form of madness: "Others who have thought themselves made of glass have used the caution necessary to preserve such brittle bodies" (Locke, 1690/1959, Book II, Chapter XI, 13).

The other great seventeenth century narrative provides a model according to which hypochondriasis can emerge gradually, in an interactional context with physicians and relatives and express deep personality needs. *Le Malade imaginaire*, the last play by Molière (1622–1673), was performed for the first time few weeks before his death. It carried a strange subtitle, *Élomire Hypocondre*, which Molière seems to have borrowed from a pamphlet published in 1660 by someone using the pseudonym of Le Boulanger de Chalussay. The theme and personages are not entirely new, and Molière seems to have borrowed some of them from earlier plays. Argan, the protagonist, finds himself at the center of a triangle constituted by his second young wife and his lawyer (who want his money), his own family, daughter by first marriage, her boyfriend, his brother, and his servant (who love him well), and his physicians and apothecary, who are self-interested and feed his hypochondriacal fears, which grow by the day. At the end of the play, and symbolizing the very essence of neurotic hypochondriasis, Argan becomes a medic himself (Hucher, 1965).

## *Hypochondriasis as a "Nervous Disorder"*

The concept of "nervous disorder" was created during the seventeenth century (Hare, 1991; López Piñero, 1983). Thomas Willis (1621–1675) regarded both hypochondriasis in men and hysteria in women as disorders of the brain: "As we have shewn before that the passions vulgarly called hysterical do not always proceed from the womb, but often from the head's being affected: so though it has been vulgarly held that the affects called hypochondriacal are caused for the most part by Vapours arising from the spleen, and running hither and thither; yet in truth those distempers are for the greatest part convulsions and contractions of the nervous parts" (Willis, 1685, p. 307).

To flatulence, indigestion, pain, and other gastrointestinal symptoms, Willis added complaints reminiscent of panic disorder: "Moreover, the diseased are wont to complain of a trembling and palpitation of the heart, with a mighty oppression of the same, also frequent failings of the spirits, a danger of swooning come upon them, that the diseased always think death at hand . . . fluctuation of thoughts, inconstancy of mind, a disturbed fancy, a dread and suspicion of everything." But also (and this is one of the earliest references to *valetudinarian* complaints): "an imaginary being affected with diseases of which they are free, and many other distractions of the spirit . . . wandering pains, also cramps and numbnesses with a sense of formication seize likewise almost all the outward parts: night sweats, flushing of blood . . ." (Willis, 1685, p. 308).

Thomas Sydenham (1624–1689) noted that symptoms "which cannot be accounted for on the common principle of investigating diseases" were often preceded by "disturbances of the mind," which he regarded as "the usual causes of this disease." Sydenham noted that these symptoms were often accompanied by depression, panic, anger or despair; sufferers were "enemies to joy and hope." Like Willis, he linked hysteria and hypochondriasis "since, however much antiquity may have laid the blame of hysteria upon the uterus, hypochondriasis [which we impute to some obstruction of the spleen or viscera] is as like it, as one egg is to another" (p. 85). Furthermore, "the affection which I have characterized in females as hysteria and in males as hypochondriasis, arises (in my mind) from a disorder (ataxy) of the animal spirits" (Sydenham, 1850, p. 90).

Sydenham (1850) then comments on the remarkable frequency and the numerous forms under which hysteria and hypochondriasis appear, "resembling most of the distempers wherewith mankind are afflicted." Moreover, "unless the physician be a person of judgement and penetration," it was easy to confuse these hysterical symptoms with symptoms of physical disease. Such symptoms included severe pain "attacking the external part of the Head, between the pericranium and the cranium"; vomiting; "terrible convulsions much like the epilepsy": and "such a palpitation that the patient makes sure that the sound of the heart beating against the ribs can be heard by the bystanders" (p. 86). Sydenham's descriptions of hysterical symptoms were widely quoted by his contemporaries (Williams, 1990).

## The "English Malady"

What George Cheyne (1671–1743) called the "English malady" overlaps only partially with contemporary notions of hypochondriasis. Be that as it may, the eighteenth century is blessed with great books on this disorder, which set the scene for all further developments. As that great century winds down, a trend can be noticed (particularly amongst the Scottish physicians) to consider hypochondriasis as a specific disturbance of the nerves (López Piñero, 1983).

In *A Treatise of the Spleen and Vapours: or, Hypochondriacal and Hysterical Affections* (1725), Sir Richard Blackmore (1654–1729) (physician to William III and Queen Anne) regarded pains and other sensory symptoms in various parts of the body, as well as the disturbed mind and imagination, as reflecting hysteria in women and hypochondriasis in men. Unfortunately, Blackmore observed, "Patients are unwilling their Disease should go by its right Name" because the public regarded their symptoms as an "imaginary and fantastick Sickness of the Brain, filled with odd and irregular ideas," and such individuals often become "an Object of Derision and Contempt." However, their "sufferings are without doubt real and unfeigned" (Blackmore, 1725).

Blackmore ridiculed the notion that such somatic complaints were caused by fumes or vapors rising up from the lower to upper regions of the body. For one thing, "there are no Passages, or proper Conveyances, by which these Streams and Exhalations may mount from the inferior to the superior Parts." Instead, Blackmore offered a psychological explanation: "Terrible ideas, formed only in the Imagination, will affect the Brain and the Body with painful Sensations." He also believed that hypochondriasis was not a form of insanity: "The Limits and Partitions that bound and discriminate . . . Hypochondriack and Hysterick Disorders, and Melancholy, Lunacy and Phrenzy, are so nice, that it is not easy to distinguish them, and set the Boundaries where one ends, and the other begins." Hypochondriasis and hysteria "sometimes affect the intellectual Faculties" but seldom result in "a State of Lunacy" (Blackmore, 1725).

In *A Treatise of the Hypochondriak and Hysterick Passions*, Bernard de Mandeville (1670–1733) reported the imaginary exchanges between Philopirio (a physician representing de Mandeville's views) and Misomedon, a *hypochondriacus confirmatus* who consults him after 12 years of gastrointestinal symptoms and countless episodes of bleeding and purging. The second dialogue discusses the etiological theories of Diocles, Sylvius, Willis, Sydenham, Highmore, Platter, Tulp, and Baglivi. De Mandeville then advances his own view: "That the disorders of the chylifications are chiefly the cause of the distempers in question, I shall endeavour to prove" (de Mandeville, 1711, p. 121).

In *The English Malady: or, a Treatise of Nervous Diseases of all Kinds, as Spleen, Vapours, Lowness of Spirits, Hypochondriacal, and Hysterical Distempers, etc.*, George Cheyne described the classical view of a disease that tended to affect persons of greater intelligence and upper social class. The "English Malady" resulted from "the Moisture of our Air, the Variableness of our Weather, (from our Situation amidst the Ocean) . . . the Richness and Heaviness of our Food, the Wealth and Abundance of the Inhabitants (from their universal Trade) the Inactivity and sedentary Occupations of the better Sort (among whom this Evil mostly rages) and the Humour of living in great, populous and consequently unhealthy Towns. . . . These nervous Disorders being computed to make almost one-third of the Complaints of the People of Condition in England . . ." (Cheyne, 1733).

Nicholas Robinson (1697–1775), a governor of London's Bethlem Hospital, wanted to account "mechanically" for mental as well as bodily diseases. Influenced by eighteenth-century "nerve fibre" neurophysiology, he argued that because mind without brain was inconceivable, psychological processes were simply expressions of physical events in "the Nerves and Fibres that compose the Brain." Thus, "Every Change of the Mind, therefore, indicates a Change in the bodily Organs; nor is it possible for the Wit of Man to conceive how the Mind can, from a chearful [sic], gay Disposition, fall into a sad and disconsolate State, without some Alterations in the Fibres, at the same Time" (Robinson, 1729).

In relation to "those Disorders we call the Spleen, Vapours, and Hypochondriack Melancholy," Robinson (1729) argued: "Neither the Fancy, nor Imagination, nor even Reason itself, the highest Faculty of the Understanding, can feign a Perception, or a Disease that has no foundation in Nature; . . . cannot feel Pain or Uneasiness in any Part, unless there be Pain or Uneasiness in that Part: The affected Nerves of that Part must strike the Imagination with the Sense of Pain, before the Mind can conceive the Idea of Pain in that Part" (p. 406).

Robert Whytt (1714–1766) is the most original writer on hypochondriasis during the eighteenth century. In his *Observations on the Nature, Causes and Cure of Those Diseases Which Are Commonly Called Nervous, Hypochondriac or Hysteric*, Whytt defended the view that "sympathy" (an old notion used to explain how bodily components came to be coordinated) was based on a network of nerves, and hence was a function of the brain. This has been aptly summarized by French (1969): "Since sympathy presupposes feeling, nerves are the mechanism of feeling, and all nerves originate in the brain and spinal marrow . . . all sympathy was to be referred to the brain" (p. 34).

Following Sydenham, Whytt (1764) believed that hysteria and hypochondriasis were identical, but the former affected females and the latter males (p. 534). Nervous disorders, in general, resulted from "a too great delicacy and sensibility of the whole nervous system" or "an uncommon weakness, or a depraved or unnatural feeling, in some of the organs of the body" (p. 537). Hysteria and "hypochondria" resulted from a combination of these two types of causes and were but the expression of pathological sympathy.


## The "Nervous Disorders" Become "Neuroses"

William Cullen (1712–1790) sponsored a version of "neuralpathology" (the view that all diseases were diseases of the nervous system). Not much has been written on Cullen's psychiatric views although he is quoted *ad nauseam* for having coined the term *neurosis* (Bowman, 1975). Cullen's taxonomic approach was synthetic in that he blended into larger groups the often over-detailed nosological conditions of his predecessors. This also applies to his views on hypochondriasis. As someone wrote in the popular *Edinburgh Practice of Physic*: "Although some of the nosological writers, particularly Sauvages, have considered this genus as consisting of different species, Dr Cullen is of the opinion that there is only one idiopathic species, the *hypochondriasis melancholica*. He considers not only the hypochondriasis hysterica, phthisica and asthmatica, but also the biliosa, sanguinea, and pituitosa, as being only symptomatic; but he views the true melancholic hypochondriasis as being a proper idiopathic disease, perfectly distinct from hysteria, with which has often been confounded" (Anonymous, 1803, p. 358; see also Cullen, 1803, pp. 291–292).

The symptoms of hypochondriasis, according to Cullen, were dyspepsia, indigestion, pain under the ribs, palpitations, sleepless nights and occasionally "depression of spirits and apprehension of danger." Among the causes the following can be listed: "plethora and preternatural thickness of the blood, suppression of customary evacuations, high and full diet, together with a sparing quantity of drink; and hereditary disposition; indolence; atony of the intestines and violent passions of the mind" (Anonymous, 1803). "The hypochondriacal affection, when left to itself, is more troublesome than dangerous" (Anonymous, 1803).

## Hypochondriasis as a Form of "Insanity"

Changes in etiological theory led to a gradual broadening of the "nervous disorders," which became "neuroses" in terms of Cullen's "neuralpathology" theory (Bynum, 1985; López Piñero, 1983). During the following century, the implementation of the *anatomo-clinical model of disease* (Ackerknecht, 1967) and the new descriptive psychopathology (Berrios, 1996) caused a progressive attrition of the "neuroses." By the second half of the nineteenth century, the group was thus much smaller than it once had been. The over-generalized nature of the Cullean definition of neuroses as "preternatural affections of sense and motion, which are without pyrexia as a part of the primary disease" (Cullen, 1827, p. 1), made little sense in the new world of specificities.

In this new climate, hypochondriasis was classified as an insanity (i.e., a disease resulting from a brain lesion). For example, Fabre (1849) wrote: "Today, and like all the other monomanias (partial insanities), hypochondria is generally and with reason considered as being caused by a disorder of brain function." When reviewing the pathological anatomy of the condition, however, Fabre ruefully states: "In the case of hypochondria this section is kept only for reasons of organization. For, in the rare cases in which it has been possible to carry out postmortems in subjects who have actually died whilst hypochondriacal (rather than on account of a complication of the disease) no lesion has been found to explain the disorder. Among recent authors, Broussais has been the only one to report 'gastric inflammation' only to recant later" (Fabre, 1849, p. 629). Indeed, Broussais had returned to the idea that there existed a "reciprocal influence between emotions and visceral irritations: for example, in the same way that fear causes palpitations, the latter—when caused by any physical cause—might trigger the memory of fear. This may explain the frequency of sensations in hypochondriacs who have developed chronic gastritis" (Broussais, 1828, p. 462).

Likewise, Jean Baptiste Parchappe, in his exhaustive collection of postmortem reports, included the case of a 51-year old married carpenter who developed an affective disorder in reaction to the insanity of his wife. This was accompanied by abdominal pains and "hypochondriacal complaints." On postmortem he was found to have "large cortical plaques and softening of the brain" (Parchappe, 1841, pp. 36–37).

Hypochondriasis was thus reconceptualized as a form of insanity. Luyer-Villermay (quoted in Fabre, 1841) even proposed a model to explain how this took place in a given individual: "During the first stage, the disorder only involves the organs of the abdomen; in the second, it extends to the chest and the head, and in the third and last the involvement of brain functions becomes predominant." Georget (quoted in Fabre, 1841) believed that Luyer-Villermay "had no basis other than his opinion." Dubois (d'Amiens) (quoted in Fabre, 1841, p. 91), in turn, also proposed a three-stage model, although his criterion was severity of the disorder rather than progressive involvement of organs: "The third stage consisted in a chronic inflammation of most organs . . . and recovery was almost impossible."

At the very end of the nineteenth century, George Savage (1892) attempted to reconcile the two views: "The word hypochondriasis has a very wide meaning, and includes forms of insanity, as well as many disorders which cannot properly be so-called. Under this name we shall have to describe a nervous disorder varying from slight over-sensitiveness to insanity with marked delusions and actively suicidal tendencies" (Savage, 1892, p. 619).

## Hypochondriasis and Melancholia

Upon returning to the United States from Edinburgh, Benjamin Rush (1745–1813) observed: First, "It would be equally proper to call every form of madness hypochondriasm . . . for they are all accompanied by abdominal symptoms"; and second, the name "has unfortunately been supposed to imply an imaginary disease" and "is always offensive to patients who are affected with it" (Rush, 1812).

Rush himself preferred "tristimania," arguing that it differed from hysteria in its symptomatology, notably in its "extremes of high and low spirits."

Along the same lines, Guislain (1852) wrote: "Sometimes, melancholia is characterized by intense valetudinarian preoccupations . . . The patient worries about having non-existent diseases. This is called melancholic hypochondria . . . Hypochondria can be bodily and mental, the latter being melancholic hypochondria proper. The former is uncommon in mental hospitals but is often found in the community. These patients only come to hospital when severely ill" (pp. 120–121).

By defining hypochondria as a "sad monomania" (*manie triste*), C.F. Michéa (1815–1882) also committed himself to the view that the condition was a form of depression in which there was "an exaggeration or exaltation of the instinct of preservation (*biophilie*)" (Michéa, 1843, p. 575). Because of this association, Michéa believed that hypochondria had a bad outcome: It could transform itself into insanity or lead to suicide.

Prone to the disease were men between 30 and 40 years of age with family history of the condition and with a nervous temperament. There were idiopathic and secondary forms, and only the former was a "true" hypochondriasis. Michéa agreed with Dubois d'Amiens' three-stage analysis: "The first stage is characterized by mental changes such as delusions and pure monomania. The second includes functional disorders and neuroses of some organs. The third includes anatomical changes (*lésions de tissu*)" (Michéa, 1843, p. 577).

For B.A. Morel (1809–1873), true hypochondriasis was a form of insanity (*folie hystérique*) that resulted from the transformation of certain neuroses (*la transformation de certaines névroses*) (Morel, 1860, p. 264). There was a *hypochondrie simple*, which affected "those who worried excessively about their health and these persons were *le désespoir des médecins*" (Morel, 1860, p. 266). It could become a veritable delusional syndrome in which case the valetudinarian symptoms always "occupied the forefront of the condition" (Morel, 1860, p. 709). This disorder was often hereditary. As Morel observed: "I have seen hereditary insanity become complicated by hypochondriacal phenomena" (Morel, 1860, p. 525).

W. Griesinger (1817–1868) also believed that "the hypochondriacal states represent the most moderate form of insanity, and have features which essentially distinguish them from the other forms of melancholia" (Griesinger, 1861, p. 215). "The hypochondriac may reason correctly—setting out from false premises, but this does not negate the fact that hypochondria is a mental disorder, any more than because hypochondria often accompanies or complicates various chronic diseases seated in different organs, it ought on that account to be confounded with these diseases" (p. 216). Griesinger's effort to integrate hypochondriasis into the continuum of insanity is a manifestation of his support for the unitary approach to insanity (Berrios and Beer, 1994).

Hypochondria, according to Griesinger, "may arise in two different ways. In the first place, as a secondary cerebro-spinal irritation, in consequence of internal, but often slight, diseases (of the intestine, the liver, the genital organs, and even kidney), which give rise more to a feeling of general discomfort. . . . In the second place, however, hypochondria may also arise via a direct psychological route (*psychischem Wege entstehen*), inasmuch as through external circumstances the ideas may be so constantly directed to the state of the general health, or of one particular organ, as to induce morbid sensations" (Griesinger, 1861, p. 221).

## Hypochondriasis as a Disorder of "Sensation"

The French clinical notion of *cénesthopathie* (Dupré, 1925; Dupré and Camus, 1907) was based on the earlier German concept of "common feeling" (*Gemeingefühl*) (Starobinski, 1977, 1990), which referred to "bodily sensations" that were not touch, temperature, pressure, and location sensations (*Tastsinn*). The common-feeling group included pain and "objectless" sensations such as well-being, pleasure, fatigue, shudder, hunger, nausea, organic muscular feeling, and so on.

In the non-German speaking countries, these sensations were named "coenaesthesis" by the middle of the nineteenth century (Hamilton, 1859) and began to be used as explanation for the "sense of existence" (Gautheret, 1961). However, why such diverse feelings converged into a common sensation of bodily "unity" needed explanation (the sort of problem that Bakal [1999] has recently tackled; for the historical origins of these ideas, see Vila, 1998; Rousseau, 1990). According to associationism, coenaesthesis resulted from a *summation* of proprioceptive and interoceptive sensations (Taine, 1890). Faculty psychology, in contrast, postulated the existence of a hypothetical *brain center* or *faculty* on which sensations converged. The latter mechanism was later invoked to explain the generation of the "body schema."

As hunger, thirst, sexual pleasure, and so on began to be studied independently, the erstwhile broad territory of coenaesthesis became eroded. In the end, all that was left were indistinct sensations common to most organs such as deep pressure, pain, and unanalyzable sensations such as "tickling" or "stuffiness" (Titchener, 1901).

Baron E. von Feuchtersleben (1806–1849) was one of the first to suggest that "hypochondriasis . . . is in its essence nothing but a coenaesthesis abnormally heightened in all directions" (Feuchtersleben, 1847, p. 222). Hypochondriasis *sine materie* resulted from a psychological heightening (e.g., persistent attention to sensations) of the *Gemeingefühl*. Hypochondriasis *cum materie* resulted from nerve hypersensitivity caused by an organic disease. Feuchtersleben (1847) commented that Dubois (1833) was not altogether right in believing that organic hypersensitivity was the *only* cause of hypochondriasis: "In nature, however, there appears a circle between psychical and physical causes." The debate on whether imagination or real sensation was the primary cause continued well into the twentieth century (Berrios, 1985).

J. L. Luys (1828–1897) advanced the similar suggestion that hypochondriasis resulted from proprioceptive hallucinations (*hallucinations viscérales*):

> "Hallucinations that originate from disorders of visceral sensibility determine the various forms of hypochondria. . . . These are delusional types which are first intermittent and then become continuous. Patients may claim that their throat is closed, that they are edentulous, that their stomach is blocked, that they have no bowels and cannot go to the toilet, etc. . . . These complaints should be considered as veritable interoceptive hallucinations mostly resulting from the gastrointestinal regions; thoracic ones are rare. When these hallucinations become associated with those from external senses, the prognosis is somber because spreading of the irritation to the cortex can be suspected. (Luys, 1881, pp. 420–421)

J. Cotard (1840–1889) proposed a variant of the coenaesthesis hypothesis, stating that hypochondriasis is "characterized by an exaggerated psychological response. Not only visceral pains are amplified but also normal sensations cause anxiety. . . . It is less a veritable hyperaesthesia than a dysaesthesia, i.e., a hyperaesthesia linked to a blunting of sensation (*léger degré d'obtusion sensorielle*). . . . But it is mainly in the cortical site where sensations are transformed into extraordinary notions that insanity can begin" (Cotard, 1888, pp. 141–142).

Richard von Krafft-Ebing (1840–1902) also sponsored a form of sensorial theory: "Hypochondria may be called a neurosis of the general feeling (*Gemeingefühlneurose*), with effects on the psychological sphere." The important psychological manifestations of hypochondriacal neuropsychosis (*hypochondrische Neuro(psycho)se*) are "a facilitated power of apperception (*Apperceptionsfähigkeit*) of the psychological organs, as a result of which the exciting processes (often causal) in the nerves of other organs become conscious. At the same time they become colored by lively feelings of displeasure. The state of consciousness of the patient may extend from ideas of severe disease to the most absurd interpretations of sensations that are actually experienced" (Krafft-Ebing, 1893).

The concept of coenaesthesis entered in French psychiatry in the now neglected concept of *cénesthopathie*, which referred to a "local alteration of the common sensibility in the sphere of general sensation, corresponding to hallucinosis in the sphere of sensorium" (Dupré, 1913). "Painful" and "paraesthesic" coenaesthopathies were recognized, and each, in turn, divided into cephalic, thoracic and abdominal areas. Patients in the "painful" group felt their organs "stretched, torn, twisted"; in the "paraesthesic" group, they experienced itching, hyperaesthesiae, paraesthesiae, and so on. Some coenaesthopathies were treated as separate syndromes. For example, *topalgie* (or cephalic coenaestopathy) was reclassified as a "neurovegetative dystonia" (Bernard and Trouvé, 1977) and as a psychosomatic syndrome (Ey, 1950).

The coenaesthopathies were never fully recognized in Anglo-Saxon psychiatry, and the very complaints were named *hypochondriasis*, *neurasthenia*, or *dysmorphophobia* (Reilly and Beard, 1976). In other countries, similar phenomena were classified as "disorders of sensibility" or "psychoneuroses" (Ladee, 1966).


## Conclusion

Although now it seems to have been relegated to the sad position of being just an "order" of a higher class—"the somatoform disorders" (ICD-10)—hypochondriasis still offers rich pickings as an object of historical research. Stemming from the "convergence" (probably first occurring in classical Greece) among a *word* coined to refer to an anatomical locus, a *theory* of emotions (which is no more), and *utterances* by worthy Greek citizens who worried about sensations in their abdomens, *hypochondriasis* has since those halcyon days soldiered on, regardless, and remains a challenge to medicine.

Ever since the seventeenth century, two allegorical descriptions of hypochondriasis have governed thinking on the subject. According to one, hypochondriacal beliefs and preoccupations overtake the individual like a storm and are alien to his being; hence, as in the case of Cervantes's "Licenciado Vidriera," there is the hope of a cure. According to the other description, such preoccupations are part of the psychological makeup and grow inside the individual as he or she fails to negotiate a stressful environment; such worries are difficult to get rid of, and as in the case of Molière's (*Le Malade imaginaire*), the patient has to learn to live with them.

This old literary dichotomy is reflected in the differentiation between hypochondriasis as insanity and as nervous disorder. As the seventeenth-century concept of nervous disorder became "neurosis" during the eighteenth century, hypochondriasis became diluted out by the many other conditions that constituted the noble Cullean category. During the nineteenth century, all nervous disorders related to identifiable and localized lesions were gradually separated off (to contribute to the foundation of neurology) and this, once again, emphasized the fact that there were no explanations for hypochondriasis.

Some chose to explain it as reflecting the right reading of exaggerated bodily sensations; others as the wrong reading of normal sensations; yet others, like Freud, created narratives to account for the manner in which the obscure parts of the self interacted with symbols and with the environment. Structurally, however, all accounts have remained within the framework once set by the seventeenth-century writers. The reader, however, should go through the remainder of this book before deciding whether things have improved since.

## References

Ackerknecht E. 1967. *Medicine at the Paris Hospital 1794–1848*. Baltimore: Johns Hopkins University Press.

Anonymous. 1803. *The Edinburgh Practice of Physic, Surgery, and Midwifery. Vol. 2: Medicine*. London: Kearsley.

Bakal D. 1999. *Minding the Body*. New York: Guilford Press.

Bernard P., Trouvé S. 1977. *Sémiologie Psychiatrique*, Paris: Masson.

Berrios G.E. 1985. Delusional parasitosis and physical disease. *Comprehensive Psychiatry* 26: 395–403.

Berrios G.E. 1988. Melancholia and depression during the 19th century: a conceptual history. *British Journal of Psychiatry* 153: 298-304.

Berrios G.E. 1996. *The History of Mental Symptoms: Descriptive Psychopathology Since the 19th Century*. Cambridge: Cambridge University Press.

Berrios G.E., Beer D. 1994. The notion of unitary psychosis: a conceptual history. *History of Psychiatry* 5: 13–36.

Berrios G.E., Mumford D. 1995. Somatoform disorders. In *The History of Clinical Psychiatry* (eds. Berrios G.E., Porter R.), London: Athlone Press.

Bevir M. 1999. *The Logic of the History of Ideas*. Cambridge: Cambridge University Press.

Blackmore R. 1725. *A Treatise of the Spleen and Vapours: or, Hypochondriacal and Hysterical Affections With Three Discourses on the Nature and Cure of Cholick, Melancholy, and Palsies*. London: Pemberton.

Bowman I.A. 1975. *William Cullen (1710–90) and the Primacy of the Nervous System*. Indiana University doctoral thesis, History of Science, Ann Arbor, MI: Xerox University Microfilms.

Broussais F.J.V. 1828. *De l'irritation et de la folie*. Paris: Delaunay.

Burton R. 1883. *The Anatomy of Melancholy*. London: Chatto and Windus (Original work published 1621).

Bynum W.F. 1985. The nervous patient in eighteenth- and nineteenth-century Britain: the psychiatric origins of British neurology. In *The Anatomy of Madness*, Vol. 1 (eds. Bynum W.F., Porter R., Shepherd M.), London: Tavistock.

Campbell R. 1992. *Truth and Historicity*. Oxford: Clarendon Press.

Celsus. 1935. *De Medicina, Vol. 1* (transl. by W.G. Spencer). London: Heinemann.

Cervantes M. 1916. *El Licenciado Vidriera*. Edition by Alonso Cortés. Valladolid: Imprenta Castellana.

Cheyne G. 1733. *The English Malady: or, a Treatise of Nervous Diseases of all Kinds, as Spleen, Vapours, Lowness of Spirits, Hypochondriacal, and Hysterical Distempers, etc.* London: J. Strachan.

Cotard J. 1888. Hypocondrie. In *Dictionnaire Encyclopédique des Sciences Médicales, Vol. 51* (eds. Dechambre A., Lereboullet A.), Paris: Masson.

Cullen W. 1803. *Synopsis Nosologiae Methodicae, Sixth Edition.* Edinburgh: W. Creech.

Cullen W. 1827. *The works of William Cullen,* 2 vols., (ed. by Thomson J.) Edinburgh: William Blackwood.

Dubois E.F. (d'Amiens) 1833. *Histoire philosophique de l'hypocondrie et de l'hystérie.* Paris: Cavelin, Librairie de Deville.

Dupré E. 1913. Les cénestopathies. *Mouvement Médical* 23: 3–22.

Dupré E. 1925. *Pathologie de l'imagination et de l'émotivité.* Paris: Payot.

Dupré E., Camus P. 1907. Les cénesthopathies. *L'Encéphale* 2: 616-631.

Ey H. 1950. Hypochondrie. Étude No 17. In *Études Psychiatriques, Vol. 2.* Paris: Desclée de Brouwer.

Fabre D. (ed.). 1841. Hypochondrie. In *Dictionnaire des Dictionnaires de Médecine, Vol 5.* Paris: Béthune et Plon.

Fabre D. (ed.). 1849. Maladies de l'encéphale, maladies mentales, maladies nerveuses. *Bibliothèque du Médecin-Practicien, Vol. 9.* Paris: Baillière.

Fischer-Homberger E. 1983. Hypochondriasis. In *Handbook of Psychiatry, Vol. 1* (eds. Shepherd M., Zangwill O.L.), Cambridge: Cambridge University Press.

French R.K. 1969. *Robert Whytt: The Soul and Medicine.* London: The Wellcome Institute of the History of Medicine.

Gautheret F. 1961. Historique et Position Actuelle de la Notion de Scheme Corporel. *Bulletin de Psychologie* 11: 41–49.

Griesinger W. 1861. *Die Pathologie und Therapie der psychischen Krankheiten,* Second Edition. Stuttgart: Krabbe.

Guislain J. 1852. *Leçons orales sur les phrénopathies, ou traité théorique et pratique des maladies mentales,* 3 vols. Gand, Belgium: L. Hebbelynck.

Hamilton W. 1859. *Lectures on Logic and Metaphysics.* 4 vols. Edinburgh: William Blackwood and Sons.

Hare E. 1991. The history of "nervous disorder" from 1600 to 1840 and a comparison with modern views. *British Journal of Psychiatry* 159: 37-45.

Hippocrates. 1972. *Works* (with English translation by W.H.S. Jones). London: Loeb Classical Library, William Heinemann.

Hucher Y. (ed.). 1965. *Molière's Le Malade Imaginaire.* Paris: Larousse.

Kenyon F.E. 1965. Hypochondriasis: a survey of some historical, clinical and social aspects. *British Journal of Medical Psychology* 38: 117–133.

Krafft-Ebing R. 1893. *Lehrbuch der Psychiatrie, Fifth Edition.* Stuttgart: Enke.

Ladee G.A. 1966. *Hypochondriacal Syndromes.* Amsterdam: Elsevier.

Leuret. 1834. Quoted in Brusset B. 1998 *L'hypocondrie.* Paris: Presses Universitaires de France.

Locke J. 1959. *An Essay Concerning Human Understanding,* 2 vols. New York: Dover. (Original work published 1690).

López Piñero J.M.L. 1983. *Historical Origins of the Concept of Neurosis* (trans. by D. Berrios). Cambridge: Cambridge University Press.

Lovejoy A.O. 1936. *The Great Chain of Being.* Cambridge, MA: Harvard University Press.

Luys J. 1881. *Traité clinique et pratique des maladies mentales.* Paris: Delahaye et Lecrosnier.

Mandeville de B. 1711. *A Treatise of the Hypochondriack and the Hysterick Passions. Vulgarly Called the Hypo in Men and Vapours in Women.* London: Dryden Learb.

Meister R. 1980. *Hypochondria.* New York: Taplinger.

Michéa F. 1843. Du siége, de la nature intime, des symptomes et du diagnostic de l'hypocondrie. *Mémoires de l'Académie Royale de Médicine* 2: 573–654.

Morel B.A. 1860. *Traité des Maladies Mentales.* Paris: Masson.

Parchappe J.B. 1841. *Traité théorique et pratique de la folie.* Paris: Béchet et Labé.

Place J.L. 1986. L'Hypocondrie. Éloge de Dubois d'Amiens. *L'Evolution Psychiatrique* 51: 567–586.

Plato. 1973. *The Collected Dialogues of Plato* (eds. Hamilton E, Cairns H.), Princeton, NJ: Princeton University Press.

Reilly T M., Beard A.W. 1976. Monosymptomatic hypochondriasis. *British Journal of Psychiatry* 129:191–192.

Robinson N. 1729. A new System of the Spleen, Vapours, and Hypochondriack Melancholy: wherein all the decays of the nerves, and lownesses of the spirits, are mechanically accounted for. In *Three Hundred Years of Psychiatry 1535–1860* (eds. Hunter R., Macalpine I.), London: Oxford University Press, 1963.

Rousseau G.S. (ed.). 1990. *The Languages of Psyche. Mind and Body in Enlightenment Thought.* Berkeley: University of California Press.

Rush B. 1812. *Medical Inquiries and Observations upon the Diseases of the Mind.* New York: Hafner, 1962.

Sampayo J.R. 1986. *Rasgos erasmistas de la locura del Licenciado Vidriera de Miguel de Cervantes.* Kassel: Reichenberger.

Savage G. 1892. Hypochondriasis and insanity. In *A Dictionary of Psychological Medicine, Vol. 1.* (ed. Tuke D.H.), London: J & A Churchill.

Speak G. 1990. An odd kind of melancholy: reflections on the glass delusion in Europe (1440–1680). *History of Psychiatry* 1: 191–206.

Starobinski J. 1977. Le concept de cénesthésie et les idées neuropsychologiques de Moritz Schiff. *Gesnerus* 34: 2–19.

Starobinski J. 1990. A short history of bodily sensation. *Psychological Medicine* 20: 23–33.

Sydenham T. 1850. *The Works of Thomas Sydenham M.D.* (transl. by G. Latham), 2 vols. London: Printed for the Sydenham Society.

Taine H. 1890. *De l'Intelligence, Vol 2.* Paris: Hachette.

Titchener E.B. 1901. Common sensation. In *Dictionary of Philosophy and Psychology, Vol. 1* (ed. Baldwin J.W.), London: Macmillan.

Vila A.C. 1998. *Enlightenment and Pathology: Sensibility in the Literature and Medicine of Eighteenth Century France.* Baltimore: The Johns Hopkins University Press.

von Feuchtersleben Baron E. 1847. *The Principles of Medical Psychology* (transl. by H.E. Evand, B.G. Babington). London: The Syndenham Society.

Warrington N. 1965. *Plato's Timaeus*. Edited and translated with an introduction. London: Dent.

Whytt R. 1764. *Observations on the Nature, Causes and Cure of Those Diseases Which Are Commonly Called Nervous, Hypochondriac or Hysteric, First Edition*. In *The Works of Robert Whytt*, MD. Published by his son. Edinburgh: T. Becket and P.A. Dehondt, pp. 487–745. (Reprint, The Classics of Neurology & Neurosurgery Library, 1984.)

Williams K.E. 1990. Hysteria in seventeenth-century case records and unpublished manuscripts. *History of Psychiatry* 1: 383–401.

Willis Th. 1685. *The London Practice of Physick*. London: Thomas Basset.

World Health Organization. 1992. *The ICD-10 Classification of Mental and Behavioural Disorders*. Geneva: Author.

# 2

# Clinical Features and Diagnosis of Hypochondriasis

## VLADAN STARCEVIC

The term "hypochondriasis" has been in use for more than 2,000 years. However, its meaning throughout this time has been changing (see also Chapter 1). Today, it seems more difficult to agree on the defining characteristics of hypochondriasis than on its negative interpersonal and social implications. As a result, hypochondriasis is still frequently used as a derogatory label, and not as a medical diagnosis *per se*. In this respect, the situation does not seem to change: In the 1970s, "hypochondriac" was a "term of abuse" (Kenyon, 1976), and in the 1990s, hypochondriasis is associated with a "strong social stigma" (Rief and Hiller, 1998). To many, hypochondriasis continues to imply exaggeration and "imaginary sickness" at best, and feigning and fabrication at worst. Hypochondriasis is also a disqualifying label in the sense that no further questions are asked because of the assumption that everyone accepts the unfavorable implications of the label.

But what *is* hypochondriasis? As Table 2.1 shows, many definitions of hypochondriasis exist, with more than one given by the same author. Each definition of hypochondriasis attempts to capture its essential features. Hypochondriasis can be succinctly defined as excessive and persistent preoccupation with health, disease, and body, which is associated with a fear and suspicion that one is a victim of serious disease.

An important and early factor analytic study of hypochondriasis (Pilowsky, 1967) identified three dimensions of hypochondriasis: bodily preoccupation, disease phobia, and conviction of the presence of disease with nonresponse to reassurance. The elements common to various definitions of hypochondriasis, as well as empirical studies and clinical experience, all converge to suggest that sev-

**Table 2.1.** Various definitions of hypochondriasis

- "Mental preoccupation with a real or supposititious physical or mental disorder; a discrepancy between the degree of preoccupation and the grounds for it so that the former is far in excess of what is justified; and an affective condition best characterized as interest with conviction and consequent concern, and with indifference to the opinion to the environment, including irresponsiveness to persuasion" (Gillespie, 1929)
- "An obsessive kind of preoccupation with physical symptoms or body processes which is often accompanied by the development of various, and often shifting, somatic complaints" (Laughlin, 1956)
- "Unfounded fear of suffering from a disease" (Stenbäck and Rimón, 1964, p. 379)
- "Persistent preoccupation with disease despite reassurance given after thorough medical examination" (Pilowsky, 1967, p. 90)
- "Morbid preoccupation with mental or bodily functions or state of health" (Kenyon, 1976, p. 11)
- "Form of abnormal illness behaviour (dysnosognosia) in which the individual experiences and manifests a degree of concern over his state of health, which is out of proportion to the amount considered appropriate to the degree of objective evidence for the presence of disease" (Pilowsky, 1983, p. 319)
- "Concern with symptoms and with illness that the outside observer regards as excessive" (Sims, 1988, p. 171)
- "Pervasive and excessive concern about disease and a preoccupation with one's health" (Barsky, 1992, p. 791)
- "General propensity to worry about health, focus on one's body, and amplify discomfort" (Barsky et al., 1992, p. 107)
- "Constellation of health-related attitudes, a perceptual style, and a set of beliefs, which are experienced as ego syntonic and an integral part of the individual's identity" (Barsky et al., 1992, p. 102)

eral key components exist in the clinical presentation of patients with hypochondriasis. These components are as follows:

1. Bodily symptoms
2. Bodily preoccupation
3. Fear that a serious disease is already present
4. Suspicion that a serious disease is already present
5. Resistance to *routine* medical reassurance
6. Hypochondriacal behaviors

There is a question of whether a single diagnosis (of hypochondriasis) should "cover" such a broad range of phenomena. In addition, these components of hypochondriasis are not present to the same degree in all patients, which further contributes to its heterogeneity. Moreover, some components are not encountered in certain patients. For example, patients whose bodily symptoms are so over-shadowed by other characteristics of hypochondriasis may seem to be without symptoms. Some authors (Noyes et al., 1992) found that somatic symptoms were absent in certain patients with hypochondriasis. Likewise, some hypochondria-cal patients are predominantly afraid of having a life-threatening disease, with-out expressing a striking suspicion that they are already ill. Others may be so preoccupied with suspicions about the presence of a disease that the extent of their fear of that disease is not readily apparent. A reaction to medical reassur-ance may also vary significantly, and reassurance is not necessarily rejected; how-ever, hypochondriacal patients usually resist it.

Another important characteristic of hypochondriasis is persistence of its fea-tures, albeit with a fluctuating intensity, over a period of many months and, of-ten, many years. The usual onset of hypochondriasis is in the third and fourth decade of life, but the illness can appear in adults of any age. The features of hy-pochondriasis in the elderly are usually not significantly different from those in younger patients (Barsky *et al.*, 1991a), except that at a later age, they may be more frequently associated with depression (Brown *et al.*, 1984; de Alarcon, 1964; Kramer-Ginsberg *et al.*, 1989).

## Bodily Symptoms

Hypochondriacal patients usually complain of various bodily symptoms. The symptoms either have no demonstrable organic basis ("functional somatic symp-toms") or, if patients do have a medical condition, the symptoms are experienced as far more intense than what could be expected on the basis of the objectively existing, organic pathology. Patients might complain of one or more symptoms at a time, with symptoms arising from various organ systems. They often talk about their symptoms in great detail, but the overall description of symptoms may be vague. The more ambiguous the symptoms are to patients, the greater is their distress and concern about health, often because such symptoms are likely to be interpreted negatively (Hitchcock and Mathews, 1992; Robbins and Kir-mayer, 1996).

There are no symptoms typical of hypochondriasis. However, some symptoms (in the head, hair, neck, abdomen, and chest and in the musculoskeletal, gas-trointestinal, dermatologic, and central nervous systems) were found more fre-quently among patients with hypochondriasis (Kenyon, 1964, 1976; Pilowsky, 1970). Various pains, headache, and cardiovascular symptoms are also encoun-tered frequently. Patients with chronic pain may be prone to developing hypo-chondriasis. A positive correlation was found between the number of symptoms and the diagnosis of hypochondriasis (Barsky *et al.*, 1986), and hypochondriacal patients tend to report more symptoms than do healthy control subjects (Haenen *et al.*, 1996).

It is not known if there is anything—other than the association between certain symptoms and specific diseases—that determines the "choice" of symptoms *reported* by patients with hypochondriasis. In other words, although patients experience many sensations and symptoms, they may report only those they attribute to a disease with which they are preoccupied. Thus, headache may be "singled out" and reported because it is attributed to a brain tumor; in the same vein, palpitations might be attributed to heart disease and reported as most distressing. The characteristics of symptom reporting style in hypochondriasis are reviewed in Chapter 10.

The intensity of symptoms usually varies over time. Patients often have a peculiar attitude toward their symptoms: They are not so distressed by symptoms *per se* as they are by their implications and meaning (Barsky and Klerman, 1983). Haenen *et al.* (1997a) speculate that there is a relationship between perception of bodily symptoms and hypochondriacal patients' reaction to them, so that "whenever these patients feel something inexplicable to them inside their bodies, it is likely to evoke fear and irritation. Not being able to differentiate between actual cancer warning signals and non-warning signals causes a situation in which all bodily sensations are potentially threatening and, therefore, deserve full attention" (p. 131). When patients feel their symptoms "deserve full attention," it is understandable that they easily become preoccupied with their bodies.

## Bodily Preoccupation

Bodily preoccupation is one of the defining, enduring, and most conspicuous characteristics of hypochondriasis. Indeed, it can be regarded as a crucial component of the hypochondriacal patient's identity, a *sine qua non* of hypochondriasis. Bodily preoccupation pertains to the excessive awareness of and interest in bodily symptoms and bodily functioning in general. It is manifested through a constant and careful "listening" to and examining of one's own body, with the consequent tendency to report more symptoms. Patients are preoccupied not only with their symptoms, but also with the *meaning* of the symptoms (Avia, 1999). In a wider sense, bodily preoccupation refers to an enduring attention to, interest in, and vigilant attitude toward a variety of health- and illness-related matters.

In addition to being excessive, bodily preoccupation is also characterized by a large decrease in attention paid to and interest shown in other people, other objects, and other matters. As a result, patients may be preoccupied with the activities related to the suspected disease and health and illness in general, to the exclusion of almost all other activities. Hypochondriasis is seen as a "thematic restriction of experience and behavior on to the body alone" (Schäfer, 1982, p. 239). Indeed, patients may be so preoccupied with their fears of and suspicions about disease that they sometimes appear withdrawn from the outside world.

Hypochondriacal patients manifest bodily preoccupation in many ways. Thus, they pay inordinate attention to bodily sensations that others usually find innocuous and insignificant (e.g., peristalsis). They are often troubled by minor or expected variations in their normal bodily functioning (e.g., changes in the heart rate in response to physical exertion) or by minor physical symptoms (e.g., sore throat). Their bodily symptoms are so disturbing and patients so concerned about health that the disease- and health-related topics are a dominant feature in almost all of their conversations and interactions with others. Likewise, patients with hypochondriasis are exquisitely sensitive to all illness- and health-relevant information, and they may literally absorb all such information. It is usually difficult for them to be distracted when they experience the symptoms and when their attention is directed to matters of health and illness. Patients also frequently examine their bodies for signs of disease. When they hear or read about a particular dreaded disease, they often become aware of bodily symptoms, suggesting to them that they may be suffering from that disease.

The bodily preoccupation in hypochondriasis is often obsessional in nature, with emphasis on details and minutiae of the patients' somatic experience, along with a desperate attempt to attain total control over the body. The latter can be seen in their persistent pattern of reassurance-seeking and health-checking. The hypochondriacal patients' locus of control with respect to illness may be basically external (Avia, 1999), which intensifies their health anxiety and strengthens the obsessional pursuit of control. Another obsessional feature of hypochondriacal patients is their intolerance of somatic uncertainty, along with relentless insistence on certainty with regard to their state of health (Slavney, 1987). The extent to which hypochondriacal patients are anxiously preoccupied with health and disease suggests that they perceive the body as threatening and locate the danger "within," that is, in the body. Indeed, they expect to be "betrayed" by the body or feel that such a "betrayal" has already occurred.

Patients are usually immersed in thoughts and fears of one disease at a time, but they may be preoccupied with different diseases in the course of hypochondriasis. Thus, a patient who suspected having multiple sclerosis may be afraid of having developed a brain tumor at another stage of the disorder. Cancer is the disease that is probably most feared by hypochondriacal patients, but the usual focus of such patients' preoccupations has been changing over the years, depending largely on social factors and scientific and treatment advances. Whereas patients with hypochondriasis had frequently been preoccupied with tuberculosis and syphilis a century ago, nowadays they are more preoccupied with a possibility of having contracted AIDS.

## Fear That a Serious Disease Is Already Present

Most people are afraid of life-threatening and debilitating diseases, and so are patients with hypochondriasis. However, most people do not regard such diseases as a direct, current threat to them. They see diseases as either a threat in the distant future ("If it happens to me, it won't be now") or a danger with a low probability of affecting them ("It will not be me"). "Allocation" of the threat of a serious disease to the distant future and/or a sense that the disease will not strike helps most people dismiss fears of such diseases. Hypochondriacal patients, in contrast, are unable to do that and, as a result, are afraid of already having a disease.

In a more general sense, hypochondriacal patients are unable to protect themselves from fears involving dangers that they cannot prevent, and they do not tolerate low-risk threats to their health—threats to which everyone is exposed, but also threats that most people are able to "live with" and ultimately dismiss (Barsky, 1996; Mechanic, 1972).

The meaning of the disease of which hypochondriacal patients are afraid may be quite specific and may have symbolic significance. For example, the feared disease may be the same as that from which a significant other died. This may be experienced and interpreted by patients in very different ways, ranging from guilt over the loss of the loved one to identification with the deceased. In other cases, patients are afraid of a particular disease because it is disfiguring or because the handicap caused by the disease might have a devastating effect on their careers.

Fear of disease in patients with hypochondriasis has certain characteristics. It is like phobic fear in that it has a clear and specific focus: disease and, ultimately, death. Patients are afraid of a specific disease, such as cancer. According to some authors (Salkovskis and Clark, 1993), hypochondriacal patients are more likely to be afraid of the presence of serious disease with a chronic course and fatal outcome in the relatively distant future (e.g., multiple sclerosis). On rare occasions, patients with hypochondriasis are afraid of mental illness. This is referred to as "mental hypochondriasis," but it is doubtful that such a condition has anything substantial in common with hypochondriasis in which somatic disease is the focus of preoccupation.

Hypochondriacal fear of disease differs from phobic fear, and especially from "simple" disease phobia, in the following respects:

- Hypochondriacal patients do not consider their fear excessive and/or unreasonable.
- Hypochondriacal patients are not as afraid of becoming seriously ill in the future as they are of already having a serious disease that has not yet been detected.

- Hypochondriacal patients do not have a marked tendency to avoid physicians and hospitals.
- Hypochondriacal patients usually do not show an immediate anxiety response to encounters with physicians, because they regard such encounters as an opportunity to seek medical reassurance and thus alleviate their fears.

Patients with hypochondriasis are usually distressed by thoughts and images of death. The excessive fear of death seems to be one of the fundamental, underlying characteristics of hypochondriasis. The fear of death and hypochondriasis have been linked both empirically and on philosophical grounds. Thus, phenomenological philosophy considers hypochondriasis a consequence of an inability to "come to terms with the finiteness" of life, and the consequent "deep-rooted unresolved fear of death" (Schäfer, 1982, p. 237). In psychodynamic terms, hypochondriasis has been seen as a defense against the fear of death (Wahl, 1963).

Although studies have consistently shown an association between fear of death and hypochondriasis (Barsky and Wyshak, 1989; Hollifield et al., 1999a; Kellner et al., 1987a), the direction of potential causality in this relationship remains uncertain: Does excessive fear of death precede or even cause hypochondriasis or is it a consequence of hypochondriasis? Some authors (e.g., Kellner, 1986, p. 294) regard hypochondriacal features as primary, and fear of death as secondary.

## Suspicion That a Serious Disease Is Already Present

The terms "disease belief" and "disease conviction" are often used to describe the hypochondriacal patients' attitudes toward the disease with which they are preoccupied. However, these terms may be misleading, because of their implication of delusion, especially when the "belief" and "conviction" are resistant to medical reassurance and to all evidence that disease is not present. Therefore, the term "disease suspicion" seems more appropriately described as a cognitive component of the hypochondriacal experience (Starcevic, 1988). Patients with hypochondriasis typically suspect that they have a serious disease that physicians have not yet detected.

There is a crucial distinction between suspicion and belief/conviction. Suspicion reflects uncertainty, whereas a belief/conviction denotes certainty. The uncertainty of hypochondriacal patients pertains to their central dilemma: "Am I ill or not?" As long as such uncertainty persists, there is no delusion. Hypochondriacal patients find it particularly difficult to tolerate uncertainty, which compels them to look for "final" evidence or "perfect" proof that the disease is either present or not; however, the lack of such evidence or proof maintains their suspicion and strengthens their disbelief in a physician's diagnosis.

If there is no uncertainty, and patients are *sure* and *know* that they are ill, de-

**Table 2.2.** Characteristics of the disease suspicion as an overvalued idea

- An unfounded, abnormal idea ("I am ill") dominates the person's life.
- The idea is not held on the basis of delusional evidence (the explanation for having it may be plausible).
- The idea is acceptable and reasonable (ego-syntonic) to the person.
- The idea is usually associated with particularly strong emotions (fear of the disease and/or death).
- Although the person does not tend to test the validity of the idea, he or she may eventually abandon it, especially when presented with sufficient and convincing evidence that it is abnormal.
- The person experiences distress as a result of this idea or it causes disturbances in functioning.
- The idea leads to the activities (e.g., repeated reassurance-seeking, numerous medical examinations), which often have untoward effects on the person and an adverse impact on significant others and people in the person's immediate surroundings.

spite all evidence that the disease is not present, they are not likely to seek reassurance and look for "proofs" that they are not ill. Such a false and persistent belief/conviction that cannot be corrected should most appropriately be regarded as delusion. And the presence of a delusion is incompatible with a diagnosis of hypochondriasis. Hypochondriacal delusions suggest a psychotic illness, often a delusional disorder, somatic type according to the *Diagnostic and Statistical Manual of Mental Disorders DSM-IV* (American Psychiatric Association, 1994) or delusional disorder, hypochondriacal/somatic type according to the *International Classification of Diseases* ICD-10 (World Health Organization, 1992).

The disease suspicion can be conceptualized as a consequence of "morbid preoccupation" with health (Rachman, 1974; Salkovskis and Warwick, 1986) or as an overvalued (or "fixed") idea about the presence of disease. Other authors (Pilowsky, 1970; Sims, 1988) have also linked hypochondriasis to an overvalued idea. The characteristics of the disease suspicion as an overvalued idea, based on the works of McKenna (1984), Starcevic (1988), and Sims (1988), are presented in Table 2.2.

## Resistance to *Routine* Medical Reassurance

Patients with hypochondriasis are resistant to *routine* medical reassurance (i.e., reassurance that is *ordinarily* given to patients after physical examination and diagnostic tests have found no organic basis for their symptoms). It is important to emphasize the routine nature of such reassurance, because response to reassurance depends on several factors that are unrelated to hypochondriasis (e.g., the manner in which patients are reassured). Thus, if hypochondriacal patients are reassured carefully, with greater attention paid to their particular situation and personality characteristics, and if they are provided with all necessary and relevant information, they do not necessarily reject such reassurance (see Chapter 13).

Reactions of hypochondriacal patients to routine medical reassurance can vary greatly (Starcevic, 1990a). Some patients easily become irritated and angry by any attempt at reassurance. In such cases, there is usually an associated personality disorder, or hypochondriasis itself may be regarded as a personality disturbance.

Other patients do not respond to routine medical reassurance in a way that indicates they have accepted it, and it may seem that such reassurance has been rejected. However, the effects of reassurance in some patients may not be apparent if they are reassured only once. In many cases of hypochondriasis, reassurance is actually accepted, but its "amount" is never sufficient, which gives the impression that it has no effect.

Effects of reassurance in hypochondriasis may be connected to the sense of being accepted and understood by the reassurance-giving physician; it is difficult for hypochondriacal patients to feel accepted and understood after routine medical reassurance; hence, such reassurance may have little or no effect. The role of reassurance in the psychopathology and treatment of patients with hypochondriasis is discussed in more detail in Chapter 13.

Why is it difficult for hypochondriacal patients to accept routine reassurance? Possible explanations have only recently been investigated. One may have to do with distrust of physicians and suspicious attitudes toward them (Avia, 1999). A study by Haenen *et al.* (1997b) showed that hypochondriacal patients were less suggestible and proposed that "this lack of 'suggestibility' causes patients to distrust medical reassurance and to continue worrying" (p. 546). If so, this "insusceptibility" to suggestion might be a reflection of the obsessive character structure of hypochondriacal patients, of their general lack of trust, and of their unrelatedness to histrionic personality disturbance. Other authors (Barsky *et al.*, 1993a) have suggested that hypochondriacal phenomena, including resistance to medical reassurance, are a consequence of a peculiar belief that good health is akin to an ideal state in which there are no symptoms and no discomfort at all. Any deviation from such a state is interpreted by patients as an indication of the presence of illness; thus, it is understandable that with such a belief, medical reassurance is not likely to be effective.

## Hypochondriacal Behaviors

Typical hypochondriacal behaviors are repetitious health-checking (including checking the diagnosis) and seeking reassurance that one is not ill. Both are a

consequence of disease fears and disease suspicion. Examples of such patient behaviors include undergoing numerous physical examinations, laboratory tests, and
other diagnostic investigations; undergoing unnecessary surgical procedures and
hospitalizations; and repeatedly asking family members, friends, or physicians to
reassure them that they do not have the dreaded and/or suspected disease. In addition, patients may attempt to diagnose themselves and conduct their own treatment, often with the help of medical books and encyclopedias. Thus, various
activities related to health and disease become a characteristic lifestyle for
hypochondriacal patients.

Hypochondriacal patients collect their medical reports, pay much attention to
them, and examine them carefully. They compare reports made by different physicians to check whether there are any disagreements or inconsistencies. Patients
usually interpret any such discrepancies as another sign that physicians are also
puzzled by their condition and that their life-threatening disease has not been detected by physicians. One study (Hadjistavropoulos et al., 1998) found that individuals prone to hypochondriasis usually seek additional information about the
results of medical tests, "regardless of the diagnostic feedback they received"
(p. 161).

A need to obtain an "adequate" explanation for one's condition is the basis for
many hypochondriacal behaviors. It was found that, unlike nonhypochondriacal
patients, patients with hypochondriasis and hypochondriacal tendencies are not
so interested in being treated as they are in obtaining a "good enough" explanation for their illness (Starcevic et al., 1992): how and why they got ill, what exactly is the nature of their illness, what brings it on, and so on. Other authors
(e.g., Schmidt, 1994) also drew attention to the hypochondriacal patients' propensity to constantly look for an explanation of their complaints, and some (MacLeod
et al., 1998; Shaklee and Fischoff, 1982) suggested that this might result from
the patients' discontent with the lack of "fit" between explanations and symptoms for which these explanations had been given. Barsky and Klerman (1983)
expressed a similar view: "Hypochondriacal patients seem more concerned with
the authenticity, meaning, and etiological significance of their symptoms than
they are with the unpleasant physical sensations per se" (p. 275).

This peculiar feature—seeking explanation, rather than treatment—causes
much misunderstanding in the relationship between hypochondriacal patients and
health professionals. Physicians are primarily trained to offer advice, help, and
treatment. They usually do not provide detailed, etiologic explanations of disease
to patients, because most patients do not seek such explanations. It is difficult
for physicians to understand hypochondriacal patients, because patients need explanations for their illness instead of what physicians are most likely to offer—
medical advice and treatment suggestions. In other words, these patients may be
sending us a message that "although they seek help and caring, they will not eas-

ily accept what we have to offer" (Lipsitt, 1997, p. 313). The patients' frustrating pattern of requesting help and rejecting it at the same time becomes understandable in light of their underlying needs: They do not reject help that they need, only what physicians usually offer them, because the latter is not what they had asked for and expected.

Hypochondriacal patients are often disappointed both because they feel that physicians have not recognized their needs, and because whatever explanation they might have received does not satisfy them. Such disappointment is even more likely if the physicians (as is often the case) tell the patients that they are in good health and that there is no need for further consultation. Patients may interpret this as physicians' rejection of them. Furthermore, patients may feel and complain that their symptoms have not been taken seriously, and that they have been examined superficially. Such feelings pave the way for requests for repeated examinations and, ultimately, for a pattern often referred to as "doctor shopping." Going from one physician to another often makes the hypochondriacal patients more and more resentful, and they "end up" seeing themselves as victims of the medical establishment and of physicians' ignorance or neglect. They continue asking for help, yet complain that no one is helping and that no one understands them (see also Chapter 12).

Studies have shown that health care utilization is increased among hypochondriacal patients. In comparison with nonhypochondriacal individuals, they see more physicians (Noyes *et al.*, 1993), visit their physicians more often (Barsky *et al.*, 1991b; Noyes *et al.*, 1993), and have more emergency medical visits (Barsky *et al.*, 1991b). Some authors (Noyes *et al.*, 1993) reported more hospitalizations among patients with hypochondriasis, but others (Barsky *et al.*, 1991b) could not confirm this.

Not surprisingly, studies have also shown that hypochondriacal patients are not satisfied with their medical care (Barsky *et al.*, 1991b; Noyes *et al.*, 1993). More specifically, hypochondriacal patients felt that their health problems were not "thoroughly evaluated" and that their physicians were "not interested or concerned about their health problems" (Noyes *et al.*, 1993, p. 968). It is interesting, but quite in keeping with the dynamics of these patients, that although they distrusted physicians more, they were found to seek medical care more frequently (Kellner *et al.*, 1987a).

It is somewhat paradoxical that hypochondriacal patients may not be particularly cautious about behaviors that increase a real risk of becoming ill. Thus, one study (Kellner *et al.*, 1987a) found that in comparison with a group of family practice patients, hypochondriacal patients did not smoke less and did not take other health precautions, such as avoiding food that may not be healthy. This finding, if replicated, will illuminate better the behavior of hypochondriacal patients. More specifically, it is important to test a hypothesis (Kellner *et al.*, 1987a) that the patient's behavior is more determined by the perception of a direct and more immediate threat from the suspected disease than by any possible benefit from disease-prevention strategies in the relatively remote future.

The impairment in functioning is largely a consequence of hypochondriacal behaviors. All aspects of functioning might be affected. Family and intimate relationships are disrupted, because it is usually difficult for hypochondriacal patients' significant others to tolerate these patients' self-centeredness, overwhelming and exclusive attention paid to their bodies, and lack of interest in the matters of concern and significance to the couple's or family's well-being. Persistent and demanding requests from such patients' family members to be more involved in their plight is also frustrating. Relationships with friends and with others in the patients' social milieu may be disrupted for similar reasons. Finally, hypochondriacal patients are often unable to take up their responsibilities at work as a result of their all-encompassing preoccupation with their health and their symptoms, and the constant health-checking and reassurance-seeking behaviors that follow.

## The Spectrum of Hypochondriacal Manifestations

The range of hypochondriacal manifestations is very wide (Table 2.3). It has been suggested that hypochondriacal phenomena are distributed along a continuum of severity and that differences between hypochondriacal and nonhypochondriacal persons may be quantitative rather than qualitative (Barsky and Klerman, 1983; Barsky et al., 1986; Kenyon, 1976; Schmidt, 1994).

Such a dimensional conceptualization of hypochondriasis postulates that on one side of its psychopathological spectrum are states and behaviors that are usually not considered abnormal, and that may be even reinforced by social factors. Thus, with current emphasis on personal responsibility for prevention of disease, people are flooded with information that prescribes what to eat, how to avoid toxic substances, how to stay "fit," and how to minimize the risk for specific diseases. Taking this information and the corresponding advice too seriously or too

**Table 2.3.** The spectrum of hypochondriacal manifestations

- Excessive "health consciousness," with health-promoting and disease-preventing "rituals"
- Transient hypochondriasis
- Secondary hypochondriasis (e.g., in the course of panic disorder or a major depressive episode as the principal disorder)
- Primary hypochondriasis ("true" hypochondriasis)
- Hypochondriacal delusions (e.g., as part of delusional disorder, hypochondriacal/somatic type)

literally may contribute to preoccupation with eating "natural" food, living a "healthy" life, exercising vigorously, and having one's body in "perfect shape" (Barsky and Klerman, 1983). Although individuals with such preoccupation do not have fears or suspicions that they have succumbed to a serious disease, their health-promoting and disease-preventing behaviors are clearly excessive. However, it is unknown whether such behaviors and attitudes predispose to clinically significant hypochondriasis. Some research (Lecci *et al.*, 1996) has found a correlation between hypochondriacal tendencies on one hand and illness-prevention and health-promotion orientation on the other.

Transient hypochondriasis (lasting under 6 months) can occur in various situations. For example, it is encountered in the context of somatic illness, during recovery from an acute, life-threatening disease such as myocardial infarction, among people who care for terminally ill family members or friends, as part of the process of bereavement, or after some other stressful life event. One study (Barsky *et al.*, 1990) found that hypochondriacal phenomena were less intense in patients with transient hypochondriasis than in those with "classical" chronic hypochondriasis. When compared to the nonhypochondriacal patients (Barsky *et al.*, 1990), those with transient hypochondriasis had more lifetime psychiatric comorbidity and more personality disorders, and they were more sensitive to various bodily sensations (with higher levels of somatosensory amplification). These findings supported a notion that presence of an Axis I mental disorder and personality disorder, as well as a tendency toward somatosensory amplification, might predispose to hypochondriacal manifestations in the context of somatic disease (Barsky *et al.*, 1990). At a 2-year follow-up, patients with transient hypochondriasis were found to exhibit some hypochondriacal features, but they were not more likely to develop a chronic form of hypochondriasis (Barsky *et al.*, 1993b).

When patients with chronic and transient hypochondriacal tendencies were compared (Robbins and Kirmayer, 1996), the former were more likely to have a serious lifetime history of medical morbidity and impairment, higher rates of lifetime and current psychiatric comorbidity (especially with major depression and anxiety disorders), higher levels of vulnerability to serious emotional problems, and stronger feelings that they had very little support from others in their attempts to cope with disease fears.

Transient and recurrent hypochondriasis can be seen in medical students. The recurrent nature of hypochondriacal concerns in medical students and different diseases with which they are often preoccupied may be accounted for by the students' exposure to different disease-related information and to people ill with serious diseases at various times during their medical studies. Two studies (Hunter *et al.*, 1964; Woods *et al.*, 1966) reported high proportions (70%–79%) of medical students with hypochondriacal manifestations, also referred to as "medical students' disease" (Woods *et al.*, 1966). However, when medical students and law students were systematically compared in terms of hypochondriacal features (Kellner *et al.*, 1986a), it was found that medical students took only slightly more precautions about their health and paid more attention to somatic symptoms, but did not exhibit more hypochondriacal fears and beliefs. These findings suggest that it takes more than exposure to disease-relevant information and to seriously ill people for significant hypochondriacal features to appear, and that any manifestations of hypochondriasis in medical students are rather limited in scope. For some students, medical studies may represent a part of their "counterphobic strategy," intended to overcome excessive fear of death to which medical students are prone (Howells and Field, 1982); insofar as excessive fear of death is associated with hypochondriasis, it may explain the propensity to hypochondriasis in some medical students.

Secondary hypochondriasis occurs in the course of a principal psychiatric condition and is more likely to be encountered in psychiatric settings. The principal condition is the one that causes greatest distress and impaired functioning and/or the one for which help is sought. It is usually panic disorder or major depression. Secondary hypochondriasis is apparently more frequent than primary hypochondriasis, and its manifestations are usually less severe. It is usually transient and disappears or diminishes greatly with the successful treatment of the principal condition. The latter was demonstrated by Noyes *et al.* (1986) in the treatment of panic disorder and by Kellner *et al.* (1986b) in the treatment of depression.

Primary hypochondriasis is defined as a *principal* disorder, and so that it is in the focus of clinical attention, even when other mental disorders are also present. It is usually seen in primary care or general medical settings. Primary hypochondriasis is a disorder for which patients seek treatment and/or which causes greatest distress or impaired functioning. It is usually associated with other mental disorders. Indeed, studies suggest that in the majority (62%–88%) of hypochondriacal patients, there is at least one comorbid mental disorder (Barsky *et al.*, 1992; Noyes *et al.*, 1994b). Hypochondriasis was found to co-occur most frequently with depressive and anxiety disorders, and somatization disorder.

It should be noted that the terms *primary* and *secondary hypochondriasis* are used here with a meaning different from the one espoused by some authors (e.g., by Barsky *et al.*, 1992). They define primary hypochondriasis as a condition unaccompanied by any other mental disorder, and secondary hypochondriasis as a disorder with concurrent psychiatric disturbance.

The presence of hypochondriacal delusions denotes psychotic illness. These delusions are encountered as relatively isolated in delusional disorder, somatic type. This condition has been commonly referred to as "monosymptomatic hypochondriacal psychosis" or "monosymptomatic hypochondriasis." Monosymptomatic hypochondriacal psychosis was reviewed by Munro (1988), who observed the following forms of its presentation: (*1*) delusions of infestation or parasitosis (delusions of being infested with parasites, insects, worms, or foreign bodies under the skin); (*2*) dysmorphic delusions (delusions of being ugly or of having a bodily deformity); (*3*) delusions of body odor or halitosis or "olfactory reference syndrome" (delusions that one is emitting unpleasant body odors that are noticed by others). Although monosymptomatic hypochondriacal psychosis may be generally common in developing countries (Osman, 1991), it is in Japan that the delusions of body odor are frequently encountered as part of the syndrome *Taijin Kyofusho*, characterized by fears that one's body is in various ways offensive to other people (Kirmayer, 1991; Tanaka-Matsumi, 1979).

If accompanied by other prominent psychotic symptoms (e.g., other delusions and/or hallucinations), hypochondriacal delusions are usually a part of the clinical picture of schizophrenia or major depressive disorder with psychotic features.

## Diagnosis of Hypochondriasis

Hypochondriasis is classified among the somatoform disorders in *DSM-IV*, and among the neurotic, stress-related, and somatoform disorders in ICD-10 as well as in the ICD-10 modification for use in research, ICD-10-DCR (Diagnostic Criteria for Research; World Health Organization, 1993). The diagnostic criteria for hypochondriasis in *DSM-IV* and ICD-10-DCR are presented in Tables 2.4 and 2.5.

**Table 2.4.** *DSM-IV* diagnostic criteria for hypochondriasis*

A. Preoccupation with fears of having, or the idea that one has, a serious disease based on the person's misinterpretation of bodily symptoms.
B. The preoccupation persists despite appropriate medical evaluation and reassurance.
C. The belief in Criterion A is not of delusional intensity (as in Delusional Disorder, Somatic Type) and is not restricted to a circumscribed concern about appearance (as in Body Dysmorphic Disorder).
D. The preoccupation causes clinically significant distress or impairment in social, occupational, or other important areas of functioning.
E. The duration of the disturbance is at least 6 months.
F. The preoccupation is not better accounted for by Generalized Anxiety Disorder, Obsessive-Compulsive Disorder, Panic Disorder, a Major Depressive Episode, Separation Anxiety, or another Somatoform Disorder.

*Specify* if:
*With Poor Insight*: if, for most of the time during the current episode, the person does not recognize that the concern about having a serious illness is excessive or unreasonable

*Reprinted with permission from the *Diagnostic and Statistical Manual of Mental Disorders,* Fourth Edition. Copyright © 1994 American Psychiatric Association.

**Table 2.5.** ICD-10-DCR diagnostic criteria for hypochondriacal disorder*

---

A. Either of the following must be present:
   (*1*) A persistent belief, of at least 6 months' duration, of the presence of a maximum of two serious physical diseases (of which at least one must be specifically named by the patient);
   (*2*) A persistent preoccupation with a presumed deformity or disfigurement (body dysmorphic disorder).
B. Preoccupation with the belief and the symptoms causes persistent distress or interference with personal functioning in daily living, and leads the patient to seek medical treatment or investigations (or equivalent help from local healers).
C. There is persistent refusal to accept medical reassurance that there is no physical cause for the symptoms or physical abnormality. (Short-term acceptance of such reassurance—i.e., for a few weeks during or immediately after investigations—does not exclude this diagnosis.)
D. *Most commonly used exclusion clause.* The symptoms do not occur only during any of the schizophrenic and related disorders (particularly persistent delusional disorders) or any of the mood [affective] disorders.

---

*Reprinted with permission from the ICD-10 *Classification of Mental and Behavioural Disorders, Diagnostic Criteria for Research.* World Health Organization, Geneva, 1993.

In both the *DSM-IV* and ICD-10-DCR, hypochondriasis is described as a chronic disorder (lasting for at least 6 months) and characterized by the idea or belief that there is a serious physical disease which persists despite medical evaluation and reassurance. The main difference between the two classification systems is in the relationship between hypochondriasis and body dysmorphic disorder: In *DSM-IV*, body dysmorphic disorder is a separate diagnostic entity; in ICD-10-DCR, it is a part of hypochondriasis. In addition, the fear of having a disease and the underlying mechanism of misinterpretation of bodily symptoms are not mentioned among the diagnostic criteria in ICD-10-DCR.

Both the *DSM-IV* and ICD-10-DCR postulate a partial diagnostic hierarchy between hypochondriasis and other mental disorders. In clinical practice, this means that a diagnosis of hypochondriasis can very rarely, if ever, be made along with a diagnosis of chronic psychotic disorder, such as schizophrenia, because it would be extremely difficult to see hypochondriasis occurring independently from the simultaneously present schizophrenia. But in cases of co-occurrence of hypochondriasis and mood, anxiety, and other somatoform disorders, the main task is to determine whether hypochondriasis is, in fact, a part of these disorders, so that it occurs only during the episodes of panic disorder, major depressive disorder, and so on. If so, the diagnosis of hypochondriasis is not warranted. In all other cases of co-occurrence with mood, anxiety, and other somatoform disorders, there is no hierarchy, and diagnoses of hypochondriasis and another such disorder can both be made at the same time.

It should be emphasized that a diagnosis of hypochondriasis is to be used only after a complete physical examination and necessary diagnostic tests have shown that the patient's health concerns are unjustified or excessive. In this endeavor, it is important for the physician to realize that "there is never an absolute end to the process of ruling out organic disease" (Kirmayer and Robbins, 1991, p. 211). Such an attitude paves the way for the physician's acceptance of the true limitations of medical knowledge, and of the consequent, inevitable uncertainty. Only then will it be possible for the physician gradually and carefully to address these limitations and uncertainty in the course of treating a hypochondriacal patient.

## Validity of the Diagnosis of Hypochondriasis

The concept of hypochondriasis has been criticized on grounds that it possesses very little, if any, validity. In particular, some authors (e.g., Kenyon, 1964) did not consider hypochondriasis a distinct nosologic entity, but always secondary to other mental disorders. In the same vein, hypochondriasis was regarded merely as a "reaction ranging from normality to totally disabling severity" (Mayou, 1976, p. 59) and as "an entirely arbitrary syndrome defined more by consultation behavior than by true phenomenology" (Mayou, 1976, p. 59). Others viewed hypochondriasis as an "amplifying somatic style" (Barsky and Klerman, 1983, p. 280) and "dimension rather than a disorder" (Lipowski, 1988, p. 1364), or conceptualized hypochondriasis as a defense mechanism, and not an illness *per se* (Vaillant, 1977). Henri Ey (1966) wondered whether an imaginary illness could be considered a "true" illness.

In response to such profound doubts about the validity of the diagnostic concept of hypochondriasis, several studies have examined various aspects of the validity of the diagnosis of hypochondriasis. These studies appeared relatively late, only after the operationalized diagnostic criteria had been introduced by the *DSM-III* (American Psychiatric Association, 1980). In the first such study (Barsky *et al.*, 1986), it was found that several elements of the *DSM-III*-based diagnosis of hypochondriasis (bodily symptoms, bodily preoccupation, disease fear, and disease conviction) are significantly intercorrelated, and that they cluster together. The authors suggested that hypochondriasis had considerable internal validity and consistency, and that it might constitute a distinct mental disorder. Noyes *et al.* (1993) subsequently confirmed the internal validity of hypochondriasis, diagnosed on the basis of the *DSM-III-R* criteria (American Psychiatric Association, 1987).

Studies conducted by Barsky and Wyshak (1989), Noyes *et al.* (1993), and Gureje *et al.* (1997) examined external validity of hypochondriasis, which pertains to extrinsic, associated characteristics of this disorder. These studies identified several indicators of external validity of the diagnosis of hypochondriasis: prominent fears of aging and death; great importance placed on health and on one's physical appearance; strong sense of bodily vulnerability to illness and injury; negative perception of one's overall health; an amplifying perceptual style; high levels of distress due to bodily symptoms; multiple comorbid psychiatric diagnoses and syndromes (especially those of depression, anxiety, and somatization); frequent diagnoses of "functional somatic syndromes" (such as fibromyalgia, irritable bowel syndrome, chronic fatigue syndrome, and temporomandibular joint syndrome); increased health care utilization; decrease in usual activities; impairment in work performance and physical functioning; and disability. Two recent studies (Hollifield et al., 1999b; Jyväsjärvi et al., 1999) have confirmed a significant association between hypochondriasis and frequent use of health services, although in a study by Hollifield et al. (1999b) this association was accounted for more by somatization than by hypochondriasis.

Three studies have addressed aspects of predictive validity of the diagnosis of hypochondriasis. This type of validity refers to the ability of the diagnosis to predict accurately the course, treatment response, and outcome of illness. A 1-year follow-up study of patients with hypochondriasis (Noyes et al., 1994a) provided some evidence for predictive validity of hypochondriasis as a chronic condition: The study showed that this diagnosis was stable over time (with two-thirds of the patients continuing to meet criteria for hypochondriasis and most of the remaining one-third still reporting hypochondriacal symptoms but failing to meet criteria for the diagnosis of hypochondriasis); in addition, although symptoms waxed and waned, characteristic features of the disorder persisted after a year.

Another study (Robbins and Kirmayer, 1996) showed that at 1-year follow-up, one-half of patients who were initially considered hypochondriacal on the basis of their response to a questionnaire continued to be more concerned about their health than were nonhypochondriacal patients. A prospective 4- to 5-year study of patients with hypochondriasis (Barsky et al., 1998) provided further support for the stability of the diagnosis of hypochondriasis and the associated chronicity of the condition: two-thirds of patients continued to meet diagnostic criteria for hypochondriasis after a long interval, although hypochondriacal symptoms and disability generally decreased. Even in patients who experienced hypochondriacal concerns less frequently and less intensely, the improvement was considered unstable, because it was seen as a result of favorable external factors rather than as a result of any fundamental change in the patients' attitudes toward illness and health (Barsky et al., 1998).

The hypochondriacal patients' response to treatment was traditionally considered poor, but it is now recognized as highly variable. However, a response to treatment is not predicted by the diagnosis itself. The diagnosis of hypochondriasis also appears to be of little value in predicting remissions in the course of illness and its outcome. Predictors of a more favorable outcome of hypochondriasis include shorter duration of illness; absence of personality disorders and of past psychiatric history; lower level of neuroticism; generally less Axis I comorbidity (although some authors have found presence of more symptoms of anxiety and depression to be associated with better outcome); and more medical comorbidity (Barsky *et al.*, 1998; House, 1989; Kellner, 1983; Noyes *et al.*, 1994a; Pilowsky, 1968; Robbins and Kirmayer, 1996).

There continue to be some conflicting findings regarding the overall validity of hypochondriasis. Thus, the validity of the diagnosis was not supported by Noyes *et al.* (1997), because there was no evidence of family aggregation of hypochondriasis. The authors concluded that hypochondriasis might not be an independent disorder, and that it might be a "variable feature of other mental disorders, most notably somatization disorder" (Noyes *et al.*, 1997, p. 231). In addition, two studies (Barsky *et al.*, 1992; Noyes *et al.*, 1994b) showed high comorbidity rates (ranging from 62% to 88%) in patients with a principal diagnosis of hypochondriasis, suggesting that hypochondriasis is relatively rarely encountered in the absence of other psychopathology, and raising some doubt about the validity of hypochondriasis as an entity in its own right.

It could be argued that the absence of family aggregation and high comorbidity rates do not necessarily indicate that hypochondriasis is not an independent disorder. The comorbidity criterion may be particularly troublesome, in view of the fact that many mental disorders, including those that are more firmly established and whose validity is questioned far less often (e.g., panic disorder), do have high rates of comorbidity. Nevertheless, a discriminant validity of hypochondriasis (i.e., the extent to which hypochondriasis can be described by features that reliably and consistently distinguish it from other disorders) requires further study.

Hypochondriasis is similar to most mental disorders in that the construct validity of the diagnosis of hypochondriasis is lacking. In other words, the diagnosis of hypochondriasis is not based on a clear understanding of etiology and pathogenesis, and cannot be confirmed by independent validators such as biological markers or laboratory tests.

In conclusion, studies suggest that the diagnosis of hypochondriasis does have greater overall validity than was previously believed. This also includes increasing evidence that hypochondriasis is an independent disorder, albeit with high rates of comorbidity with other disorders. Further research into various aspects of the validity of the diagnosis of hypochondriasis is clearly warranted.

## Critical Review of the Diagnostic Criteria for Hypochondriasis

Although introduction of the operationalized diagnostic criteria for hypochondriasis represented a significant advance, these criteria did not provide a completely satisfying description of hypochondriasis. As a result, there are several problems with the criteria, which also reflect some of the unresolved conceptual dilemmas about hypochondriasis. This section will critically examine the *DSM-IV* and ICD-10-DCR criteria for hypochondriasis.

1. In the *DSM-IV*, the key criterion for defining hypochondriasis is "preoccupation with fears of having, or the idea that one has, a serious disease based on the person's misinterpretation of bodily symptoms" (American Psychiatric Association, 1994, p. 465). Thus, hypochondriasis refers to an unreasonable fear or a "false" belief, and according to the *DSM-IV*, both qualify equally well for the diagnosis of hypochondriasis. This proposition is controversial, because there may be a hierarchical relationship between the disease fear and disease suspicion. The fear appears to be a more fundamental characteristic of hypochondriasis, as it is common to all patients with this diagnosis. This is supported by an observation that there are hypochondriacal patients who are only afraid that they are ill, but who do not have a strong suspicion (or a "false" belief) that they are ill. Such patients may suffer from a less severe form of hypochondriasis than do those with both a fear and suspicion. Conversely, the hypochondriacal suspicion usually subsumes hypochondriacal fear, and hypochondriacal patients who suspect having a serious disease such as cancer, without being afraid that they are ill, are a true rarity.

Other authors (e.g., Schmidt, 1994) noted the same problem with an almost identical *DSM-III-R* criterion for hypochondriasis. More specifically, Schmidt (1994) suggested that the fear of disease and belief that one has a disease should not be "treated as being of equal importance" (p. 307), and that fear was a primary phenomenon, whereas belief represented a secondary phenomenon in this condition.

Fears and beliefs are certainly not the same psychopathological phenomena, and they should not be treated interchangeably. Moreover, disease fears may have primacy over disease suspicions, and especially over disease beliefs, in that they identify more patients with hypochondriasis. This issue needs to be tested, for example, by comparing the proportion of patients with hypochondriasis who are identified on the basis of the positive responses to the two "screening" questions:

- "Are you afraid you have a serious illness that doctors have not discovered yet?"
- "Do you believe (suspect) you have a serious illness that doctors have not discovered yet?"

Another key question with respect to the fear versus suspicion/belief issue pertains to the possibility of two discrete subtypes of hypochondriasis: One would be characterized predominantly by disease fears, whereas disease suspicions (or beliefs) would predominate in the other. There are reports and observations that hypochondriacal fears may be associated more with symptoms of anxiety, obsessional features, and anxiety disorders in general, whereas hypochondriacal beliefs may be related more to somatic symptoms and comorbid depression (Barsky, 1992; Fallon, 1999; Kellner *et al.*, 1992). It has also been suggested that phobialike disease fears in hypochondriasis may be treated effectively with specific modalities such as psychopharmacotherapy (Wesner and Noyes, 1991) and behavior therapy (Warwick and Marks, 1988). However, the current lack of systematic data fails to support the notion that there are two distinct and valid subtypes of hypochondriasis. It also appears that there are more hypochondriacal patients with various mixtures of disease fears and disease suspicions than there are patients with pure disease fears and pure disease suspicions.

**2.** A careful reading of the diagnostic criteria for hypochondriasis (preoccupation with the "wrong" or "false" idea/belief that persists despite appropriate medical evaluation and reassurance) makes one wonder whether hypochondriacal (somatic) delusion has been incorporated into a definition of hypochondriasis. Elsewhere in this chapter, attention was drawn to confusion arising from failure of current diagnostic criteria for hypochondriasis to make a clearer distinction between delusional and nondelusional beliefs. Guidelines for making this distinction are presented in the sections "Suspicion That a Serious Disease Is Already Present" and "Differential Diagnosis of Hypochondriasis" of this chapter.

**3.** Failure to respond to medical reassurance as a diagnostic criterion for hypochondriasis is controversial for several reasons. First, it is often assumed that reassurance is a simple act, which is provided uniformly. Second, the "appropriate" medical reassurance is not defined precisely, and its meaning is subject to various interpretations. Third, the pattern of response to medical reassurance by hypochondriacal patients has a tendency to vary. Fourth, to make a diagnosis of hypochondriasis on the basis of resistance to medical reassurance, it is imperative that the physician and the patient disagree (Pilowsky, 1992), and the definitive diagnosis has to be "postponed until the response to medical information can be fully appraised" (Pilowsky, 1996, p. 116) (see also Chapter 11). Fifth, it is not logical to define a disorder in terms of the (in)ability of the person from whom help is sought to reassure and thus reduce anxiety (Salkovskis and Clark, 1993). Finally, a large, cross-national study of hypochondriasis in primary care (Gureje *et al.*, 1997) found that the adherence to the criterion of a failure (or refusal) to respond to medical reassurance led to an underdetection of hypochondriasis in primary care and to the spuriously decreased prevalence of hypochondriasis. Gureje *et al.* (1997) suggested criteria for "abridged" hypochondriasis (consisting of illness worry or disease conviction, associated distress or interference with functioning, and medical help-seeking), which would contribute to a better recognition of hypochondriacal patients and to a more accurate estimate of the prevalence of hypochondriasis in primary care.

There is no easy way to resolve this problem. Pilowsky (1992) proposed diagnostic criteria for hypochondriasis, in which he split the "reassurance criterion" into two more detailed and more phenomenological criteria: "(*1*) An awareness of an inability to accept reassurance from doctors who have offered clear information, associated with the concern that doctors have not done everything possible to detect disease or are withholding information and/or treatment which could be helpful; (*2*) An awareness of an inability to accept the suggestion that non-physical, i.e. psychosocial, factors may be relevant to one's condition, and marked emotional discomfort when this possibility is raised" (p. 215).

Another possibility is to state the following among the diagnostic criteria: (*1*) Resistance to medical reassurance occurs when reassurance is given "routinely" and (*2*) routine reassurance can be defined as the physician's provision of brief and anxiety-alleviating medical information on a single occasion. If patients do not respond to carefully planned and more elaborate medical reassurance, given over a longer period of time (so that this approximates the notion of "appropriate" medical reassurance), it is likely that they have a more severe form of hypochondriasis (see also Chapter 13).

**4.** A diagnosis of hypochondriasis may be made if organic disease is present, but the patients' degree of bodily preoccupation, disease fear, and other features of hypochondriasis should be out of proportion with respect to the extent of organic pathology. This suggestion might be confusing because of the lack of clarity (i.e., how much organic pathology is necessary to make a diagnosis of hypochondriasis redundant). It also leads to important conceptual questions, such as whether hypochondriasis can be diagnosed in someone suffering from verified heart disease. No guidelines are given as to whether and how a diagnosis of hypochondriasis is to be made when a discrepancy between the objective findings and subjective account exists; indeed, it appears that a diagnosis of hypochondriasis can then be made quite arbitrarily.

Schmidt (1994) has offered several useful criteria by which it would be possible to make a diagnosis of hypochondriasis in patients with serious organic disease. These criteria include propositions that hypochondriacal tendencies were present before the onset of organic disease, that what the patients are afraid of or preoccupied with has no relationship whatsoever with the objectively existing disease, and that patients are not comforted or reassured by any alleviation in, or even disappearance of, the symptoms of their organic disease.

**5.** The specifier "with poor insight" in the *DSM-IV* is somewhat confusing because it implies that there are two kinds of hypochondriacal patients: those who recognize that their concern about having a serious illness is excessive or unreasonable, and those who do not. However, most hypochondriacal patients do not have that kind of insight, and, by and large, they consider their fears and suspicions quite reasonable. Therefore, most hypochondriacal patients would, according to the *DSM-IV*, have "poor insight," but it is questionable how those with "preserved" insight should be diagnosed and classified.

The hypothesized distinction between hypochondriasis with good and poor insight has had another implication. Patients with good insight have been considered to have a related condition, or a subtype of hypochondriasis (Schmidt, 1994), referred to as "disease phobia" (Bianchi, 1971) or "illness phobia" (Marks, 1987). There is some evidence (Warwick and Marks, 1988; Wesner and Noyes, 1991) that patients with "disease phobia" or "illness phobia" may benefit from a different treatment approach than those with pure hypochondriasis (and poor insight). However, a treatment response cannot serve as the basis for introducing new diagnostic categories or for dividing those already existing into subtypes.

**6.** The *DSM-IV* diagnostic criteria presume a mechanism—misinterpretation of bodily symptoms—by which hypochondriacal patients develop fears and ideas of having a serious disease. Although this cognitive mechanism may play a role in the development and/or maintenance of hypochondriasis, we still do not know enough about the pathogenesis of hypochondriasis to suggest that misinterpretation is the only pathway to the occurrence of this disorder.

**7.** The ICD-10-DCR contains a rather "clumsy" diagnostic criterion, namely that the hypochondriacal patient must have a belief in "the presence of a maximum of two serious physical diseases (of which at least one must be specifically named by the patient)" (World Health Organization, 1993, p. 106). This criterion seems arbitrary and redundant: It is arbitrary because it is not clear why the number of suspected serious diseases should be limited to two at a time. The criterion is redundant because it is understood by definition that hypochondriacal patients are able to name a serious disease that they are afraid of having or whose presence they suspect.

**8.** A proposition by the ICD-10-DCR to treat body dysmorphic disorder as a "variant" of hypochondriasis is controversial and not supported by clinical observation and research data.

## Differential Diagnosis of Hypochondriasis

It is important to perform differential diagnosis of hypochondriasis in the sequence of the decreasing importance and/or the decreasing likelihood of occurrence of the disorders that are to be taken into consideration. This sequence is presented in Table 2.6.

### Organic Diseases

The first step in the differential diagnosis of hypochondriasis is to consider a physical basis for the patient's symptoms, even if organic disease has been pre-

**Table 2.6.** Differential diagnosis of hypochondriasis

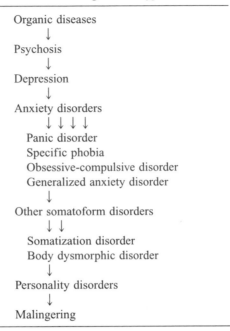

Organic diseases
↓
Psychosis
↓
Depression
↓
Anxiety disorders
↓ ↓ ↓ ↓
    Panic disorder
    Specific phobia
    Obsessive-compulsive disorder
    Generalized anxiety disorder
    ↓
Other somatoform disorders
↓ ↓
    Somatization disorder
    Body dysmorphic disorder
    ↓
Personality disorders
↓
Malingering

viously excluded. Many anecdotal reports of hypochondriacal patients whose fears and suspicions turned out to be justified and who were eventually diagnosed with a tumor or some other organic disease serve as a powerful reminder that organic disease must never be overlooked.

Most patients who are referred to the psychiatrist have already had numerous diagnostic examinations that excluded organic disease, and it is rarely necessary to order additional diagnostic tests. Such investigations are justified only if new symptoms appear and if the psychiatrist suspects the presence of another disease (see also Chapter 13). Naturally, in the course of hypochondriasis, patients do become ill from organic disease, which may or may not be related to their original somatic complaints. A complicating factor in managing such cases adequately is that people in the immediate surroundings of these patients (including their doctors) may not take their complaints seriously, because over many months or years they have become accustomed to such patients' "excessive" complaints and bodily preoccupation.

There are no typical organic diseases that should be considered in the differential diagnosis of hypochondriasis. However, some diseases with insidious onset and chronic or intermittent course, especially if their presentation is atypical, varied, and involving several organ systems, may be relevant to hypochondriasis.

Examples of such diseases are some occult malignancies, and endocrine, neurologic, and autoimmune diseases (American Psychiatric Association, 1994).

It should be emphasized again that a diagnosis of hypochondriasis is not incompatible with the presence of organic disease. If there is organic disease, a diagnosis of hypochondriasis can be made if it is established that the patient's complaints and degree of bodily preoccupation are disproportionate to the extent of the verified pathology, seriousness, and implications of organic disease. However, without precise criteria to make this judgment, it remains somewhat arbitrary.

## Psychosis

The next step in the differential diagnosis of hypochondriasis is to determine whether there is a delusion about the presence of a serious disease (hypochondriacal or somatic delusion). Sometimes it is difficult to make a clear distinction between disease suspicion, which characterizes hypochondriasis, and false disease belief that should be conceptualized as a delusion. However, an effort to make such a distinction is always warranted, as emphasized in other sections of this chapter.

The distinguishing feature of hypochondriacal delusion is a firm, unfounded, and false belief about the presence of serious disease, which persists despite adequate medical reassurance and all evidence to the contrary. Such a belief is usually held on the basis of delusional evidence, so that the person's explanation for having it indicates gross impairment of reality testing. For example, the patient may be convinced of having cancer as a result of being poisoned with carcinogens. In addition, hypochondriacal delusions may be accompanied by bizarre features, such as beliefs that intestines have been moved to the chest by some external agency or that a liver has been "pierced" by X-rays and made "hollow."

Hypochondriacal delusions are usually seen in delusional disorder (somatic/hypochondriacal type), schizophrenia, or major depressive disorder with psychotic features. Except for delusional disorder, hypochondriacal delusions represent an associated characteristic in these conditions, so that other, more fundamental features of these psychotic disorders dominate patients' clinical presentations.

## Depression

Hypochondriacal manifestations frequently accompany depression. In such cases, features of a depressive syndrome dominate patients' clinical presentations, and they may even color hypochondriacal phenomena. For example, the disease that is suspected may be experienced as punishment for wrongdoing. If hypochondriacal manifestations occur for the first time later in life, the diagnosis of a major depressive disorder is more likely. The intensity of hypochondriacal manifestations secondary to depression usually decreases substantially with the recovery from a depressive episode (Kellner et al., 1986b).

The diagnosis of hypochondriasis is compatible with that of major depressive disorder if the features of the former are not confined to depressive episodes, and if hypochondriacal manifestations are not considered a part of the clinical presentation of depression. In such cases, the treatment of depression has little effect on the underlying and enduring hypochondriacal characteristics (Demopulos et al., 1996). In one study (Noyes et al., 1994b), hypochondriasis was found to be more likely to precede depression.

The link between hypochondriasis and depression does not appear as strong as once believed, although a significant association between them continues to be reported (Barsky et al., 1986; Escobar et al., 1998). In some studies, hypochondriacal features were found to be associated with depression as much as they were with anxiety (Barsky et al., 1986; Gureje et al., 1997; Kellner et al., 1987b), but other studies showed a stronger relationship with anxiety than with depression (Demopulos et al., 1996; Kellner et al., 1989, 1992; von Scheele et al., 1990). Kellner et al. (1992) conclude that the "association of hypochondriasis with depression is secondary because of the frequent coexistence of depression with anxiety" (p. 531).

## Panic Disorder

The relationship between panic disorder and hypochondriasis is complex (see also Chapters 4, 6, and 9). Hypochondriasis can be a secondary feature of panic disorder, and many patients (45%–50%) with panic disorder exhibit significant hypochondriacal features (Benedetti et al., 1997; Furer et al., 1997; Starcevic et al., 1992). Conversely, panic disorder and hypochondriasis may coexist, with neither condition considered principal or chronologically primary. Hypochondriasis was also reported to precede panic attacks in some patients (Fava et al., 1990). Panic disorder was found in as many as 59% of patients with hypochondriasis (Warwick and Salkovskis, 1990). An important step in the differential diagnosis of hypochondriasis is to establish whether features such as excessive bodily preoccupation, disease fear, and disease suspicion are better accounted for by panic disorder—that is, whether or not they occur exclusively during panic attacks and/or as part of anticipatory anxiety between the attacks.

From the cognitive perspective, the most conspicuous similarity between panic disorder and hypochondriasis is that both are based on or associated with catastrophic misinterpretation of innocuous bodily sensations and symptoms. However, one study (Barsky et al., 1994) concluded that, despite some similarity and diagnostic overlap, panic disorder and hypochondriasis are distinct conditions that "occur separately far more often than together in the same individual" (p. 924), and which are "phenomenologically and functionally differentiable and distinguishable" (p. 924).

Differences between panic disorder and hypochondriasis pertain to the nature of threat that is anticipated. The threat in panic disorder is experienced as more direct and immediate than the threat in hypochondriasis (Salkovskis and Clark, 1993), with panic disorder patients feeling they are about to die from suffocation, heart attack or stroke. Hence, they are more likely than are patients with hypochondriasis to seek help promptly—for example, by calling the ambulance or by rushing to an emergency room, whenever they have a panic attack. The pattern of medical help-seeking in hypochondriacal patients is not characterized by such urgency, because the danger from the disease with which they are usually preoccupied (e.g., cancer) is not experienced as immediate. Noyes (1999) has aptly suggested that panic patients fear dying, while hypochondriacal patients fear death.

Another difference between panic disorder and hypochondriasis concerns the symptoms that are misinterpreted by patients (Salkovskis and Clark, 1993). Panic disorder patients typically misinterpret symptoms of autonomic hyperactivity and arousal (e.g., tachycardia and shortness of breath), whereas the range of symptoms misinterpreted by patients with hypochondriasis is much wider.

## Specific Phobia (Disease Phobia Subtype, "Nosophobia")

The distinction between the disease phobia subtype of specific phobia and hypochondriasis has been addressed in the chapter section titled "Fear That a Serious Disease Is Already Present."

## Obsessive-Compulsive Disorder

Certain similarities exist between hypochondriasis and obsessive-compulsive disorder (OCD). Bodily preoccupation in hypochondriasis and obsessions in OCD are recurrent, uncontrollable, and distressing. Both are associated with intolerable uncertainty and anxiety. There is also similarity in the content of patients' preoccupations: Patients with hypochondriasis are often preoccupied with illness, germs, and contamination, whereas those with OCD often have contamination obsessions. Hypochondriacal disease suspicions are resistant to routine medical reassurance just as obsessions and compulsions are resistant to explanation and persuasion. In view of an apparently strong link among worrying, doubting, and checking (Tallis and de Silva, 1992), worries about and preoccupation with disease in hypochondriasis may take the form of obsessional doubts. In turn, these doubts lead to specific compulsions—checking the health status and presence of disease through self-examination, reassurance-seeking, and medical help-seeking. Both repeated health-checking in hypochondriasis and compulsions in OCD (especially checking rituals) alleviate anxiety, at least in the short term (Salkovskis and Warwick, 1986).

For these reasons, as well as on the basis of some hypochondriacal patients' favorable response to treatment with selective serotonin reuptake inhibitors and to certain techniques of behavior therapy (exposure and response prevention), hypochondriasis has been considered an "OCD spectrum disorder" (Hollander, 1993a, 1993b). More specifically, hypochondriasis was conceptualized as being "closer" to the compulsive, risk-avoidance, harm-overestimating end of the compulsive-impulsive continuum (Hollander, 1993a, 1993b). Josephson and associates (1996) considered OCD, body dysmorphic disorder, and hypochondriasis "three variations on a theme." However, the concept of "OCD spectrum disorders" has been recently criticized (Crino, 1999) on the grounds that important differences exist among the conditions included in the spectrum, and that many of the spectrum disorders (including hypochondriasis) have a broader relationship with anxiety and depressive disorders in general, rather than with OCD in particular (see also Chapter 4).

The differential diagnosis of hypochondriasis and OCD may be aided by the reported significant differences between these conditions. In contrast to bodily preoccupation and other features of hypochondriasis that are not resisted by patients (regardless of how unpleasant they may be), obsessions and compulsions in OCD are usually experienced by patients as intrusive, unreasonable, senseless, and/or alien; therefore, obsessions and compulsions are resisted, particularly the obsessions. Unlike patients with hypochondriasis, those with OCD are usually ashamed of their obsessive thoughts and compulsive behavior, and they attempt to conceal them; they are also far less likely to have somatic symptoms (Barsky, 1992).

There is another, more subtle, but important difference between OCD and hypochondriasis: Obsessions are "disconnected" and "discrete" thoughts and ideas that "disrupt one's underlying train of thought," whereas health-related thoughts and ideas of hypochondriacal patients are a coherent "way of viewing health, of thinking about disease, and of interpreting bodily sensation" (Barsky, 1992, p. 793). Finally, in comparison with OCD patients, hypochondriacal patients were found to have significantly more symptoms of anxiety, and they scored significantly higher on measures of somatization (Aigner, 1999).

### Generalized Anxiety Disorder

Generalized anxiety disorder (GAD) is characterized by chronic, excessive, and uncontrollable worry, along with the symptoms of apprehension, vigilance, and motor tension. The worry content in GAD is wide and may include matters of health and disease. In patients with hypochondriasis, almost all worries are focused on health and disease. Therefore, it comes as no surprise that the overlap between GAD and hypochondriasis is relatively small, especially in patients with GAD. Even GAD patients who worry a lot about health and disease relatively rarely have clinically significant hypochondriacal features (Starcevic *et al.*, 1994), which suggests significant psychopathological differences between the more *general* health worries and the more *specific* disease fears.

If patients with hypochondriasis have additional worries (unrelated to health) and other features of GAD, they may qualify for a comorbid diagnosis of GAD. In one study, the current comorbidity rate for GAD among patients with hypochondriasis was 24% (Barsky *et al.*, 1992), while another study (Noyes *et al.*, 1994b) found no hypochondriacal patients at all with a comorbid diagnosis of GAD. It may be concluded that a distinction between hypochondriasis and GAD is relatively easy, and that GAD is rarely a problem in the differential diagnosis of hypochondriasis.

### Somatization Disorder

Both somatization disorder and hypochondriasis are characterized by multiple functional (idiopathic, unexplained) somatic symptoms, and there appears to be some conceptual and diagnostic overlap between them. Owing to different diagnostic criteria and use of "syndromal" and "subsyndromal" concepts of somatization disorder, the comorbidity rates for somatization disorder among patients with hypochondriasis varied from 7.4% (Noyes *et al.*, 1994b) to 39% (Tyrer *et al.*, 1980). Patients with both hypochondriasis and somatization disorder were found to have a more severe illness (Noyes *et al.*, 1994b).

However, there are important differences between the two conditions: Patients with somatization disorder are more distressed by the symptoms themselves, whereas patients with hypochondriasis are more concerned about the interpretation, meaning, and implications of the symptoms. Patients with hypochondriasis are also more likely than are patients with somatization disorder to have specific disease fears (Schmidt, 1994). In addition, somatization disorder is far more likely to begin before age 30, and it is more frequently encountered in women and in first-degree relatives of patients with this condition; hypochondriasis, is common in age groups above 30, approximately equally distributed between men and women, and without a strong familial component. Finally, patients with somatization disorder are more likely to have histrionic features, in contrast to patients with hypochondriasis, who appear more obsessional.

A recent study (Escobar *et al.*, 1998) supports the notion that hypochondriasis and somatization disorder constitute distinct diagnostic entities, whereas another study (Hollifield *et al.*, 1999a) found significant differences between patients with hypochondriasis and those with "high somatic concern," whose condition was considered to belong to "somatization spectrum disorders." In comparison with patients with "high somatic concern," those with hypochondriasis showed less bodily preoccupation, tended to have fewer abnormal personality characteristics, had fewer mood and anxiety disturbances, and were less likely to seek treatment. In contrast, hypochondriacal patients were significantly more afraid of death. These differences appear subtle and to a certain extent surprising, and they should be examined in further research.

## Body Dysmorphic Disorder

Body dysmorphic disorder ("dysmorphophobia") and hypochondriasis share a preoccupation with the body, which is often of an obsessional nature and associated with specific overvalued ideas. Along with hypochondriasis, body dysmorphic disorder has also been considered one of the "OCD spectrum disorders" (Hollander, 1993a, 1993b; Josephson et al., 1996). The key difference is in the focus of preoccupation, for patients with body dysmorphic disorder are excessively concerned about their appearance and presumed deformity of the body. They are also more likely to consult certain medical specialists, particularly dermatologists and plastic surgeons, often seeking cosmetic or reconstructive surgery from the latter.

## Personality Disorders

Clinical manifestations of hypochondriasis, such as persistent bodily preoccupation, can also be construed as the most conspicuous personality characteristics of hypochondriacal patients. Furthermore, features of hypochondriasis have been considered crucial components of the patients' identity (with suffering from illness being their most important "theme"), their "interpersonal language," "basis for forming and breaking relationships and for social intercourse," and a "way of reacting to life stress" (Barsky and Klerman, 1983; Barsky and Wyshak, 1989; Barsky et al., 1992).

Although the importance of the relationship between hypochondriasis and personality disorders is recognized by many clinicians, there is no agreement on how best to conceptualize that relationship (see also Chapter 5). It seems likely that the relationship between hypochondriasis and personality disturbance differs from one patient to another. What is common to all discussions of this relationship is the observation that the features of hypochondriasis typically persist over prolonged periods of time, and that they usually permeate every aspect of the patient's behavior, which makes hypochondriasis "look like" a personality disturbance. This is the main reason that one form of hypochondriasis was called "hypochondriac personality" (Stenbäck and Jalava, 1961), and why, almost 30 years later, hypochondriasis itself was conceptualized as a distinct personality disturbance and termed "hypochondriacal personality disorder" (Tyrer *et al.*, 1990).

It is not clear when hypochondriasis *without* an associated specific personality disturbance might be considered a "pure" mental state disorder, and when it might be better conceptualized as a personality disorder. Even Tyrer *et al.* (1990) state that "the diagnosis of hypochondriacal personality disorder should be regarded in most cases as an additional diagnosis rather than as an alternative to a mental state one" (p. 641), and they go on to suggest that hypochondriacal personality disorder might be a more appropriate diagnosis for hypochondriacal patients whose disorder begins in early adult life and persists throughout most of adult life. A lifestyle characterized by constant pursuit of health maintenance may be more a feature of hypochondriacal personality disorder than a characteristic of hypochondriasis as a mental state disorder. In fact, the criteria for diagnosing hypochondriacal personality disorder, spelled out by Tyrer *et al.* (1990), resemble a condition closer to the "normality-end" of the spectrum of hypochondriacal manifestations, as described in another section of this chapter.

Even when it is not considered a distinct personality disturbance, hypochondriasis is very often associated with various personality disorders. In one study (Barsky *et al.*, 1992), two-thirds of patients with hypochondriasis had an associated personality disturbance. The severity of hypochondriasis was linked to the severity of an associated personality disturbance (Noyes *et al.*, 1994b). Although no one type of personality disorder is uniquely associated with hypochondriasis, some may be found more frequently among hypochondriacal patients—for example, obsessive-compulsive, narcissistic, avoidant, borderline, and paranoid personalities (Kenyon, 1964; 1976; Pilowsky, 1970; Starcevic, 1988, 1989, 1990b).

In some cases, hypochondriacal features can be conceptualized as part of a personality disorder—that is, as a way through which a specific personality disorder is manifested. A typical example of such a personality disturbance is narcissistic personality disorder (Starcevic, 1989). If it is clear that hypochondriasis is no more than a reflection of an underlying specific personality disorder or a form of decompensation of an enduring personality disturbance, a formal diagnosis of hypochondriasis is redundant. In such cases, the recognition of specific, maladaptive personality traits and behaviors offers a clue to an underlying personality disorder. Hypochondriasis can also appear as a consequence of the longstanding personality disturbance (Barsky *et al.*, 1992; Kellner, 1986), in which case both diagnoses (of hypochondriasis and of a specific personality disorder) can be made if the corresponding diagnostic criteria have been met.

## Malingering

Malingering is rarely considered in the differential diagnosis of hypochondriasis because it is relatively easy to distinguish between genuine distress (caused by disease fears and suspicions) and specific illness-related behaviors of the hypochondriacal patients on one hand and simulation of hypochondriacal manifestations on the other. In this context, it may be more important to remember that the exaggerated reporting of symptoms and simulation of distress are often the "core" components of the public perception of hypochondriasis. Such a perception should remind physicians that their hypochondriacal patients sometimes need to be protected from being treated as malingerers. Conversely, physicians who do not take the time to clarify the diagnosis may be too quick to mislabel hypochondriacal patients malingerers.

## Conclusion

This chapter has presented essential clinical features of hypochondriasis, grouped into components. These components are as follows: (1) usually multiple, often vague, but sometimes quite specific bodily symptoms; (2) preoccupation with one's body, bodily symptoms, and matters of health and disease; (3) fear that a serious disease is already present; (4) suspicion that a serious disease is already present; (5) resistance to routine medical reassurance; and (6) hypochondriacal behaviors, most typical of which are persistent reassurance-seeking and health-checking.

The heterogeneity of the clinical presentation of hypochondriacal patients is largely a consequence of the fact that the components of hypochondriasis are not present to the same degree in all patients. Thus, some hypochondriacal patients are characterized more by excessive disease worries and fears, while hypochondriacal suspicions are more prominent in other patients. Although disease fears and disease suspicions may warrant a somewhat different treatment approach, it is premature to consider them as two distinct diagnostic subtypes of hypochondriasis.

Likewise, there is little justification for substitution of the term "health anxiety disorder" for the term "hypochondriasis," as proposed by Rief and Hiller (1998, 1999). Although the term "hypochondriasis" is often used in a pejorative context, and although its etymological underpinnings have little to do with its present-day meaning, the abandonment of hypochondriasis is not advocated here both because of respect for its long history and the associated, easy name-recognition, and because a more conceptually sound, widely accepted, and evidence-based substitution has not yet been found. Instead of "dropping" the term, it might be more worthwhile investing in a clearer conceptualization of hypochondriasis and in a greater effort to reach better agreement about its meaning. In addition, it is appropriate at this point to remember the wisdom of Aubrey Lewis (1975), who observed that some psychiatric terms have a tendency to outlive their obituarists.

Some support exists for a dimensional conceptualization of hypochondriasis and hypochondriasis-related behaviors and disorders. According to this conceptualization, hypochondriacal phenomena are placed on a continuum of increasing severity from heightened awareness of bodily sensations and greater attention directed to matters of body, health, and illness—through transient, secondary, and primary hypochondriasis—to hypochondriacal delusions. However, for both nosologic reasons and for greater convenience of use in clinical practice, a categorical formulation of hypochondriasis (in terms of either its presence or absence) has been "officially" favored over its dimensional conceptualization. Future research should establish a usefulness of the combined, dimensional–categorical approach to the diagnosis of hypochondriasis, so that a minimum number of specific, dimensionally distributed, and correspondingly scored hypochondriacal features would qualify for a categorical diagnosis of hypochondriasis.

The *DSM-IV* and ICD-10-DCR diagnostic criteria for hypochondriasis have been criticized on several accounts. Of these, most important are the following: (*1*) a failure to define disease belief in nonambiguous terms so as to make a better distinction between nondelusional and delusional disease belief; (*2*) proposition of an "interchangeable" relationship between a fear of disease and idea/belief that one has a disease; and (*3*) inclusion of a failure to respond to appropriate medical reassurance as a diagnostic criterion, without defining such a reassurance. In addition, the diagnostic concept of hypochondriasis is too heterogeneous, and criteria for making a diagnosis in the presence of organic disease need to be spelled out more clearly. Despite these shortcomings, studies suggest that the diagnosis of hypochondriasis has a measure of internal and external validity, and they generally support the notion that hypochondriasis is an independent disorder.

The nosologic status of hypochondriasis remains somewhat uncertain, even though it is officially classified among somatoform disorders in the *DSM-IV*. Although some justification exists to include hypochondriasis among the anxiety disorders, as suggested by several authors (Noyes, 1999; Salkovskis and Clark, 1993; Wolpe, 1986), hypochondriasis is nosologically "located" in the vast and insufficiently explored territory among somatoform, anxiety, and personality disorders.

The differential diagnosis of hypochondriasis encompasses organic diseases and many mental disorders, including psychoses, depressive illness, several anxiety disorders (panic disorder, specific phobia, and obsessive-compulsive disorder), personality disorders, other somatoform disorders (somatization disorder and body dysmorphic disorder), and malingering.

Finally, because the psychopathology of hypochondriasis may overlap with that of numerous other conditions, a wide range of disorders needs to be taken into account when making a diagnosis of hypochondriasis (Fig. 2.1). Indeed, making this diagnosis entails a "promenade" through and a sound knowledge of the psychiatric nosology (Starcevic, 1988).

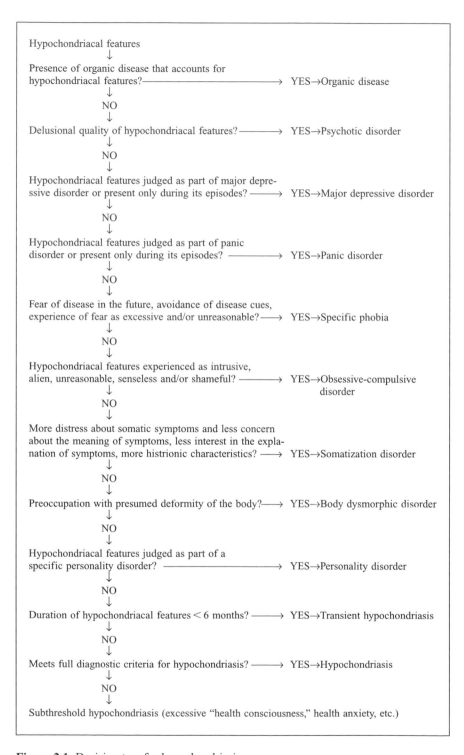

**Figure 2.1.** Decision tree for hypochondriasis

## References

Aigner M. 1999. The obsessive compulsive spectrum—differences between hypochondriasis and obsessive compulsive disorder. *XI World Congress of Psychiatry, Abstracts, Vol. II*, p. 214.

American Psychiatric Association. 1980. *Diagnostic and Statistical Manual of Mental Disorders, Third Edition (DSM-III)*. Washington, DC: American Psychiatric Association.

American Psychiatric Association. 1987. *Diagnostic and Statistical Manual of Mental Disorders, Third Edition Revised (DSM-III-R)*. Washington, DC: Author.

American Psychiatric Association. 1994. *Diagnostic and Statistical Manual of Mental Disorders, Fourth Edition (DSM-IV)*. Washington, DC: American Psychiatric Association.

Avia M.D. 1999. The development of illness beliefs. *Journal of Psychosomatic Research* 47: 199–204.

Barsky A.J. 1992. Hypochondriasis and obsessive compulsive disorder. *Psychiatric Clinics of North America* 15: 791–801.

Barsky A.J. 1996. Hypochondriasis: medical management and psychiatric treatment. *Psychosomatics* 37: 48–56.

Barsky A.J., Klerman G.L. 1983. Overview: hypochondriasis, bodily complaints, and somatic styles. *American Journal of Psychiatry* 140: 273–283.

Barsky A.J., Wyshak G. 1989. Hypochondriasis and related health attitudes. *Psychosomatics* 30: 412–420.

Barsky A.J., Wyshak G., Klerman G.L. 1986. Hypochondriasis: an evaluation of the DSM-III criteria in medical outpatients. *Archives of General Psychiatry* 43: 493–500.

Barsky A.J., Wyshak G., Klerman G.L. 1990. Transient hypochondriasis. *Archives of General Psychiatry* 47: 746–752.

Barsky A.J., Frank C.B., Cleary P.D., Wyshak G., Klerman G.L. 1991a. The relation between hypochondriasis and age. *American Journal of Psychiatry* 148: 923–928.

Barsky A.J., Wyshak G., Latham K.S., Klerman G.L. 1991b. Hypochondriacal patients, their physicians, and their medical care. *Journal of General Internal Medicine* 6: 413–419.

Barsky A.J., Wyshak G., Klerman G.L. 1992. Psychiatric comorbidity in DSM-III-R hypochondriasis. *Archives of General Psychiatry* 49: 101–108.

Barsky A.J., Coeytaux R.R., Sarnie M.K., Cleary P.D. 1993a. Hypochondriacal patients' beliefs about good health. *American Journal of Psychiatry* 150: 1085–1089.

Barsky A.J., Cleary P.D., Sarnie M.K., Klerman G.L. 1993b. The course of transient hypochondriasis. *American Journal of Psychiatry* 150: 484–488.

Barsky A.J., Barnett M.C., Cleary P.D. 1994. Hypochondriasis and panic disorder: boundary and overlap. *Archives of General Psychiatry* 51: 918–925.

Barsky A.J., Fama J.M., Bailey E.D., Ahern D.K. 1998. A prospective 4- to 5-year study of DSM-III-R hypochondriasis. *Archives of General Psychiatry* 55: 737–744.

Benedetti A., Perugi G., Toni C., Simonetti B., Mata B., Cassano G.B. 1997. Hypochondriasis and illness phobia in panic-agoraphobic patients. *Comprehensive Psychiatry* 38: 124–131.

Bianchi G.N. 1971. The origins of disease phobia. *Australian and New Zealand Journal of Psychiatry* 5: 241–257.

Brown R.P., Soveeney J., Loutsch E., Kocsis J., Frances A. 1984. Involutional melancholia revisited. *American Journal of Psychiatry* 141: 24–28.

Crino R.D. 1999. Obsessive-compulsive spectrum disorders. *Current Opinion in Psychiatry* 12: 151–155.

de Alarcon R. 1964. Hypochondriasis and depression in the aged. *Gerontology Clinics* 6: 266–277.

Demopulos C., Fava M., McLean N.E., Alpert J.E., Nierenberg A.A., Rosenbaum J.F. 1996. Hypochondriacal concerns in depressed outpatients. *Psychosomatic Medicine* 58: 314–320.

Escobar J.I., Gara M., Waitzkin H., Silver R.C., Holman A., Compton W. 1998. DSM-IV hypochondriasis in primary care. *General Hospital Psychiatry* 20: 155–159.

Ey H. 1966. Hypochondriasis. *International Journal of Psychiatry* 2: 332–334.

Fallon B. 1999. Hypochondriasis vs. anxiety disorders: why should we care? *General Hospital Psychiatry* 21: 5–7.

Fava G.A., Grandi S., Saviotti F.M., Conti S. 1990. Hypochondriasis with panic attacks. *Psychosomatics* 31: 351–353.

Furer P., Walker J.R., Chartier M.J., Stein M.B. 1997. Hypochondriacal concerns and somatization in panic disorder. *Depression and Anxiety* 6: 78–85.

Gillespie R.D. 1929. *Hypochondria*. London: Kegan Paul.

Gureje O., Üstün T.B., Simon G.E. 1997. The syndrome of hypochondriasis: a cross-national study in primary care. *Psychological Medicine* 27: 1001–1010.

Hadjistavropoulos H.D., Craig K.D., Hadjistavropoulos T. 1998. Cognitive and behavioral responses to illness information: the role of health anxiety. *Behaviour Research and Therapy* 36: 149–164.

Haenen M-A., Schmidt A.J.M., Kroeze S., van den Hout M.A. 1996. Hypochondriasis and symptom reporting—the effects of attention versus distraction. *Psychotherapy and Psychosomatics* 65: 43–48.

Haenen M-A., Schmidt A.J.M., Schoenmakers M., van den Hout M.A. 1997a. Tactual sensitivity in hypochondriasis. *Psychotherapy and Psychosomatics* 66: 128–132.

Haenen M-A., Schmidt A.J.M., Schoenmakers M., van den Hout M.A. 1997b. Suggestibility in hypochondriacal patients and healthy control subjects: an experimental case-control study. *Psychosomatics* 38: 543–547.

Hitchcock P., Mathews A. 1992. Interpretation of bodily symptoms in hypochondriasis. Behaviour *Research and Therapy* 30: 223–234.

Hollander E. 1993a. *Obsessive-Compulsive Related Disorders*. Washington, DC: American Psychiatric Press.

Hollander E. 1993b. Obsessive-compulsive spectrum disorders: an overview. *Psychiatric Annals* 23: 355–358.

Hollifield M., Tuttle L., Paine S., Kellner R. 1999a. Hypochondriasis and somatization related to personality and attitudes toward self. *Psychosomatics* 40: 387–395.

Hollifield M., Paine S., Tuttle L., Kellner R. 1999b. Hypochondriasis, somatization, and perceived health and utilization of health care services. *Psychosomatics* 40: 380–386.

House A. 1989. Hypochondriasis and related disorders: assessment and management of patients referred for a psychiatric opinion. *General Hospital Psychiatry* 11: 156–165.

Howells K., Field D. 1982. Fear of death and dying among medical students. *Social Science and Medicine* 11: 1421–1424.

Hunter R.C.A., Lohrenz J.G., Schwartzman A.E. 1964. Nosophobia and hypochondriasis in medical students. *Journal of Nervous and Mental Disease* 139: 147–152.

Josephson S.C., Hollander E., Fallon B., Stein D.J. 1996. Obsessive-compulsive disorder, body dysmorphic disorder, and hypochondriasis: three variations on a theme. *CNS Spectrums* 1(2): 24–31.

Jyväsjärvi S., Joukamaa M., Väisänen E., Larivaara P., Kivelä S-L., Keinänen-Kiukaanniemi S. 1999. Alexithymia, hypochondriacal beliefs, and psychological distress among frequent attenders in primary health care. *Comprehensive Psychiatry* 40: 292–298.

Kellner R. 1983. Prognosis of treated hypochondriasis: a clinical study. *Acta Psychiatrica Scandinavica* 67: 69–79.

Kellner R. 1986. *Somatization and Hypochondriasis*. New York: Praeger.

Kellner R., Wiggins R.G., Pathak D. 1986a. Hypochondriacal fears and beliefs in medical and law students. *Archives of General Psychiatry* 43: 487–489.

Kellner R., Fava G.A., Lisansky J., Perini G.I., Zielezny M. 1986b. Hypochondriacal fears and beliefs in DSM-III melancholia: changes with amitriptyline. *Journal of Affective Disorders* 10: 21–26.

Kellner R., Abbott P., Winslow W.W., Pathak D. 1987a. Fears, beliefs, and attitudes in DSM-III hypochondriasis. *Journal of Nervous and Mental Disease* 175: 20–25.

Kellner R., Slocumb J.C., Wiggins R.J., Abbott P.J., Romanik R.L., Winslow W.W., Pathak D. 1987b. The relationship of hypochondriacal fears and beliefs to anxiety and depression. *Psychiatric Medicine* 4: 15–24.

Kellner R., Abbott P., Winslow W.W., Pathak D. 1989. Anxiety, depression, and somatization in DSM-III hypochondriasis. *Psychosomatics* 30: 57–64.

Kellner R., Hernandez J., Pathak D. 1992. Hypochondriacal fears and beliefs, anxiety, and somatisation. *British Journal of Psychiatry* 160: 525–532.

Kenyon F.E. 1964. Hypochondriasis: a clinical study. *British Journal of Psychiatry* 110: 478–488.

Kenyon F.E. 1976. Hypochondriacal states. *British Journal of Psychiatry* 129: 1–14.

Kirmayer L.J. 1991. The place of culture in psychiatric nosology: Taijin Kyofusho and DSM-III-R. *Journal of Nervous and Mental Diseases* 179: 19–28.

Kirmayer L.J., Robbins J.M. 1991. Conclusion: prospects for research and clinical practice. In *Current Concepts of Somatization: Research and Clinical Perspectives* (eds. Kirmayer L.J., Robbins J.M.), Washington, DC: American Psychiatric Press.

Kramer-Ginsberg E., Greenwald B.S., Aisen P.S., Brod-Miller C. 1989. Hypochondriasis in the elderly depressed. *Journal of the American Geriatric Society* 37: 507–510.

Laughlin H.P. 1956. *The Neuroses in Clinical Practice*. Philadelphia: WB Saunders.

Lecci L., Karoly P., Ruehlman L.S., Lanyon R.I. 1996. Goal-relevant dimensions of hypochondriacal tendencies and their relation to symptom manifestation and psychological distress. *Journal of Abnormal Psychology* 105: 42–52.

Lewis A.J. 1975. The survival of hysteria. *Psychological Medicine* 5: 9–12.

Lipowski Z.J. 1988. Somatization: the concept and its clinical application. *American Journal of Psychiatry* 145: 1358–1368.

Lipsitt D.R. 1997. The challenge of the "difficult patient" (déjà vu all over again—only more so). *General Hospital Psychiatry* 19: 313–314.

MacLeod A.K., Haynes C., Sensky T. 1998. Attributions about common bodily sensations: their associations with hypochondriasis and anxiety. *Psychological Medicine* 28: 225–228.

Marks I.M. 1987. *Fears, Phobias and Rituals*. London: Oxford University Press.

Mayou R. 1976. The nature of bodily symptoms. *British Journal of Psychiatry* 129: 55–60.

McKenna P.J. 1984. Disorders with overvalued ideas. *British Journal of Psychiatry* 145: 579–585.

Mechanic D. 1972. Social psychologic factors affecting the presentation of bodily complaints. *New England Journal of Medicine* 286: 1132–1139.

Munro A. 1988. Monosymptomatic hypochondriacal psychosis. *British Journal of Psychiatry* 153 (Suppl. 2): 37–40.

Noyes R., Jr. 1999. The relationship of hypochondriasis to anxiety disorders. *General Hospital Psychiatry* 21: 8–17.

Noyes R., Jr., Reich J., Clancy J., O'Gorman T.W. 1986. Reduction in hypochondriasis with treatment of panic disorder. *British Journal of Psychiatry* 149: 631–635.

Noyes R., Jr., Wesner R.B., Fisher M.M. 1992. A comparison of patients with illness phobia and panic disorder. *Psychosomatics* 33: 92–99.

Noyes R., Jr., Kathol R.G., Fisher M.M., Phillips B.M., Suelzer M.T., Holt C.S. 1993. The validity of DSM-III-R hypochondriasis. *Archives of General Psychiatry* 50: 961–970.

Noyes R., Jr., Kathol R.G., Fisher M.M., Phillips B.M., Suelzer M.T., Woodman C.L. 1994a. One-year follow-up of medical outpatients with hypochondriasis. *Psychosomatics* 35: 533–545.

Noyes R., Jr., Kathol R.G., Fisher M.M., Phillips B.M., Suelzer M.T., Woodman C.L. 1994b. Psychiatric comorbidity among patients with hypochondriasis. *General Hospital Psychiatry* 16: 78–87.

Noyes R., Jr., Holt C.S., Happel R.L., Kathol R.G., Yagla S.J. 1997. A family study of hypochondriasis. *Journal of Nervous and Mental Disease* 185: 223–232.

Osman A.A. 1991. Monosymptomatic hypochondriacal psychosis in developing countries. *British Journal of Psychiatry* 159: 428–431.

Pilowsky I. 1967. Dimensions of hypochondriasis. *British Journal of Psychiatry* 113: 89–93.

Pilowsky I. 1968. The response to treatment in hypochondriacal disorders. *Australian and New Zealand Journal of Psychiatry* 2: 88–94.

Pilowsky I. 1970. Primary and secondary hypochondriasis. *Acta Psychiatrica Scandinavica* 46: 273–285.

Pilowsky I. 1983. Hypochondriasis. In *Handbook of Psychiatry, Vol. 4* (eds. Russell G.E., Hersov L.), Cambridge: Cambridge University Press.

Pilowsky I. 1992. Somatic symptoms/somatization. *Current Opinion in Psychiatry* 5: 213–218.

Pilowsky I. 1996. Diagnostic criteria and classification in psychosomatic research. *Psychotherapy and Psychosomatics* 65: 115–116.

Rachman S.J. 1974. Some similarities and differences between obsessional ruminations and morbid preoccupations. *Canadian Psychiatric Association Journal* 18: 71–73.

Rief W., Hiller W. 1998. Somatization—future perspectives on a common phenomenon. *Journal of Psychosomatic Research* 44: 529–536.

Rief W., Hiller W. 1999. Toward empirically based criteria for the classification of somatoform disorders. *Journal of Psychosomatic Research* 46: 507–518.

Robbins J.M., Kirmayer L.J. 1996. Transient and persistent hypochondriacal worry in primary care. *Psychological Medicine* 26: 575–589.

Salkovskis P.M., Warwick H.M.C. 1986. Morbid preoccupations, health anxiety and reassurance: a cognitive-behavioural approach to hypochondriasis. *Behaviour Research and Therapy* 24: 597–602.

Salkovskis P.M., Clark D.M. 1993. Panic disorder and hypochondriasis. *Advances in Behaviour Research and Therapy* 15: 23–48.

Schäfer M.L. 1982. Phenomenology and hypochondria. In *Phenomenology and Psychiatry* (eds. De Koning A.J.J., Jenner F.A.), New York: Grune & Stratton.

Schmidt A.J.M. 1994. Bottlenecks in the diagnosis of hypochondriasis. *Comprehensive Psychiatry* 35: 306–315.

Shaklee H., Fischoff B. 1982. Strategies of information search in causal analysis. *Memory and Cognition* 10: 520–530.

Sims A. 1988. *Symptoms in the Mind: An Introduction to Descriptive Psychopathology.* London: Baillière Tindall.

Slavney P.R. 1987. The hypochondriacal patient and Murphy's "law." *General Hospital Psychiatry* 9: 302–303.

Starcevic V. 1988. Diagnosis of hypochondriasis: a promenade through the psychiatric nosology. *American Journal of Psychotherapy* 42: 197–211.

Starcevic V. 1989. Contrasting patterns in the relationship between hypochondriasis and narcissism. *British Journal of Medical Psychology* 62: 311–323.

Starcevic V. 1990a. Role of reassurance and psychopathology in hypochondriasis. *Psychiatry* 53: 383–395.

Starcevic V. 1990b. Relationship between hypochondriasis and obsessive-compulsive personality disorder: close relatives separated by nosological schemes? *American Journal of Psychotherapy* 44: 340–347.

Starcevic V., Kellner R., Uhlenhuth E.H., Pathak D. 1992. Panic disorder and hypochondriacal fears and beliefs. *Journal of Affective Disorders* 24: 73–85.

Starcevic V., Fallon S., Uhlenhuth E.H., Pathak D. 1994. Generalized anxiety disorder, worries about illness, and hypochondriacal fears and beliefs. *Psychotherapy and Psychosomatics* 61: 93–99.

Stenbäck A., Jalava V. 1961. Hypochondria and depression. *Acta Psychiatrica Scandinavica* 37 (Suppl. 162): 240–246.

Stenbäck A., Rimón R. 1964. Hypochondria and paranoia. *Acta Psychiatrica Scandinavica* 40: 379–385.

Tallis F., de Silva P. 1992. Worry and obsessional symptoms: a correlational analysis. *Behaviour Research and Therapy* 30: 103–105.

Tanaka-Matsumi J. 1979. Taijin kyofusho: diagnostic and cultural issues in Japanese psychiatry. *Culture, Medicine and Psychiatry* 3: 231–245.

Tyrer P., Lee I., Alexander J. 1980. Awareness of cardiac function in anxious, phobic, and hypochondriacal patients. *Psychological Medicine* 10: 171–174.

Tyrer P., Fowler-Dixon R., Ferguson B., Kelemen A. 1990. A plea for the diagnosis of hypochondriacal personality disorder. *Journal of Psychosomatic Research* 34: 637–642.

Vaillant G.E. 1977. *Adaptation to Life*. Boston: Little, Brown.

von Scheele C., Nordgren L., Kempi V., Hetta J., Hallborg A. 1990. A study of so-called hypochondriasis. *Psychotherapy and Psychosomatics* 54: 50–56.

Wahl C.W. 1963. Unconscious factors in the psychodynamics of the hypochondriacal patient. *Psychosomatics* 4: 9–14.

Warwick H.M.C., Marks I.M. 1988. Behavioural treatment of illness phobia. *British Journal of Psychiatry* 152: 239–241.

Warwick H.M.C., Salkovskis P.M. 1990. Hypochondriasis. *Behaviour Research and Therapy* 28: 105–117.

Wesner R.B., Noyes R., Jr. 1991. Imipramine: an effective treatment for illness phobia. *Journal of Affective Disorders* 22: 43–48.

Wolpe J. 1986. Individualisation: the categorical imperative of behaviour therapy practice. *Journal of Behaviour Therapy and Experimental Psychiatry* 17: 145–153.

Woods S.M., Natterson J., Silverman J. 1966. Medical students' disease: hypochondriasis in medical education. *Journal of Medical Education* 41: 785–790.

World Health Organization. 1992. The *ICD-10 Classification of Mental and Behavioural Disorders: Clinical Descriptions and Diagnostic Guidelines*. Geneva: World Health Organization.

World Health Organization. 1993. *The ICD-10 Classification of Mental and Behavioural Disorders: Diagnostic Criteria for Research*. Geneva: World Health Organization.

# 3

# Assessment of Hypochondriasis

## ANNE E. M. SPECKENS

Before considering the available instruments to assess hypochondriasis and related illness behaviors, general problems regarding the assessment of hypochondriasis need to be addressed. According to *DSM-IV* criteria (American Psychiatric Association, 1994), hypochondriasis is characterized by a preoccupation with the fear or idea of having a serious illness, based upon a false interpretation of bodily sensations. This fear or idea must persist despite appropriate medical examination and reassurance. Several authors have pointed to the problems associated with these criteria (Pilowsky, 1990; Schmidt, 1994). The nature of the medical examination and the extent to which laboratory or other investigations are to be conducted are not clearly spelled out. Moreover, a medical examination does not necessarily preclude the existence of a (still) undiagnosed illness.

A second difficulty emerges in the required medical reassurance. Again, a definition of the nature of the reassurance, the data on which it should be based, and the mode of its communication are lacking. In many studies, hypochondriasis is diagnosed solely on history or self-report questionnaires, without any medical examination and reassurance. When a medical examination and reassurance were provided, they were often not adequately described or assessed.

## Psychometric Concepts

### Reliability and Validity

Before discussing the psychometric properties of the different instruments, the main concepts used will be described briefly.

By *reliability* is meant the degree to which an instrument yields consistent results under varying circumstances (MacDowell and Hewell, 1987). Reliability is assessed by the internal consistency, the test–retest reproducibility (reliability), and the interrater agreement (reliability). Internal consistency is calculated by estimating the correlations between all possible pairs of items belonging to a scale or subscale. A test with high inter-item correlations is homogeneous and is also likely to produce consistent responses. Cronbach's coefficient alpha is a frequently used indicator of internal consistency. Test–retest reliability is estimated by applying the measurement twice and comparing the results. Interrater reliability is assessed by comparing the ratings of the same subject by two or more raters. Reliability is usually expressed numerically as some kind of correlation coefficient ranging from 0 to 1.0, with 0 signifying total unreliability and 1.0 indicating 100% reliability. Reliability coefficients above 0.85 are generally regarded as high and between 0.60 and 0.85 as moderate (Williams, 1988). Another way of expressing the agreement between two examinations or examiners is to calculate the proportion of cases in which one clinician agreed with another (Sackett *et al.*, 1991). Because part of this agreement will occur by chance alone, a more useful index of clinical agreement is *kappa*, the ratio of the actual agreement beyond chance to the potential agreement beyond chance.

*Validity* usually means the degree to which an instrument measures what it intends to measure. There are many types of validity. In *concurrent* or *criterion validity* the instrument is compared with a criterion or "gold standard." For example, a new measure of hypochondriasis is compared with either a diagnosis made by a clinician, a standardized diagnostic interview, or already established hypochondriasis questionnaires. A variant of this approach is known as *predictive validation*. Predictive validity of the hypochondriasis instrument is tested in a prospective study in which patient outcomes—for example, physical symptoms or frequency of physician visits—are compared to measurements made at the start of the study.

## Sensitivity and Specificity

Related to concurrent validity are the concepts of sensitivity and specificity. *Sensitivity* is defined as the proportion of patients with hypochondriasis who have a positive test result (Sackett *et al.*, 1991). The *specificity* is the proportion of patients without hypochondriasis who have a negative test result. In clinical practice, the positive and negative predictive values of a test are more relevant. The *positive predictive value* (PPV) of an instrument for assessing hypochondriasis is the proportion of patients with positive test results who are hypochondriacal. Correspondingly, the *negative predictive value* (NPV) is the proportion of patients with negative test results who do not have the target disorder.

*Receiver operating characteristic* (ROC) analyses are used to determine the overall discriminative ability of instruments. A ROC curve is a graph of the pairs of true positive rates (sensitivity) and false positive rates (100%-specificity) that correspond to each possible cutoff for the diagnostic test result. The test whose ROC curve encloses the largest area is the most accurate one. For example, the ROC curve of a perfect diagnostic test will include the upper left-hand corner of the figure with a true positive rate of 1.00 (all patients with the target disorder are detected) and a false positive rate of 0 (no one without the target disorder is falsely labeled) and enclose an area of 1.0. It follows that the ROC curve that lies farthest to the "northwest" is the most accurate (Sackett *et al.*, 1991).

In cases where a measurement is designed to reflect an abstract, conceptual definition of health, evidence from several validation procedures must be assembled. This process is known as *construct validation*. Construct validity can be divided in convergent and divergent validity. *Convergent validity* is assessed by correlating a measure of hypochondriasis with other concepts thought to be related to hypochondriasis. For example, hypochondriasis may be associated with somatic symptoms, frequency of physician visits, anxiety and depression, and functional disability. *Divergent validity* is the ability of the instrument to distinguish different categories of subjects.

## Selection of Available Instruments

Instruments assessing hypochondriasis and related illness behavior were selected by examining all papers identified by Medline, using the keyword "hypochondriasis." Any relevant papers that were referred to were examined as well. The following instruments were identified: the Structured Diagnostic Interview for Hypochondriasis, the Whiteley Index, the Illness Behaviour Questionnaire, the Illness Attitude Scales, and the Somatosensory Amplification Scale. The psychometric properties of these five instruments will be discussed in detail below. The less commonly used instruments, such as the Illness Coping Strategies Scale (Jones *et al.*, 1989), the Maastrichter Eigen Gezondheids-Attitude en Hypochondrie-scale (de Jong *et al.*, 1998; Schmidt *et al.*, 1993), and visual analogue scales as used in some treatment studies of hypochondriasis (Clark *et al.*, 1998; Warwick *et al.*, 1996), will not be discussed further. The Minnesota Multiphasic Personality Inventory (MMPI) Hypochondriasis Scale, consisting of a wide variety of vague and nonspecific complaints about bodily functioning rather than hypochondriacal symptoms (Greene, 1991), is also excluded from this chapter.

### *The Structured Diagnostic Interview for Hypochondriasis (SDIH)*

In 1992, Barsky *et al.* (1992a) developed the Structured Diagnostic Interview for *DSM-III-R* Hypochondriasis (Appendix 1). The SDIH begins with four probe questions. An affirmative answer to any one triggers the rest of the interview, which consists of five sections, one for each of the five *DSM-III-R* diagnostic criteria. The interviewer judges whether each criterion is satisfied, based upon the information elicited by all of the questions in that section.

**Reliability.** Using the joint assessment method, interrater agreement on individual questions ranged from 88% to 97%, agreement on individual diagnostic criteria ranged from 92% to 96%, and agreement on the diagnosis was 96% (Barsky *et al.*, 1992a). No kappa values for interrater reliability were given. Nor was any information provided about the interrater agreement between two different interviewers using the SDIH in the same patient.

**Concurrent and predictive validity.** Barsky *et al.* (1992a) administered the instrument to 88 general medical outpatients who scored above a predetermined cutoff on a hypochondriacal symptom questionnaire (the Whiteley Index), and to 100 comparison patients randomly chosen from among those below the cutoff. Interview-positive patients scored higher on the Whiteley Index and physician ratings of hypochondriasis than did interview-negative patients. However, the Whiteley Index was also used as a screening instrument to identify the medical outpatients who were to undergo the interview. In a 4- to 5-year study of 120 patients with hypochondriasis according to the SDIH, 54 (64%) still met *DSM-III-R* diagnostic criteria at follow-up (Barsky *et al.*, 1998).

Noyes *et al.* (1993) tried to replicate the findings of Barsky *et al.* (1992a) in a study of 50 patients with hypochondriasis and 50 matched controls. Hypochondriacal subjects scored higher on the Whiteley Index, the Health Worry/Concern subscale of the Health Perception Questionnaire, and the Somatosensory Amplification Scale. However, in this study, the Whiteley Index had also been part of the screening procedure to identify hypochondriacal patients. Noyes *et al.* (1994a) followed the study patients after 1 year. At follow-up, 32 subjects (67%) still met criteria for current hypochondriasis. They tended to make more visits to doctors, saw more different doctors, and took more medicine than did nonhypochondriacal control subjects in the year after their medical clinic evaluation.

In a study of 183 patients with medically unexplained physical symptoms (Speckens *et al.*, 1996a), hypochondriacal patients according to the SDIH had higher scores on the Whiteley Index and the Health Anxiety subscale of the Illness Attitude Scales. At 1-year follow-up, hypochondriacal patients according to the diagnostic interview had a poorer outcome in terms of recovery than did nonhypochondriacal patients. No significant difference was found between hypochondriacal and nonhypochondriacal patients in the frequency of visits to their general practitioners.

**Convergent and divergent validity.** In comparison with interview-negative patients, interview-positive patients had more nonspecific complaints in their medical records, more disability, and more medical outpatient visits (Barsky *et al.*, 1992a). They did not differ in the degree to which their physicians judged their somatic symptoms to be due to medical disease. In the study by Noyes *et al.* (1993), clinic physicians did rate hypochondriacal subjects as having less physical disease with which to explain their symptoms and as having more unrealistic fear of illness. Record audits showed that more laboratory tests and treatments were recommended for hypochondriacal subjects and that they were taking a greater number of medications at the time of their clinic visit. They reported more impairment in work performance according to the Functional Status Questionnaire. Hypochondriacal subjects utilized more medical care in the 6 months prior to their medical clinic appointment and reported substantially higher levels of both psychiatric and somatic symptoms. More hypochondriacal subjects (62%) had lifetime comorbidity than did controls (30%) (Noyes *et al.*, 1994b)

In another study (Barsky *et al.*, 1995), medical outpatients meeting the SDIH criteria for hypochondriasis reported significantly more functional somatic symptoms and had significantly higher scores on the Somatosensory Amplification Scale than did a comparison group of nonhypochondriacal patients. However, they did not show a more accurate awareness of resting heartbeat. These findings were confirmed in two studies by Haenen *et al.* (1996, 1997), in which patients with hypochondriasis according to the SDIH showed higher levels of symptom reporting and higher scores on the Somatosensory Amplification Scale, but did not show a lower tactual sensitivity. Patients with hypochondriasis according to the SDIH also did not show a particular proneness to selectively search for danger-confirming information in the context of health threats (de Jong *et al.*, 1998).

The SDIH appeared to have discriminant validity in that patients diagnosed as hypochondriacal had several other clinical features that distinguished them from the patients who scored above the cutoff on hypochondriacal symptomatology but failed to be diagnosed as hypochondriacal with the SDIH (Barsky *et al.*, 1992a). The SDIH also discriminated between patients with panic disorder without comorbid hypochondriasis and "pure" hypochondriasis (Barsky *et al.*, 1994a).

### The Whiteley Index (WI)

In 1967, Pilowsky developed the first questionnaire to assess hypochondriasis (Appendix 2). One hundred members of the medical, nursing, and ancillary staff of a hospital were asked to define "hypochondriasis" and to write the definition on a card. These definitions were broken down into a number of separate statements. Questions representing the statements made most frequently were included in the questionnaire, named the "Whiteley Index" (WI). The WI was then given to 200 psychiatric patients. Of these, 100 had been diagnosed as manifesting hypochondriacal features, and the other 100 as showing little or no evidence of hypochondriasis. Hypochondriasis was defined as a persistent preoccupation with disease despite reassurance given after thorough medical examination. Of the 20 questions included to tap hypochondriacal attitudes, 17 discriminated significantly between the two groups. For technical reasons this number had to be reduced to 14. The questionnaire was scored by giving one point for each of the 14 questions answered in the specified direction.

**Reliability.** Factor analysis of the responses of the psychiatric patients to the WI yielded three factors (subscales), which were labeled Bodily Preoccupation, Disease Phobia, and Disease Conviction (Pilowsky, 1967). Seventy-one psychiatric patients filled in the questionnaire on a second occasion. The test–retest reliability was 0.81 over a mean interval of 18.4 (range: 2 to 44) weeks.

In a study by Barsky et al. (1986a) of 92 medical outpatients, the subscales appeared to be highly correlated. Barsky and his associates used the WI in several studies of general medical outpatients and scored the responses on an ordinal scale from 1 to 5 (Barsky et al., 1990a). One WI item that was similar to an item on a checklist of somatic symptoms (bodily awareness) was eliminated to obviate the possibility of covariance (Barsky et al., 1990b). The intrascale consistency of the 13-item WI varied between 0.84 and 0.95 (Barsky and Wyshak, 1989; Barsky et al., 1990c, 1992a, 1992b, 1998). The test-retest reliability was 0.84, with a mean interval of 24 (Barsky et al., 1992a) or 25.6 days (Barsky et al., 1990c, 1992b).

Speckens et al. (1996b) conducted exploratory principal components analysis of all items of the WI in 130 general medical outpatients, 113 general practice patients, and 204 subjects from the general population. A one-factor solution emerged in all of the populations. The Cronbach's alpha of the total WI was 0.80 in medical outpatients, 0.78 in general practice patients, and 0.76 in the general population. The test–retest reliability as assessed in medical outpatients was 0.90, with a mean interval of 42 (SD = 4.3) weeks.

**Concurrent validity.** To examine evidence of validity of the WI, Pilowsky (1967) compared the scores of the patients with information about the patients from their relatives. The correlation between the scores of 118 newly referred patients and their spouses was 0.59 (P < 0.001). In two studies in general practice, patient scores on the WI were not related to the diagnosis of hypochondriasis made by the physician. In a study of 109 family practice patients, none of 6 patients with a WI score greater than 10 had hypochondriasis as a problem listed in their medical records. (Beaber and Rodney, 1984). In a later study in primary care, only

29 (14%) of 210 patients scoring above an established cutoff on the WI were rated by their physicians as hypochondriacal (Gerdes *et al.*, 1996). General medical outpatients diagnosed as hypochondriacal had significantly higher WI scores than did patients who scored above the cutoff on the hypochondriacal symptomatology but failed to be diagnosed as hypochondriacal (Barsky *et al.*, 1990a, 1992a). In a later study by Speckens *et al.* (1996a) of 183 general medical outpatients with unexplained physical symptoms, scores on the WI were also significantly higher in hypochondriacal than in nonhypochondriacal patients. Using a cutoff level of 5 or more, the sensitivity and specificity of the WI were 87% and 72%, respectively. The PPV of the WI was 46%, and the NPV 93%. The area under the ROC curve was 0.88.

The scores of the WI appear to be confirmatory of the scores on other questionnaires assessing hypochondriasis or related illness behavior. In 177 medical outpatients, the zero-order correlation between scores on the WI and those on the 5-item Somatosensory Amplification Scale was 0.56 (Barsky and Wyshak, 1990). In 75 randomly chosen patients from a medical outpatient clinic, the WI was highly correlated with amplification (Barsky *et al.*, 1990b). In 100 general practice patients and matched nonpsychotic psychiatric outpatients, Kellner *et al.* (1992) found the Disease Phobia and Disease Conviction subscales of the WI to be significantly intercorrelated with the Hypochondriacal Beliefs and Disease Phobia scales of the Illness Attitude Scales. In a survey of 130 general medical outpatients, 113 general practice patients, and 204 subjects from the general population, Speckens *et al.* (1996b) found high associations between the WI scores and those on the Illness Attitude Scales and the Somatosensory Amplification Scale.

**Predictive validity.** Several studies found scores on the WI to be related with a poor outcome in terms of hypochondriasis, physical symptoms, or health care utilization. In a study on the longitudinal course of patients known to have had a previous episode of transient hypochondriasis, baseline WI scores were closely related to somatization and WI scores at follow-up (Barsky *et al.*, 1993a). In a 1-year follow-up study of 50 patients with hypochondriasis, Noyes *et al.* (1994a) found that remittance of hypochondriasis was predicted by the scores on the WI at original assessment. In a 4- to 5-year follow-up study of 120 hypochondriacal patients, Barsky *et al.* (1998) also found that remitting patients had significantly lower scores on the Disease Conviction subscale of the WI than did nonremitters.

In a small 3-year follow-up study of general practice patients with functional somatic symptoms, patients with a score of 6 or more on the 13-item WI visited their general practitioners more often than did patients without hypochondriasis (mean 17.1 vs. 9.6) (Palsson, 1988). In a study of medical patients referred for ambulatory electrocardiographic monitoring, the WI predicted the number of emergency and walk-in visits at 3 months. It did not predict persistence of palpitations (Barsky et al., 1996). In 183 general medical patients with unexplained physical symptoms, scores on the WI were negatively associated with recovery at 1-year follow-up (Speckens et al., 1996a). However, no association was found between the scores on the WI and medical care utilization in the following year (Speckens et al., 1996a).

**Convergent validity.** Scores on the WI were found to be correlated with somatic symptoms both in the general population (Roht et al., 1985; Simon et al., 1990; Stone and Neale, 1981) and in medical patients (Barsky and Wyshak, 1990; Barsky et al., 1986a, 1992b; Hiller et al., 1995; Noyes et al., 1993). In neurological inpatients (Ewald et al., 1994) and patients with dyspeptic symptoms (Andersson et al., 1994), those with unexplained physical symptoms had higher scores on the WI than did those with underlying organic disease. In medical patients who do not have *DSM-III-R* hypochondriasis, however, Barsky et al. (1991) found the WI to be significantly associated with the extent of medical morbidity.

In the general population, in general practice, and in medical patients, WI scores were found to be related to other characteristics of somatizing patients. In 109 family practice patients, the WI scores significantly correlated with the number of no-shows at the center, the number of symptoms listed as problems in the record, the notation of psychological problems, the ordering of laboratory tests, and total symptoms enumerated as problems (Beaber and Rodney, 1984). In the same study, however, hypochondriasis as identified by the WI did not appear to be significantly related to the total number of visits.

In a later study of primary care patients (Gerdes et al., 1996), physicians identified more unexplained somatic complaints, lack of response to treatment, personal psychiatric history, current psychiatric syndrome, excessive impairment, and unstable lifestyle among patients scoring above an established cutoff on the WI. Moreover, more diagnoses were made and more medications were prescribed (Gerdes et al., 1996). In a random sample of 177 outpatients at a general medical clinic, WI scores correlated highly with aversion to death and aging, value placed on health, value placed on physical appearance, and sense of bodily vulnerability (Barsky and Wyshak, 1989). Scores on the WI were significantly correlated with patient self-rating of global health and, to a lesser extent, their satisfaction with care (Barsky et al., 1992c). The WI score was found to be inversely related to the number of symptoms medical patients believed to be compatible with good health (Barsky et al., 1993b).

In 100 general medical inpatients, the WI score moderately correlated with the discrepancy between the physician's and patient's views of the severity of the patient's illness (Mabe et al., 1988). The WI score was not related to the physician ratings of the extent to which the presentation of the patient's illness was disproportionate to demonstrable disease. Self-reports of serious illness in the past, acceptance of illness as being part of life, and affective disturbance were positively associated with hypochondriasis as identified by the WI (Mabe *et al.*, 1988).

Although several studies found the WI score related to medical care utilization (Barsky and Wyshak, 1989; Noyes *et al.*, 1993), other studies found no such relationship (Beaber and Rodney, 1984). Kasteler *et al.* (1976) concluded that the WI score, contrary to hypothesized expectation, was not related to "doctor-shopping," although some difference existed between those with high and low hypochondriasis scores in tendency to "shop." Barsky *et al.* (1986b) did not find any significant correlation between WI score and medical utilization in 92 general medical outpatients.

The scores on the WI were also found to be related to psychiatric disorders and various psychopathological phenomena. Kellner *et al.* (1992) found the Disease Phobia and Disease Conviction subscale scores of the WI to be correlated to anxiety, depression, and somatization in general practice and matched nonpsychotic psychiatric outpatients. To a limited extent, scores on the WI have been shown to be associated with coping strategies, functional impairment, and alexithymia. In medical inpatients, the WI was associated with illness coping strategies such as symptom vigilance, limiting activity, and obsessive worry (Jones *et al.*, 1989). Mabe *et al.* (1996) found an association between the WI scores and the presence of angry feelings and interpersonal friction for medical inpatients referred for psychiatric evaluation. Wise *et al.* (1990) demonstrated that the WI scores were related to alexithymia, especially in a group of medical inpatients evaluated by a psychiatric consultation service.

**Divergent validity.** Scores on the Disease Phobia and Disease Conviction subscales of the WI appeared to discriminate between psychiatric patients and family practice patients (Hernandez and Kellner, 1992; Kellner *et al.*, 1992). The WI scores did not differ between general medical inpatients and medical inpatients referred for psychiatric evaluation (Mabe *et al.*, 1996). The mean scores on the WI declined significantly from medical outpatients through general practice patients to subjects from the general population (Speckens *et al.*, 1996b).

Barsky *et al.* (1992b) found that the Disease Phobia subscale of the WI differentiated patients with primary and secondary hypochondriasis (i.e., hypochondriasis accompanied by depressive, anxiety, or somatization disorder). In contrast with Barsky's findings, Noyes *et al.* (1994b) did not find the WI to differentiate between medical hypochondriacal outpatients with and without comorbid depression, nor between subjects with and without somatization disorder. Hypochondriacal patients appeared to have significantly higher WI scores than did panic disorder patients without hypochondriasis (Barsky *et al.*, 1994a).

Among palpitation patients referred for ambulatory electrocardiographic (ECG) monitoring, those with panic disorder scored higher on the WI than did those without panic disorder (Barsky *et al.*, 1994b).

The WI was shown to be sensitive to change in a controlled trial of alprazolam versus placebo for the treatment of panic disorder: Among improved subjects, the mean score on the WI at 6 weeks was significantly lower than that at baseline (Noyes *et al.*, 1986). In a controlled study of cognitive-behavioral therapy for unexplained physical symptoms, patients in the intervention group had lower WI scores at 6 months and 1 year than did those in the control group, although this difference was not significant (Speckens *et al.*, 1995).

## Illness Behaviour Questionnaire (IBQ)

In 1975, Pilowsky and Spence developed the Illness Behaviour Questionnaire (IBQ; Appendix 3) as a measure of patients' attitudes and feelings about their illness, their perceptions of the reactions of significant others in the environment (including their doctors') to themselves and their illness, and the patients' own views on their current psychosocial situation. The self-report questionnaire consists of 52 yes/no items.

**Reliability.** The IBQ scores of 100 patients with intractable pain were factor-analyzed and seven factors were interpreted: General Hypochondriasis, Disease Conviction, Somatic versus Psychological Perception, Affective Inhibition, Affective Disturbance, Denial, and Irritability (Pilowsky and Spence, 1975). No internal consistency or test–retest reliabilities of these subscales were reported. Byrne and Whyte (1978) administered the IBQ to 120 survivors of myocardial infarction. They extracted eight factors, which were only marginally similar to patterns of illness behavior reported by Pilowsky and Spence (1975). Zonderman *et al.* (1985) tried to replicate the findings of Pilowsky and Spence in a sample of 1,061 subjects drawn from five pain-care facilities and a group of healthy volunteers. Three of the seven factors exactly replicated scales in the IBQ (Affective Inhibition, Denial, and Irritability), and two factors were similar (Affective Disturbance and General Hypochondriasis). In contrast, Disease Conviction was split into two factors, and Somatic versus Psychological Perception of Illness was not represented by any of the factors. The alpha reliabilities for each scale for the complete sample were all greater than 0.70.

Main and Waddell (1987) administered the 62-item IBQ to 200 patients with chronic low back pain in an orthopedic outpatient department. A randomly selected subgroup of 40 patients answered the identical questionnaire on a second occasion, between 2 and 4 weeks later. For ten variables the kappa values for reliability were not significantly higher than would be expected by chance. In addition, 15 items had too skewed a distribution for useful analysis. Thus, of the original 62 items only 37 met the criteria of reliability and incidence. Further analysis limited to the 37 statistically satisfactory items yielded a three-factor solution: Affective and Hypochondriacal Disturbance, Life Disruption, and Social Inhibition. Palsson and Kaij (1985) assessed the test–retest reliability of the IBS in 19 general practice patients. The test–retest reliability was 0.89 with an in-between period of 3 to 6 weeks.

**Concurrent validity.** Kellner and Schneider-Braus (1988) compared the IBQ scores of 29 patients referred by physicians at a general hospital for a study of hypochondriasis with those of a control group of patients who were attending the same clinic but had not been referred to the study. Affective Disturbance was higher in the referred group and Denial higher in the controls. In 100 general medical inpatients, Affective Disturbance significantly contributed to a Hypochondriacal Index, consisting of the Whiteley Index, a discrepancy score of the physician's and patient's view of the illness severity, and the extent to which the patient's presentation was disproportionate to demonstrable disease (Mabe *et al.*, 1988). Robbins *et al.* (1990) found that Illness Worry, a 10-item scale using questions adapted from the Illness Behaviour Questionnaire, correlated at $r = 0.83$ with the Whiteley Index.

**Predictive validity.** In a study of 120 survivors of acute myocardial infarction between 10 and 14 days after their admission to a coronary care unit, higher IBQ scores were found to be predictive of poorer cardiological outcome, failure to return to work, limitation of physical capacity, and poorer social interaction at 8 months after discharge from hospital (Byrne, 1982; Byrne *et al.*, 1981).

Comparing 39 general practice patients with unexplained physical symptoms with 56 patients in whom the presence of pathology was established, Pilowsky *et al.* (1987) demonstrated higher scores on several subscales of the IBQ to be predictive of the number of visits to their general practitioner over the next 6 months.

In patients without serious current medical illness, no differences were seen in the number of visits in the 12 months following the clinic visit between those with high and those with low scores on the Illness Worry Scale (Kirmayer and Robbins, 1991).

**Convergent validity.** The IBQ scale profiles were not found to be related to chronicity of pain in 100 patients with intractable pain (Pilowsky and Spence, 1976a). In chronic headache sufferers, the IBQ scores were not related to headache diagnosis, nor to topographical properties of head pain (Demjen and Bakal, 1981). Headache patients who experienced the greatest amount of headache activity had higher scores on Somatic versus Psychological Perception of Illness. Patients with continuous head pain also viewed their disorder in somatic as opposed to psychological terms and scored higher on Denial than did patients with episodic pain (Demjen and Bakal, 1981). In patients with fibromyalgia or rheumatoid arthritis, Illness Worry scores correlated highly with symptomatology (Robbins et al., 1990). In fibromyalgia patients, Illness Worry scores also correlated with physical disability. Kirmayer and Robbins (1991) demonstrated that patients without serious current medical illness, who scored high on the Illness Worry Scale, also reported more somatization and depression.

In a study of 14 organic pain patients, 14 nonorganic pain patients, 14 nonorganic pain nonpatients, and a control group, only activities related to sleep showed significant correlations with IBQ scores (Skevington, 1983). No differences were found for recreational or passive activities. Wise et al. (1990) found alexithymia to be related to scores on General Hypochondriasis, Disease Conviction, Affective Inhibition, Affective Disturbance, and Irritability subscales of the IBQ.

The IBQ scales were found to be related to anxiety and depression in many studies. Pilowsky et al. (1977) demonstrated that depression scores were significantly related to General Hypochondriasis, Disease Conviction, Affective Disturbance, and Irritability in 100 patients referred to a pain clinic. In 325 inpatients of a general hospital, Fava et al. (1982) found elevated correlations between depression and scores on Affective Disturbance, Disease Conviction, General Hypochondriasis, Somatic versus Psychological Perception of Illness, Denial, and Irritability. In a study population consisting of family practice patients, psychiatric outpatients, gynecologic outpatients with unexplained pelvic pain, matched gynecologic outpatients, medical students, matched law students, and employees, the correlation coefficients between General Hypochondriasis and Disease Conviction and self-ratings of anxiety, depression, and phobic anxiety ranged from very low to moderately high (Kellner et al., 1986a). Main and Waddell (1987), studying 200 patients with chronic low back pain, found a relation between their Affective and Hypochondriacal Disturbance Scale scores and depressive symptomatology and somatic awareness. Patients attending family medicine clinics with high scores on the Illness Worry Scale of the IBQ were more likely to be recognized by their physicians as having depression or anxiety (Kirmayer et al., 1993); they had more depressive and somatic symptoms and also reported being more aware of bodily sensations (Robbins and Kirmayer, 1996).

**Divergent validity.** Pilowsky and Spence (1976b) found that patients referred for the management of pain who had not responded adequately to conventional treatment had higher scores on Disease Conviction and Irritability than a comparison group of patients with pain attending rheumatology, radiotherapy, pulmonary, and physiotherapy clinics. Patients at a pain clinic had higher scores on

Disease Conviction, Somatic versus Psychological Perception of Illness, and Denial than did family practice patients (Pilowsky *et al.*, 1977). A discriminant function that included these dimensions correctly identified 76.7% of the patients as
belonging either to the pain clinic or the family practice clinic. When this function was applied to two independent samples of pain clinic and family practice
patients, the IBQ was found to have a sensitivity of 97%, specificity of 73.6%,
and a rate of true-positive scores of 0.70 (Pilowsky *et al.*, 1979).

Zonderman *et al.* (1985) also demonstrated in a sample of 1,061 subjects that
patients attending pain-care facilities had significantly larger scores than did a
healthy group of volunteers on the Health Worry and Illness Disruption subscales
of the IBQ. Conversely, Skevington (1983) found no differences in IBQ scores
among organic pain patients, nonorganic pain patients, nonorganic pain nonpatients, and a control group. Other researchers found differences in IBQ scores
among patients with unexplained and explained physical symptoms in general
practice (Palsson and Kaij, 1985; Pilowsky *et al.*, 1987), gynecology (Kellner *et
al.*, 1988), neurology (Metcalfe *et al.*, 1988), and rheumatology (Robbins *et al.*,
1990), with patients with unexplained symptoms scoring higher.

The responses to the IBQ did not differentiate between medical and law students (Kellner *et al.*, 1986b). Fava *et al.* (1982) found no differences in IBQ score
between wards in 325 general hospital inpatients. General Hypochondriasis, Disease Conviction, Affective Disturbance, Denial, and Irritability subscales were
found to distinguish among medically ill hospitalized patients who were evaluated by a psychiatric consultation service, psychiatric outpatients, patients who
were psychiatrically hospitalized on an acute care unit, and healthy subjects (Wise
*et al.*, 1990). Medical and surgical patients who had been referred to the
consultation-liaison service of the psychiatry department had higher scores on
Affective Disturbance and lower scores on Denial than did comparison patients
randomly selected from admission lists (Clarke *et al.*, 1991).

In a study on the effect of 8 weeks of imipramine treatment in 10 subjects with
illness phobia, the Illness Concerns Scale developed by Wesner and Noyes (1991)
showed significant change from baseline scores at 4, 6, and 8 weeks. This scale
was meant to cover the most important features of illness phobia and included
items from the Illness Behaviour Questionnaire as well as items having to do
with avoidant behavior and reassurance-seeking.

## Illness Attitude Scales (IAS)

The Illness Attitude Scales (IAS) were developed by Kellner *et al.* (1983–84) to
measure psychopathology that tends to be associated with hypochondriasis and
that can be responsible for abnormal illness behavior (Appendix 4). Questions
were constructed from statements made by patients who were either diagnosed

as having a hypochondriacal neurosis or who showed abnormal illness behavior. The scales consist of three questions and (except for the Treatment Experience Scale) each is self-rated on a 5-point scale from "no" through "sometimes" to "most of the time." The scales are: Worry about Illness, Concerns about Pain, Health Habits, Hypochondriacal Beliefs, Thanatophobia, Disease Phobia, Bodily Preoccupations, and Treatment Experience. A later version contains one more scale, namely Effects of Symptoms (Kellner, 1986).

**Reliability.** The subscales of the IAS were developed on the basis of theoretical considerations. Kellner *et al.* (1983–84) did not conduct a factor analysis and consequently did not mention any measures of internal consistency. The test–retest reliabilities in two groups of normals after 1 month and 2 weeks were 0.62 and 1.00, respectively (Kellner, 1987a). Fava *et al.* (1988) also found high test–retest correlations in normals, ranging from 0.74 to 0.99. In women, Savron *et al.* (1989) found test–retest correlations ranging from 0.44 to 0.95 after 3 months and from 0.67 to 0.94 after 6 months. In a study of Bouman and Visser (1998), the Cronbach's alpha of the total score of the IAS ranged from 0.87 to 0.90, with a test–retest reliability of 0.96 over a period of 4 weeks.

Two studies were conducted about the factor structure of the IAS in nonclinical populations. Ferguson and Daniel (1995), in a study of 101 undergraduate students, found a four-factor model that was correctly interpreted as follows: (*1*) Hypochondriacal Fears and Beliefs; (*2*) Symptoms Experience and Frequency of Treatments; (*3*) Thanatophobia; and (*4*) Fears About Coronary Heart Disease and Related Health Habits. The stability coefficient indicated that these factors were very stable; all but the fourth factor showed good internal reliability (0.81, 0.79, 0.73, and 0.52). Hadjistavropoulos *et al.* (1999), in a randomly selected population of 390 participants from a larger pool of 780 undergraduate students, identified a five-factor solution: (*1*) Fear of Illness, Death, Disease and Pain; (*2*) Effects of Symptoms; (*3*) Treatment Experiences; (*4*) Disease Conviction; and (*5*) Health Habits. According to a confirmatory factor analysis of the responses from the remaining 390 students, a four-factor structure in which the Health Habits factor was deleted received the greatest support. However, the authors argued that the model could be conceptualized as either four distinct factors or as hierarchical in nature, with four lower-order factors loading on a single higher-order factor.

Speckens *et al.* (1996b), in a study of 130 medical outpatients, 113 general practice patients, and 204 subjects from the general population, found a two-factor solution of the IAS that was interpreted as reflecting Health Anxiety and Illness Behaviour. Cronbach's alpha for Health Anxiety was good in all three populations (0.85, 0.86, 0.87), and for Illness Behaviour slightly lower but still satisfactory (0.76, 0.70, 0.80). The test–retest reliability as assessed in 80 medical outpatients (mean period between the first and second time the questionnaires were completed was 42 [$SD$ = 4.3] weeks) was very high for both Health Anxiety (0.93) and Illness Behaviour (0.87). This factor structure was replicated by Dammen *et al.* (1999) in 199 patients referred to cardiological outpatient investigation because of chest pain. In this population, Cronbach's alpha was 0.92 for Health Anxiety and 0.80 for Illness Behaviour.

**Concurrent validity.** Except for the Health Habits Scale, all scales of the IAS discriminated significantly among hypochondriacal patients and other psychiatric patients, family practice patients, and employees (Kellner *et al.*, 1987a). The responses of the IAS that discriminated most sensitively between hypochondriacal and other psychiatric patients were a score of 3 or 4 on the Hypochondriacal Beliefs or Disease Phobia scales or both. Applying this criterion to medical outpatients with unexplained physical symptoms, however, Speckens *et al.* (1996a) found low values of the sensitivity, specificity, PPV, and NPV. Scores on the Health Anxiety subscale of the IAS developed by them were significantly higher in hypochondriacal than in nonhypochondriacal patients. The sensitivity, specificity, PPV, and NPV for the Health Anxiety subscale were 79%, 84%, 53%, and 95%, respectively. According to the ROC analysis, the area under the curve was 0.88.

The Hypochondriacal Beliefs and Disease Phobia subscales of the IAS were significantly correlated with the Disease Phobia and Disease Conviction subscales of the Whiteley Index in both general practice patients and matched nonpsychotic psychiatric outpatients (Kellner *et al.*, 1992). In medical outpatients, general practice patients, and subjects from the general population, scores on the Health Anxiety and Illness Behaviour subscales of the IAS were also highly associated with the scores on the Whiteley Index (Speckens *et al.*, 1996b). Associations between the scores on the two subscales and those on the Somatosensory Amplification Scale were somewhat lower. Dammen *et al.* (1999) also demonstrated, in patients with chest pain, that the Health Anxiety and Illness Behaviour subscales of the IAS were associated with the scores on the Somatosensory Amplification Scale.

**Predictive validity.** The only study that examined the predictive validity of the IAS was that of Speckens *et al.* (1996a) in medical outpatients with unexplained physical symptoms. Scores on their Health Anxiety and Illness Behaviour subscales were negatively, but not significantly, related to recovery. The Illness Behaviour subscale was predictive of the number of medical visits.

**Convergent validity.** In family practice patients, scores on all IAS scales (except for Health Habits and Thanatophobia) were significantly correlated with somatization (Kellner et al., 1987b). Ferguson and Daniel (1995) compared the IAS scores of subjects who had a current diagnosis of an actual illness with those of subjects who did not have such a diagnosis. Only their Symptom Experience and Frequency of Treatments factor differed significantly between the groups. Speckens et al. (1996b) found that patients whose symptoms could be explained by organic abnormalities had lower scores on the Health Anxiety subscale than did those with medically unexplained symptoms, but this difference was not significant. Both the Health Anxiety and Illness Behaviour subscales were associated with somatization and pain in patients with chest pain (Dammen et al., 1999). The Health Anxiety subscale was also associated with alexithymia, and the Illness Behaviour subscale with the total number of reported somatic diseases and prescribed medications.

Kellner et al. (1986a) administered the IAS to family practice patients, psychiatric outpatients, gynecological outpatients with unexplained pelvic pain, matched gynecological outpatients, medical students, matched law students, and employees. The correlation coefficients of scores on the IAS on one hand and self-ratings of anxiety, depression, and phobic anxiety on the other hand ranged from very low to moderately high. Over one-half were statistically significant. The relationship between the IAS and anxiety or depression has also been established in patients with chronic airflow obstruction (Kellner et al., 1987b), chest pain (Dammen et al., 1999), general practice patients, and matched psychiatric outpatients (Kellner et al., 1992), psychiatric inpatients (Fava et al., 1987), panic disorder patients (Fava et al., 1988; Otto et al., 1992), and depressive patients (Demopulos et al., 1996; Otto et al., 1998). The scores on the IAS correlated poorly with obsessions and compulsions (Savron et al., 1996).

Hitchcock and Mathews (1992) found that undergraduate students with high hypochondriacal concerns according to the IAS endorsed more thoughts about illness interpretations of ambiguous bodily sensations. Individuals scoring in the upper 10% more quickly correctly identified previously exposed illness words than did those scoring in the lower 10%. Gramling et al. (1996) found objective differences in physiological reactivity between hypochondriacal subjects, as defined by a score of 4 or higher on either the Hypochondriacal Beliefs or Disease Phobia subscales of the IAS, and controls who scored 0 or 1 on both of these scales. However, other authors found no differences in physiological response, increase in perceived somatic activity, and pain sensitivity between subjects with low and high scores on the IAS (Lautenbacher et al., 1998; Steptoe and Noll, 1997). Ferguson and Cox (1997) found that IAS scores were associated with coping functions as assessed by the Functional Dimensions of Coping Scale.

**Divergent validity.** Some subscales of the IAS have been demonstrated to discriminate among nonhypochondriacal psychiatric patients, family practice patients, and employees (Hernandez and Kellner, 1992; Kellner et al., 1983–84,

1992). Fava *et al.* (1987) also found that psychiatric patients differed from normals on the Hypochondriacal Beliefs subscale of the IAS. None of the IAS scores showed significant differences between inpatients referred to a psychiatric consultation service and nonreferred patients from the same wards (Kellner *et al.*, 1987c). Melancholic patients rated themselves significantly higher on the Hypochondriacal Beliefs and Disease Phobia scales than did normals, whereas normals rated themselves higher on the Health Habits Scale (Kellner *et al.*, 1986c). Patients with agoraphobia and panic attacks rated themselves significantly higher than did normal controls on all IAS scales, except for Health Habits (Fava *et al.*, 1988). In patients with chest pain, both the Health Anxiety and the Illness Behaviour subscale of the IAS discriminated between patients with and without panic disorder (Dammen *et al.*, 1999). Patients with panic disorder scored significantly higher on all IAS scales than did patients with generalized anxiety disorder, except for Health Habits and Treatment Experience (Starcevic *et al.*, 1994). Scores on all IAS scales were significantly higher in patients with obsessive-compulsive disorder than in healthy control subjects (Savron *et al.*, 1996).

The IAS also discriminated among medical and law students (Kellner *et al.*, 1986b), pregnant patients and normals (Fava *et al.*, 1990), gynecological patients with pelvic pain syndrome and matched gynecological patients (Kellner *et al.*, 1988), medical, general practice patients, and general population subjects (Speckens *et al.*, 1996b).

In a study of 20 inpatients with *DSM-III* diagnosis of melancholia treated for 4 weeks with amitriptyline, no significant differences existed in IAS scores before and after treatment (Kellner *et al.*, 1986c). However, in an open study by Demopulos *et al.* (1996) on the effect of fluoxetine in 100 depressive patients, the IAS scores did show statistically significant decreases. Although the IAS scores improved in 10 patients with agoraphobia after exposure therapy, this change reached a significant level only for the Thanatophobia Scale (Fava *et al.*, 1988). Otto *et al.* (1992) found that the IAS scores for panic patients in various stages of recovery were lower than scores for untreated panic patients. A 6-month follow-up study on cognitive behavioral therapy for unexplained physical symptoms demonstrated that 39 patients in the intervention group had significantly lower scores on the Illness Behaviour subscale of the IAS than did 40 patients in the control group (Speckens *et al.*, 1995); however, at 1 year this difference was no longer significant. There were no significant differences between the two groups in the Health Anxiety subscale of the IAS. A study of cognitive or behavioral treatment in 17 patients with hypochondriasis (Bouman and Visser, 1998) also showed a significant decrease in the total IAS score after treatment. No differences were seen in the total IAS scores between patients treated with cognitive therapy and those treated with exposure *in vivo* plus response prevention.

## The Somatosensory Amplification Scale (SSAS)

The Somatosensory Amplification Scale (SSAS; Barsky et al., 1990b) asks the respondent about a range of unpleasant and uncomfortable bodily sensations, generally not connoting serious disease, on an ordinal scale from 1 to 5 (Appendix 5). Two of the items ("hunger contractions" and "various things happening in my body") are similar to items in Miller's Body Consciousness Questionnaire.

**Reliability.** The first version of the SSAS included only five items (Barsky et al., 1988). The reported internal consistency of the 10-item version of the scale varied between 0.70 and 0.82, and the test–retest reliability was 0.85 over an interval of 28 to 146 days (mean 72 days) and 0.79 over a median interval of 74 days (Barsky and Wyshak, 1989; Barsky et al., 1990b, 1998). In a study by Speckens et al. (1996b), the Cronbach's alpha of the SSAS was found to be somewhat lower: 0.77 in 130 general medical outpatients, 0.64 in 113 general practice patients, and 0.71 in 204 subjects from the general population. The stability as assessed in 80 medical outpatients over a mean period of 42 ($SD = 4.3$) weeks was 0.87.

**Concurrent validity.** In several studies, medical outpatients with hypochondriasis had significantly higher scores on the SSAS than did nonhypochondriacal patients (Barsky et al., 1990b, 1995; Noyes et al., 1993). The study by Speckens et al. (1996a) of patients with medically unexplained symptoms produced similar scores on the SSAS between patients with or without hypochondriasis. The sensitivity and specificity of the SSAS at a cutoff level 11 or more were only 58% and 55%, respectively. The PPV and NPV were 22% and 85%, respectively. Based on the ROC analysis, the area under the curve was only 0.55.

In two studies (Barsky and Wyshak, 1990; Barsky et al., 1990b), scores on the SSAS appeared to correlate with scores on the Whiteley Index. Gramling et al. (1996) found no significant differences in scores on the SSAS between female subjects scoring 4 or higher on either the Hypochondriacal Beliefs or Disease Phobia scales of the Illness Attitude Scales ($N = 15$) and female control subjects scoring 0 or 1 on both of these scales ($N = 15$). A study of general medical outpatients, general practice patients, and subjects from the general population showed moderate positive associations between the scores on the SSAS and the scores on the Whiteley Index and the Health Anxiety subscale of the Illness Attitude Scales (Speckens et al., 1996b).

**Predictive validity.** In a study examining the longitudinal course of transient hypochondriasis, scores on the SSAS were closely related to hypochondriacal symptoms and somatization at follow-up (Barsky et al., 1993a). Noyes et al. (1994a) also demonstrated a significant correlation between scores on the SSAS and level of hypochondriacal symptoms a year later in 50 patients with hypochondriasis and 50 control subjects. However, in the 4- to 5-year follow-up study of 120 hypochondriacal patients, remitters and nonremitters did not differ in somatic amplification at inception (Barsky *et al.*, 1998).

In a sample of medical patients referred for ambulatory electrocardiographic (ECG) monitoring, the interaction of scores on the SSAS and daily life stress at inception of the study predicted persistent palpitation at 3-months' follow-up (Barsky *et al.*, 1996). The number of emergency and walk-in visits was predicted by the Whiteley Index and the interaction of SSAS scores and daily irritants. Medical outpatients with unexplained physical symptoms had scores on the SSAS that were negatively, but not significantly, related to recovery (Speckens *et al.*, 1996a). No association was found between scores on the SSAS and medical care utilization.

**Convergent validity.** Both in subjects from the general population (Davis *et al.*, 1995; Simon *et al.*, 1990) and in medical outpatients (Barsky and Wyshak, 1990; Barsky *et al.*, 1988, 1990b) scores on the SSAS appeared to be related to somatic symptoms. Scores on the SSAS were not related to aggregate medical morbidity, whether measured by physician ratings or by a medical record audit. Speckens *et al.* (1996b), in a study of 130 general medical patients, found no association between the SSAS and whether or not their physical symptoms were explained.

Amplification, along with symptoms and discomfort, was found to be significantly associated with impairment in functioning in patients with upper respiratory tract infection (Barsky *et al.*, 1988). Furthermore, the SSAS correlated with self-reported importance of health and physical appearance, aversion to death and bodily vulnerability in a study of 177 general medical outpatients (Barsky and Wyshak, 1989). With 120 consecutive clinic attenders, scores on the Health Norms Sorting Task, which measures the number of symptoms that respondents believe are compatible with a state of good health, appeared to be inversely related to amplification (Barsky *et al.*, 1993b). Speckens *et al.* (1996b) found a moderate positive association between the SSAS and the Illness Behaviour subscale of the Illness Attitude Scales in general medical outpatients, general practice patients, and subjects from the general population.

The SSAS scores were closely correlated with depression and hostility in 115 patients presenting with an upper respiratory tract infection to an adult medical walk-in clinic (Barsky *et al.*, 1988). Comparing 41 hypochondriacal patients and 75 randomly chosen medical outpatients, Barsky *et al.* (1990b) found a significant association of the SSAS scores with aggregate psychiatric morbidity in both groups, and with depressive, anxiety, and somatization disorder in the random sample.

**Divergent validity.** Somatosensory amplification did not discriminate between patients with primary hypochondriasis and those with secondary hypochondriasis accompanied by depressive, anxiety, or somatization disorder (Barsky et al., 1992b). Noyes et al. (1994b) also found that scores on the SSAS did not differentiate between hypochondriacal patients with comorbid depression and those without. However, amplification did differentiate between palpitation patients with and without panic disorder (Barsky et al., 1994b).

A study of general medical outpatients, general practice patients, and subjects from the general population revealed that the scores on the SSAS did not decline significantly from medical outpatients to subjects from the general population (Speckens et al., 1996b).


## Conclusion

Although the Structured Diagnostic Interview for Hypochondriasis (SDIH) is considered the "gold standard" for the assessment of hypochondriasis, it does not assess the nature of the medical investigation and reassurance provided by the physician (Barsky et al., 1992a). However, the *DSM-III-R* and *DSM-IV* criteria for hypochondriasis themselves do not include any criteria about the nature of the clinical investigation and reassurance required. With regard to the interrater reliability, only the agreement with the joint assessment method is reported. No kappa values are given, nor is any information available about the interrater reliability of two different assessors interviewing the same patient. The concurrent, convergent, and divergent validity of the SDIH has been adequately established. The SDIH has been shown to be predictive of outcome in terms of somatic and psychic symptoms, but not in terms of frequency of physician visits (Noyes et al., 1994a; Speckens et al., 1996a).

The psychometric properties of the different self-report questionnaires are summarized in Table 3.1.

The three-factor structure of the Whiteley Index (WI) as developed by Pilowsky (1967), has not been confirmed by other researchers (Speckens et al., 1996b). Consequently, many researchers use the total score of the WI and employ an ordinal scale from 1 to 5 instead of the original dichotomous response (Barsky et al., 1990a). The reported internal consistency and test–retest reliability range from good to excellent. There is ample evidence for the concurrent and convergent validity of the WI. The WI appears to predict the persistence of hypochondriasis and physical symptoms (Barsky et al., 1993a; Noyes et al., 1994a; Speckens et al., 1996a). Evidence with regard to the prediction of frequency of physician visits is contradictory (Barsky et al. 1996; Palsson, 1988; Speckens et al., 1996a). The divergent validity of the WI is less often investigated, but appears to be good.

**Table 3.1.** Psychometric properties of self-report questionnaires assessing hypochondriasis and related illness behaviors

| | Internal Consistency* | Stability* | Concurrent Validity | Predictive Validity | Convergent Validity | Divergent Validity |
|---|---|---|---|---|---|---|
| Whiteley Index | Good | Good | Good | Good | Good | Good |
| Illness Behaviour Questionnaire | Good | Excellent | Moderate | Good | Good | Good |
| Illness Attitude Scales | Good | Excellent | Good | Moderate | Good | Good |
| Somatosensory Amplification Scale | Moderate | Good | Moderate | Moderate | Moderate | Poor |

*< 0.60 poor, > = 0.60 and <0.70 moderate, > = 0.70 and <0.85 good, > = 0.85 excellent.

The factor structure of the Illness Behaviour Questionnaire (IBQ) largely depends on the setting and population studied (Byrne and Whyte, 1978; Main and Waddell, 1987; Pilowsky and Spence, 1975; Zonderman et al., 1985). There is little evidence for the concurrent validity of the IBQ. It is predictive of outcome in patients who survived a myocardial infarction (Byrne, 1982; Byrne et al., 1981). Pilowsky et al. (1987) found some evidence of the IBQ to be predictive of frequency of physician visits in general practice patients. The IBQ scores have been found to be related to both psychic and somatic symptoms and capable of discriminating between different groups of patients, especially between chronic pain patients and nonpain patients.

The original nine subscales of the Illness Attitude Scales (IAS) have not been empirically determined. Studies of different populations revealed factor models with fewer factors, indicating health anxiety and illness behavior (Dammen et al., 1999; Ferguson and Daniel, 1995; Hadjistavropoulos et al., 1999; Speckens et al., 1996b). The reported internal consistency and test–retest reliability are good to excellent. Although the criterion for hypochondriasis postulated by Kellner et al. (1987a) does not result in good discrimination between hypochondriacal and nonhypochondriacal patients, the Health Anxiety subscale of the IAS does (Speckens et al., 1996a). In medical patients with unexplained physical symptoms, the Illness Behaviour subscale of the IAS appears to be predictive of frequency of physician visits (Speckens et al., 1996a). Found to be related to anxiety, depression, and coping, the IAS also discriminate among different groups of patients with psychiatric or somatic disorders. They have been shown to be sensitive to change in two treatment studies (Bouman and Visser, 1998; Speckens et al., 1995).

The internal consistency of the Somatosensory Amplification Scale (SSAS) is moderate, its test–retest reliability good. Evidence regarding the concurrent validity is conflicting. Although Barsky *et al.* (1990b), Noyes *et al.* (1993), and Barsky *et al.* (1995) found differences in SSAS scores between hypochondriacal and nonhypochondriacal patients, Speckens *et al.* (1996a) did not. There is limited evidence that the SSAS is predictive of hypochondriasis and somatization (Barsky *et al.*, 1993a; Noyes *et al.*, 1994a; Speckens *et al.*, 1996a). The SSAS has been found to be related to somatic and psychic symptoms. There is little evidence for the discriminative ability of the SSAS.

Table 3.1 and this summary might help clinicians and researchers select the instrument that would best help their research goals. Instruments that are most suitable to screen for hypochondriasis in a certain population are those with the best concurrent validity, namely the Whiteley Index and the Health Anxiety subscale of the Illness Attitude Scales. Instruments, of which the predictive validity has been established, such as the Whiteley Index and the Illness Behaviour Questionnaire (IBQ), will be most useful in follow-up studies. The sensitivity of change is important for instruments that are needed to evaluate the effect of interventions. In this regard, there is some empirical support for the Whiteley Index, the Illness Concerns Scale of the IBQ, and the Illness Attitude Scales.

## References

American Psychiatric Association. 1994. *Diagnostic and Statistical Manual of Mental Disorders, Fourth Edition (DSM-IV)*. Washington, DC: American Psychiatric Association.

Andersson S.I., Hovelius B., Molstad S., Wadstrom T. 1994. Dyspepsia in general practice: psychological findings in relation to *Helicobacter pylori* serum antibodies. *Journal of Psychosomatic Research* 38: 241–247.

Barsky A.J., Wyshak G. 1989. Hypochondriasis and related health attitudes. *Psychosomatics* 30: 412–420.

Barsky A.J., Wyshak G. 1990. Hypochondriasis and somatosensory amplification. *British Journal of Psychiatry* 157: 404–409.

Barsky A.J., Wyshak G., Klerman G.L. 1986a. Hypochondriasis: an evaluation of the DSM-III criteria in medical outpatients. *Archives of General Psychiatry* 43: 493–500.

Barsky A.J., Wyshak G., Klerman G.L. 1986b. Medical and psychiatric determinants of outpatient medical utilization. *Medical Care* 24: 548–560.

Barsky A.J., Goodson J.D., Lane R.S., Cleary P.D. 1988. The amplification of somatic symptoms. *Psychosomatic Medicine* 50: 510–519.

Barsky A.J., Wyshak G., Klerman G.L. 1990a. Transient hypochondriasis. *Archives of General Psychiatry* 47: 746–752.

Barsky A.J., Wyshak G., Klerman G.L. 1990b. The somatosensory amplification scale and its relationship to hypochondriasis. *Journal of Psychiatric Research* 24: 323–334.

Barsky A.J., Wyshak G., Klerman G.L., Latham K.S. 1990c. The prevalence of hypochondriasis in medical outpatients. *Social Psychiatry and Psychiatric Epidemiology* 25: 89–94.

Barsky A.J., Wyshak G., Latham K.S., Klerman G.L. 1991. The relationship between hypochondriasis and medical illness. *Archives of Internal Medicine* 151: 84–88.

Barsky A.J., Cleary P.D., Wyshak G., Spitzer R.L., Williams J.B., Klerman G.L. 1992a. A structured diagnostic interview for hypochondriasis: a proposed criterion standard. *Journal of Nervous and Mental Disease* 180: 20–27.

Barsky A.J., Wyshak G., Klerman G.L. 1992b. Psychiatric comorbidity in DSM-III-R hypochondriasis. *Archives of General Psychiatry* 49: 101–108.

Barsky A.J., Cleary P.D., Klerman G.L. 1992c. Determinants of perceived health status of medical outpatients. *Social Science and Medicine* 34: 1147–1154.

Barsky A.J., Cleary P.D., Sarnie M.K., Klerman G.L. 1993a. The course of transient hypochondriasis. *American Journal of Psychiatry* 150: 484–488.

Barsky A.J., Coeytaux R.R., Sarnie M.K., Cleary P.D. 1993b. Hypochondriacal patients' beliefs about good health. *American Journal of Psychiatry* 150: 1085–1089.

Barsky A.J., Barnett M.C., Cleary P.D. 1994a. Hypochondriasis and panic disorder: boundary and overlap. *Archives of General Psychiatry* 51: 918–925.

Barsky A.J., Cleary P.D., Sarnie M.K., Ruskin J.N. 1994b. Panic disorder, palpitations, and the awareness of cardiac activity. *Journal of Nervous and Mental Disease* 182: 63–71.

Barsky A.J., Brener J., Coeytaux R.R., Cleary P.D. 1995. Accurate awareness of heartbeat in hypochondriacal and non-hypochondriacal patients. *Journal of Psychosomatic Research* 39: 489–497.

Barsky A.J., Ahern D.K., Bailey E.D., Delamater B.A. 1996. Predictors of persistent palpitations and continued medical utilization. *Journal of Family Practice* 42: 465–472.

Barsky A.J., Fama J.M., Bailey E.D., Ahern D.K. 1998. A prospective 4- to 5-year study of DSM-III-R hypochondriasis. *Archives of General Psychiatry* 55: 737–744.

Beaber R.J., Rodney W.M. 1984. Underdiagnosis of hypochondriasis in family practice. *Psychosomatics* 25: 39–46.

Bouman T.K., Visser S. 1998. Cognitive and behavioural treatment of hypochondriasis. *Psychotherapy and Psychosomatics* 67: 214–221.

Byrne D.G. 1982. Illness behaviour and psychosocial outcome after a heart attack. *British Journal of Clinical Psychology* 21: 145–146.

Byrne D.G., Whyte H.M. 1978. Dimensions of illness behaviour in survivors of myocardial infarction. *Journal of Psychosomatic Research* 22: 485–491.

Byrne D.G., Whyte H.M., Butler K.L. 1981. Illness behaviour and outcome following survived myocardial infarction: a prospective study. *Journal of Psychosomatic Research* 25: 97–107.

Clark D.M., Salkovskis P.M., Hackmann A., Wells A., Fennell M., Ludgate J., Ahmad S., Richards H.D., Gelder M. 1998. Two psychological treatments for hypochondriasis: a randomised controlled trial. *British Journal of Psychiatry* 173: 218–225.

Clarke D.M., Minas I.H., McKenzie D.P. 1991. Illness behaviour as determinant of referral to a psychiatric consultation/liaison service. *Australian and New Zealand Journal of Psychiatry* 25: 330–337.

Dammen T., Friis S., Ekeberg O. 1999. The Illness Attitude Scales in chest pain patients: a study of psychometric properties. *Journal of Psychosomatic Research* 46: 335–342.

Davis C., Ralevski E., Kennedy S.H., Neitzert C. 1995. The role of personality factors in the reporting of side effect complaints to moclobemide and placebo: a study of healthy male and female volunteers. *Journal of Clinical Psychopharmacology* 15: 347–352.

de Jong P.J., Haenen M.A., Schmidt A., Mayer B. 1998. Hypochondriasis: the role of fear-confirming reasoning. *Behaviour Research and Therapy* 36: 65–74.

Demjen S., Bakal D. 1981. Illness behavior and chronic headache. *Pain* 10: 221–229.

Demopulos C., Fava M., McLean N.E., Alpert J.E., Nierenberg A.A., Rosenbaum J.F. 1996. Hypochondriacal concerns in depressed outpatients. *Psychosomatic Medicine* 58: 314–320.

Ewald H., Rogne T., Ewald K., Fink P. 1994. Somatization in patients newly admitted to a neurological department. *Acta Psychiatrica Scandinavica* 89: 174–179.

Fava G.A., Pilowsky I., Pierfederici A., Bernardi M., Pathak D. 1982. Depressive symptoms and abnormal illness behavior in general hospital patients. *General Hospital Psychiatry* 4: 171–178.

Fava G.A., Molnar G., Zielezny M. 1987. Health attitudes of psychiatric inpatients. *Psychopathology* 20: 180–186.

Fava G.A., Kellner R., Zielezny M., Grandi S. 1988. Hypochondriacal fears and beliefs in agoraphobia. *Journal of Affective Disorders* 14: 239–244.

Fava G.A., Grandi S., Michelacci L., Saviotti F., Conti S., Bovicelli L., Trombini G., Orlandi C. 1990. Hypochondriacal fears and beliefs in pregnancy. *Acta Psychiatrica Scandinavica* 82: 70–72.

Ferguson E., Daniel E. 1995. The Illness Attitudes Scales (IAS): a psychometric evaluation on a non-clinical population. *Personality and Individual Differences* 18: 463–469.

Ferguson E., Cox T. 1997. The Functional Dimension of Coping Scale: theory, reliability and validity. *British Journal of Health Psychology* 2: 109–129.

Gerdes T.T., Noyes R. Jr., Kathol R.G., Phillips B.M., Fisher M.M., Morcuende M.A., Yagla S.J. 1996. Physician recognition of hypochondriacal patients. *General Hospital Psychiatry* 18: 106–112.

Gramling S.E., Clawson E.P., McDonald M.K. 1996. Perceptual and cognitive abnormality model of hypochondriasis: amplification and physiological reactivity in women. *Psychosomatic Medicine* 58: 423–431.

Greene R.L. 1991. *The MMPI-2/MMPI: An Interpretive Manual*. Boston: Allyn & Bacon.

Hadjistavropoulos H.D., Frombach I.K., Asmundson G.J.G. 1999. Exploratory and confirmatory factor analytic investigations of the Illness Attitude Scales in a nonclinical sample. *Behaviour Research and Therapy* 37: 671–684.

Haenen M.A., Schmidt A.J., Kroeze S., van den Hout M.A. 1996. Hypochondriasis and symptom reporting—the effect of attention versus distraction. *Psychotherapy and Psychosomatics* 65: 43–48.

Haenen M.A., Schmidt A.J.M., Schoenmakers M., van den Hout M.A. 1997. Tactual sensitivity in hypochondriasis. *Psychotherapy and Psychosomatics* 66: 128–132.

Hernandez J., Kellner R. 1992. Hypochondriacal concerns and attitudes toward illness in males and females. *International Journal of Psychiatry in Medicine* 22: 251–263.

Hiller W., Rief W., Fichter M.M. 1995. Further evidence for a broader concept of somatization disorder using the somatic symptom index. *Psychosomatics* 36: 285–294.

Hitchcock P.B., Mathews A. 1992. Interpretation of bodily symptoms in hypochondriasis. *Behaviour Research and Therapy* 30: 223–234.

Jones L.R., Mabe P.A., Riley W.T. 1989. Illness coping strategies and hypochondriacal traits among medical inpatients. *International Journal of Psychiatry in Medicine* 19: 327–339.

Kasteler J., Kane R.L., Olsen D.M., Thetford C. 1976. Issues underlying prevalence of "doctor-shopping" behavior. *Journal of Health and Social Behavior* 17: 328–339.

Kellner R. 1986. *Somatization and Hypochondriasis*. New York: Praeger.

Kellner R., Schneider-Braus K. 1988. Distress and attitudes in patients perceived as hypochondriacal by medical staff. *General Hospital Psychiatry* 10: 157–162.

Kellner R., Abbott P., Pathak D., Winslow W.W., Umland B.E. 1983–84. Hypochondriacal beliefs and attitudes in family practice and psychiatric patients. *International Journal of Psychiatry in Medicine* 13: 127–139.

Kellner R., Slocumb J.C., Wiggins R.J., Abbott P.J., Romanik R.L., Winslow W.W., Pathak D. 1986a. The relationship of hypochondriacal fears and beliefs to anxiety and depression. *Psychiatric Medicine* 4: 15–24.

Kellner R., Wiggins R.G., Pathak D. 1986b. Hypochondriacal fears and beliefs in medical and law students. *Archives of General Psychiatry* 43: 487–489.

Kellner R., Fava G.A., Lisansky J., Perini G.I., Zielezny M. 1986c. Hypochondriacal fears and beliefs in DSM-III melancholia: changes with amitriptyline. *Journal of Affective Disorders* 10: 21–26.

Kellner R., Abbott P., Winslow W.W., Pathak D. 1987a. Fears, beliefs, and attitudes in DSM-III hypochondriasis. *Journal of Nervous and Mental Disease* 175: 20–25.

Kellner R., Samet J.M., Pathak D. 1987b. Hypochondriacal concerns and somatic symptoms in patients with chronic airflow obstruction. *Journal of Psychosomatic Research* 31: 575–582.

Kellner R., Robinson J., Vogel A., Winslow W.W., Pathak D. 1987c. Nonpsychotic patients referred to a consultation service. *International Journal of Psychiatry in Medicine* 17: 381–390.

Kellner R., Slocumb J.C., Rosenfeld R.C., Pathak D. 1988. Fears and beliefs in patients with the pelvic pain syndrome. *Journal of Psychosomatic Research* 32: 303–310.

Kellner R., Hernandez J., Pathak D. 1992. Hypochondriacal fears and beliefs, anxiety, and somatisation. *British Journal of Psychiatry* 160: 525–532.

Kirmayer L.J., Robbins J.M. 1991. Three forms of somatization in primary care: prevalence, co-occurrence, and sociodemographic characteristics. *Journal of Nervous and Mental Disease* 179: 647–655.

Kirmayer L.J., Robbins J.M., Dworkind M., Yaffe M.J. 1993. Somatization and the recognition of depression and anxiety in primary care. *American Journal of Psychiatry* 150: 734–741.

Lautenbacher S., Pauli P., Zaudig M., Birbaumer N. 1998. Attentional control of pain perception: the role of hypochondriasis. *Journal of Psychosomatic Research* 44: 251–259.

Mabe P.A., Hobson D.P., Jones L.R., Jarvis R.G. 1988. Hypochondriacal traits in medical inpatients. *General Hospital Psychiatry* 10: 236–244.

Mabe P.A., Riley W.T., Jones L.R., Hobson D.P. 1996. The medical context of hypochondriacal traits. *International Journal of Psychiatry in Medicine* 26: 443–459.

MacDowell L., Hewell C. (eds.). 1987. *Measuring Health: A Guide to Rating Scales and Questionnaires*. New York: Oxford University Press.

Main C.J., Waddell G. 1987. Psychometric construction and validity of the Pilowsky IBQ in British patients with chronic low back pain. *Pain* 28: 13–25.

Metcalfe R., Firth D., Pollock S., Creed F. 1988. Psychiatric morbidity and illness behaviour in female neurological in-patients. *Journal of Neurology, Neurosurgery, and Psychiatry* 51: 1387–1390.

Noyes R., Reich J., Clancy J., O'Gorman T.W. 1986. Reduction in hypochondriasis with treatment of panic disorder. *British Journal of Psychiatry* 149: 631–635.

Noyes R. Jr., Kathol R.G., Fisher M.M., Phillips B.M., Suelzer M.T., Holt C.S. 1993. The validity of DSM-III-R hypochondriasis. *Archives of General Psychiatry* 50: 961–970.

Noyes R. Jr., Kathol R.G., Fisher M.M., Phillips B.M., Suelzer M.T., Woodman C.L. 1994a. One-year follow-up of medical outpatients with hypochondriasis. *Psychosomatics* 35: 533–545.

Noyes R. Jr., Kathol R.G., Fisher M.M., Phillips B.M., Suelzer M.T., Woodman C.L. 1994b. Psychiatric comorbidity among patients with hypochondriasis. *General Hospital Psychiatry* 16: 78–87.

Otto M.W., Pollack M.H., Sachs G.S., Rosenbaum J.F. 1992. Hypochondriacal concerns, anxiety sensitivity, and panic disorder. *Journal of Anxiety Disorders* 6: 93–104.

Otto M.W., Demopulos C.M., McLean N.E., Pollack M.H., Fava M. 1998. Additional findings on the association between anxiety sensitivity and hypochondriacal concerns: examination of patients with major depression. *Journal of Anxiety Disorders* 12: 225–232.

Palsson N. 1988. Functional somatic symptoms and hypochondriasis among general practice patients: a pilot study. *Acta Psychiatrica Scandinavica* 78: 191–197.

Palsson N., Kaij L. 1985. Development of a screening method for probable somatizing syndromes. *Acta Psychiatrica Scandinavica* 72: 69–73.

Pilowsky I. 1967. Dimensions of hypochondriasis. *British Journal of Psychiatry* 113: 89–93.

Pilowsky I. 1990. The concept of abnormal illness behavior. *Psychosomatics* 31: 207–213.

Pilowsky I., Spence N.D. 1975. Patterns of illness behaviour in patients with intractable pain. *Journal of Psychosomatic Research* 19: 279–287.

Pilowsky I., Spence N.D. 1976a. Is illness behavior related to chronicity in patients with intractable pain? *Pain* 2: 167–173.

Pilowsky I., Spence N.D. 1976b. Pain and illness behaviour: a comparative study. *Journal of Psychosomatic Research* 20: 131–134.

Pilowsky I., Chapman C.R., Bonica J.J. 1977. Pain, depression, and illness behavior in a pain clinic population. *Pain* 4: 183–192.

Pilowsky I., Murrell T.G.C., Gordon A. 1979. The development of a screening method for abnormal illness behaviour. *Journal of Psychosomatic Research* 23: 203–207.

Pilowsky I., Smith Q., Katsikitis M. 1987. Illness behaviour and general practice utilization: a prospective study. *Journal of Psychosomatic Research* 31: 177–183.

Robbins J.M., Kirmayer L.J. 1996. Transient and persistent hypochondriacal worry in primary care. *Psychological Medicine* 26: 575–589.

Robbins J.M., Kirmayer L.J., Kapusta M.A. 1990. Illness worry and disability in fibromyalgia syndrome. *International Journal of Psychiatry in Medicine* 20: 49–63.

Roht L.H., Vernon S.W., Weir F.W., Pier S.M., Sullivan P., Reed L.J. 1985. Community exposure to hazardous waste disposal sites: assessing reporting bias. *American Journal of Epidemiology* 122: 418–433.

Sackett D.L., Haynes R.B., Guyatt G.H., Tugwell P. 1991. *Clinical Epidemiology: a Basic Science for Clinical Medicine*. Boston: Little, Brown & Company.

Savron G., Grandi S., Michelacci L., Saviotti F.M., Bartolucci G., Conti S., Trombini G., Bovicelli L., Orlandi C., Fava G.A. 1989. Hypochondriacal symptoms in pregnancy. *Psychotherapy and Psychosomatics* 52: 106–109.

Savron G., Fava G.A., Grandi S., Rafanelli C., Raffi A.R., Belluardo P. 1996. Hypochondriacal fears and beliefs in obsessive-compulsive disorder. *Acta Psychiatrica Scandinavica* 93: 345–348.

Schmidt A.J.M. 1994. Bottlenecks in the diagnosis of hypochondriasis. *Comprehensive Psychiatry* 35: 306–315.

Schmidt A.J.M., van Roosmalen R., van der Beek J.M.H., Lousberg R. 1993. Hypochondriasis in ENT practice. *Clinical Otolaryngology* 18: 508–511.

Simon G.E., Katon W.J., Sparks P.J. 1990. Allergic to life: psychological factors in environmental illness. *American Journal of Psychiatry* 147: 901–906.

Skevington S.M. 1983. Activities as indices of illness behaviour in chronic pain. *Pain* 15: 295–307.

Speckens A.E.M., van Hemert A.M., Spinhoven P., Hawton K.E., Bolk J.H., Rooijmans H.G.M. 1995. Cognitive behavioural therapy for medically unexplained physical symptoms: a randomised controlled trial. *British Medical Journal* 311: 1328–1332.

Speckens A.E.M., van Hemert A.M., Spinhoven P., Bolk J.H. 1996a. The diagnostic and prognostic significance of the Whiteley Index, the Illness Attitude Scales and the Somatosensory Amplification Scale. *Psychological Medicine* 26: 1085–1090.

Speckens A.E.M., Spinhoven P., Sloekers P.P.A., Bolk J.H., van Hemert A.M. 1996b. A validation study of the Whiteley Index, the Illness Attitude Scales, and the Somatosensory Amplification Scale in general medical and general practice patients. *Journal of Psychosomatic Research* 40: 95–104.

Starcevic V., Fallon S., Uhlenhuth E.H., Pathak D. 1994. Generalized anxiety disorder, worries about illness, and hypochondriacal fears and beliefs. *Psychotherapy and Psychosomatics* 61: 93–99.

Steptoe A., Noll A. 1997. The perception of bodily sensations, with special reference to hypochondriasis. *Behaviour Research and Therapy* 35: 901–910.

Stone A.A., Neale J.M. 1981. Hypochondriasis and tendency to adopt the sick role as moderators of the relationship between life-events and somatic symptomatology. *British Journal of Medical Psychology* 54: 75–81.

Warwick H.M., Clark D.M., Cobb A.M., Salkovskis P.M. 1996. A controlled trial of cognitive-behavioural treatment of hypochondriasis. *British Journal of Psychiatry* 169: 189–195.

Wesner R.B., Noyes R. Jr. 1991. Imipramine an effective treatment for illness phobia. *Journal of Affective Disorders* 22: 43–48.

Williams R.C. 1988. Toward a set of reliable and valid measures for chronic pain assessment and outcome research. *Pain* 35: 239–251.

Wise T.N., Mann L.S., Hryvniak M., Mitchell J.D., Hill B. 1990. The relationship between alexithymia and abnormal illness behavior. *Psychotherapy and Psychosomatics* 54: 18–25.

Zonderman A.B., Heft M.W., Costa P.T. Jr. 1985. Does the Illness Behavior Questionnaire measure abnormal illness behavior? *Health Psychology* 4: 425–436.

# 4

# Hypochondriasis and Anxiety Disorders

## GIOVANNI A. FAVA
## LARA MANGELLI

In contrast to the relationship between hypochondriasis and depression, which has been the focus of physicians for centuries (Chapter 1 of this volume), an interest in the relationship of hypochondriasis to specific anxiety disorders is of relatively recent origin. This is despite the fact that the acknowledgment of the link between hypochondriasis and anxiety is not "new," and is likely to be due to recent advances in the diagnosis and recognition of various anxiety disorders, their better differentiation, and increasingly frequent observations of a substantial overlap between hypochondriasis and some of these conditions.

The interest in the relationship of hypochondriasis to anxiety disorders is generally supported by two lines of evidence. One is concerned with psychiatric comorbidity in hypochondriasis. Barsky *et al.* (1992) found a lifetime prevalence of an anxiety disorder in the majority (86%) of their 42 patients. Noyes *et al.* (1994) reported on a lower (22%), but still noteworthy, percentage of anxiety disorders in their 50 hypochondriacal patients.

The other line of evidence involves the study of hypochondriacal phenomena in patients with specific anxiety disorders. This literature will be reviewed in this chapter, referring not only to the clinical syndrome of hypochondriasis and its corresponding, official diagnosis, but to a wide range of hypochondriacal phenomena. These phenomena are assessed by instruments such as Illness Attitude Scales (IAS; Kellner, 1986), and they will be described first. The clinical implications of the studies will then be discussed.

## Heterogeneity of Hypochondriasis

Any undue concern about bodily function is often labeled as "hypochondriacal." Barsky and Wyshak (1989) have described hypochondriasis primarily as an amplification of somatic sensations, not substantially different from health anxiety (Warwick and Salkovskis, 1990). In the *DSM-IV* (American Psychiatric Association, 1994), hypochondriasis is defined as preoccupation with a belief in or a fear of having a serious illness, which occurs without adequate organic pathology to account for preoccupation, and despite medical reassurance. Hypochondriasis may consist of various distinct yet ostensibly related fears, attitudes, and beliefs, such as disease conviction, bodily preoccupation, and thanatophobia (Fava, 1998).

The IAS is a widely used self-report instrument for assessing abnormal illness behavior in the setting of anxiety disorders. It provides a psychometric basis for differentiation of various hypochondriacal phenomena. The IAS derive separate scores on seven scales: (*1*) Worry about Illness; (*2*) Concern about Pain; (*3*) Health Habits; (*4*) Hypochondriacal Beliefs; (*5*) Thanatophobia; (*6*) Disease Phobia; and (*7*) Bodily Preoccupation. Two scales were added to a later version of the IAS: Treatment Experience and Effects of Symptoms (see Chapter 3).

When 21 patients with *DSM-III* (American Psychiatric Association, 1980) hypochondriasis were compared with matched family practice patients, nonpatient employees, and nonhypochondriacal psychiatric patients (Kellner *et al.*, 1987), there were significant differences in six of the original seven IAS scales. Only in Health Habits were there no significant differences—that is, hypochondriacal patients did not take better precautions about their health. The latter finding was replicated in other studies with psychiatric patients (Fava *et al.*, 1984, 1987; Kellner *et al.*, 1986a).

When the IAS scales were administered to various populations, different patterns emerged. Women with pelvic pain syndrome had higher scores than did controls on Hypochondriacal Beliefs and Bodily Preoccupation (Kellner *et al.*, 1988), while pregnant women had higher scores than controls on Hypochondriacal Beliefs and Disease Phobia in the first two trimesters of pregnancy and higher scores than did controls on Thanatophobia and Bodily Preoccupation in the last trimester (Fava *et al.*, 1990a). After receiving normal results from mammography, women reported significant decreases in worry about illness, concern about pain, and fear of dying (Bartolucci *et al.*, 1989). Finally, medical students differed from law students in having more health habits and bodily preoccupation (Kellner *et al.*, 1986b).

These studies suggest that different populations might be characterized by different IAS patterns. In turn, these patterns have been associated with specific phenomena and syndromes: health anxiety, hypochondriasis as a clinical syndrome and diagnosis, disease phobia (nosophobia), and thanatophobia.

**Table 4.1.** Diagnostic criteria for health anxiety (A and B are required)

A. Generic worry about illness, concern about pain and bodily preoccupations (tendency to amplify somatic sensations) of under 6 months' duration.
B. Worries and fears readily respond to appropriate medical reassurance, even though new worries may ensue after some time.

Revised from Fava *et al.* (1995).

## Health Anxiety

The term "health anxiety" encompasses nonspecific dimensions of abnormal illness behavior, such as generic worry about illness that may readily respond to medical reassurance, concern about pain and bodily preoccupation, with a tendency to amplify somatic sensations. Health anxiety is usually short-lived, unlike hypochondriasis, disease phobia, and thanatophobia, which tend to persist. Health anxiety was found in women undergoing medical procedures (Bartolucci *et al.*, 1989), and it appears as a reaction to life-threatening illnesses.

The features of health anxiety have been translated into diagnostic criteria (Diagnostic Criteria for Use in Psychosomatic Research; DCPR) by an international group of psychosomatic investigators (Fava *et al.*, 1995). Table 4.1 outlines these criteria.

## Hypochondriasis as a Clinical Syndrome and Diagnosis

According to the *DSM-IV*, hypochondriasis is defined as persistent preoccupation with the fear of having, or the idea that one has, a serious disease, when appropriate physical examination does not support the diagnosis of any physical disorder that could account for the patient's symptoms. However, the most distinct characteristic of hypochondriasis as a clinical syndrome is resistance of disease preoccupation to medical reassurance. In contrast, fears of patients with health anxiety who may become extremely worried about health are usually eliminated by a satisfactory medical examination.

## Disease Phobia (Nosophobia)

Bianchi (1971) defined "disease phobia" as "a persistent, unfounded fear of suffering from a disease, with some doubt remaining despite examination and reassurance" (p. 241). He described disease phobia as a variant of hypochondriasis, characterized by anxiety, inhibition of anger, and low tolerance of pain. Ryle (1948) not only observed that disease phobia could also include fear of inherit-

**Table 4.2.** Diagnostic criteria for disease phobia (A through C are required)

A. Persistent, unfounded fear of suffering from a specific disease (e.g., AIDS, cancer),
   with doubts remaining despite adequate examination and reassurance.
B. Fears tend to manifest themselves in attacks rather than in constant, chronic worries
   as in hypochondriasis. Panic attacks may be an associated feature.
C. The object of fears does not change with time, and duration of symptoms exceeds 6
   months.

Revised from Fava *et al.* (1995).

ing or acquiring a disease but charged the medical profession and mass media
with a direct responsibility for the development of these fears.

There are two main clinical characteristics of disease phobia. One is the specificity and longitudinal stability of the fears (e.g., patients who are afraid of suffering from heart disease are unlikely to "transfer" their fear to other organ
systems). The other key characteristic of disease phobia is a tendency to manifest itself through episodic attacks rather than constant, chronic worries (Fava *et
al.*, 1990b). In this sense, the relationship of disease phobia to hypochondriasis
is similar to that of panic disorder to generalized anxiety disorder (GAD).

The fear in disease phobia is chronic. In addition, patients with disease phobia do not readily respond to adequate physical examination and medical reassurance with complete disappearance of their fear. In both these aspects, patients
with disease phobia may resemble those with hypochondriasis. The DCPR criteria for disease phobia are presented in Table 4.2.

Warwick and Marks (1988) reported on seventeen cases of disease phobia,
treated with exposure to illness cues and "prevention of reassurance," that is, ban-
ning of giving reassurance to the patient after such an exposure. This procedure
resulted in rapid improvement—an outcome that is quite unlikely with hypochondriacal patients (Kellner, 1986).

## Thanatophobia

In 1928, Ryle described thanatophobia as the sense of dying (*angor animi*). About
20 years later, he provided the following lucid, autobiographical description:

> It had never occurred to me that I should have an actual opportunity of observing
> the symptom in my own person until the autumn of 1942, when I developed angina
> pectoris . . . My first manifestation . . . was a sudden and intense attack of the sense
> of dying. I had just climbed the stairs of the refectory in the medical school at Guy's
> and sat down to lunch when it swept upon me. I remember thinking to myself, in
> the very words employed over the radio by a gallant fighter pilot as he fell to his

**Table 4.3.** Diagnostic criteria for thanatophobia (A through C are required)

A. Attacks with the sense of impending death and/or conviction of dying soon, even though there is no objective medical reason for such a sense and/or conviction.
B. Marked and persistent fear and avoidance of news that reminds of death (e.g., funerals, obituary notices). Exposure to these stimuli almost invariably provokes an immediate anxiety response.
C. The avoidance of the stimuli, anxious anticipation of them, and the associated distress interfere significantly with the person's functioning.

Revised from Fava *et al.* (1995).

death, 'This is it,' and I could not doubt that I was about to die. The sensation then, as afterwards, passed within a few seconds. On several subsequent occasions I was almost as convinced that the end had come. Thereafter, I must have experienced the symptom, in very varying degree, probably on two hundred or more occasions within a period of 5 or 6 years, and I have long since come to accept it philosophically." (Ryle, 1949, p. 225)

Both disease phobia and thanatophobia are manifested through the attacks, but their cognitive "components" are different; the attacks in thanatophobia consist of the sense of an impending death and/or of the conviction of dying soon. Kell-

**Table 4.4.** Criteria for making distinctions among health anxiety, hypochondriasis, disease phobia, and thanatophobia

|  | Health anxiety | Hypochon- driasis | Disease phobia | Thanato- phobia |
|---|---|---|---|---|
| Worry about illness | ++ | ++ | ++ | 0 |
| Concern about pain | ++ | ++ | + | 0 |
| Bodily preoccupation | ++ | ++ | + | 0 |
| Unfounded fear of suffering from a serious disease | + | ++ | ++ | 0 |
| Attacks of an unfounded fear of suffering from a serious disease | 0 | 0 | ++ | 0 |
| Continuous presence of symptoms | ++ | ++ | 0 | 0 |
| The object of fear changes with time | ++ | ++ | 0 | 0 |
| Attacks with the sense of an impending death and/or conviction of dying soon | 0 | 0 | 0 | ++ |
| Fear and avoidance of reminders of death | 0 | + | + | ++ |
| Duration >6 months | 0 | ++ | ++ | ++ |
| Failure to respond to appropriate medical reassurance | 0 | ++ | + | + |

++Clearly present (or meets the criterion).
+Occasionally/partially present (or meets the criterion to a certain extent).
0Not present (or does not meet the criterion).

ner (1986) associated the conviction of dying soon (despite no objective medical reason) with the fear and avoidance of reminders of death, such as funerals or obituary notices. The latter feature is what qualifies thanatophobia as a phobia.

The DCPR criteria for thanatophobia (Fava *et al.*, 1995) are shown in Table 4.3. The criteria for making distinctions between health anxiety, hypochondriasis, disease phobia, and thanatophobia are presented in Table 4.4.

## Comorbidity Between Hypochondriasis and Specific Anxiety Disorders

Hypochondriacal symptomatology has been explored mainly in relation to panic disorder (with and without agoraphobia) and—to a much lesser degree—in GAD and obsessive-compulsive disorder (OCD).

### Panic Disorder

Hypochondriacal concerns were investigated in a number of studies in patients with panic disorder associated with agoraphobia. Noyes *et al.* (1986) found high scores on the Whiteley Index (Pilowsky, 1967, 1968) in patients with panic attacks, indicating hypochondriacal attitudes. After treatment with alprazolam, there was significant improvement in hypochondriacal attitudes, and this was limited to patients whose panic attacks had decreased with drug treatment. Fava *et al.* (1988a) administered the IAS to patients with panic disorder with agoraphobia. Compared to control subjects, the patients displayed significantly higher scores in all the IAS scales except for Health Habits. After panic disorder with agoraphobia had been treated with exposure, hypochondriacal concerns did not differ significantly from those of normals. These two studies suggest that the presence of anxiety is conducive to hypochondriacal fears and beliefs and that these tend to remit when anxiety decreases.

In another investigation (Fava *et al.*, 1988b), hypochondriacal symptoms were reported by 85% of patients as prodromal to the onset of panic attacks. When the illness attitudes were analyzed closely, they consisted of worry about illness, bodily preoccupations, thanatophobia, disease phobia, and hypochondriasis. Agoraphobia was also found to be a prodromal feature of panic disorder. As a result, it was difficult to ascertain whether hypochondriasis or anxiety had a primary role. These findings as to the prodromal appearance of hypochondriacal symptoms were subsequently replicated (Fava *et al.*, 1992; Perugi *et al.*, 1998).

Subsequent studies suggest the complexity of the relationship between hypochondriasis and panic disorder. Otto *et al.* (1992) administered the IAS and the Anxiety Sensitivity Index (Reiss *et al.*, 1986) to patients with panic disorder.

"Anxiety sensitivity" refers to beliefs that anxiety has undesirable and even harmful consequences apart from its immediate unpleasantness. Thus, a person scoring high on anxiety sensitivity may believe that rapid heart pounding portends a heart attack, whereas a person scoring low on anxiety sensitivity regards tachycardia as merely unpleasant (McNally and Lorenz, 1987). Anxiety sensitivity was found to characterize panic disorder in remission (Saviotti *et al.*, 1991). All IAS scales (except Health Habits and Hypochondriacal Beliefs) were significantly correlated with anxiety sensitivity in patients with panic disorder, and anxiety sensitivity was found to be the strongest predictor of hypochondriacal concerns in these patients (Otto *et al.*, 1992). The same association between anxiety sensitivity and hypochondriacal concerns was replicated in patients with major depression and no history of panic disorder (Otto *et al.*, 1998).

Starcevic *et al.* (1992) further explored the correlates of hypochondriacal symptoms (as measured by the IAS), which were found to characterize about half of their sample of patients with panic disorder. An association between hypochondriasis and agoraphobia was also found. Barsky *et al.* (1994) compared patients with a joint diagnosis of panic disorder and hypochondriasis with those who had hypochondriasis without comorbid panic disorder. Patients with panic disorder were less hypochondriacal, somatized less, were less disabled, and were more satisfied with their medical care than were patients with hypochondriasis.

Bach *et al.* (1996) found that slightly more than one-half of patients with panic disorder also had a lifetime diagnosis of hypochondriasis, and in most cases hypochondriasis was secondary to the onset of panic attacks. In that study, hypochondriasis was not strongly associated with agoraphobia. Benedetti *et al.* (1997) reported that about 50% of patients with panic disorder who also suffer from hypochondriasis had disease phobia before the onset of panic disorder.

Furer *et al.* (1997) assessed the presence of *DSM-IV* hypochondriasis in 21 patients with panic disorder, 23 patients with social phobia, and 22 healthy subjects. About half of the patients with panic disorder also met the *DSM-IV* criteria for hypochondriasis, whereas only one of the patients with social phobia and none of the control subjects met the criteria for this diagnosis.

Schmidt and Telch (1997) examined the relationship among medical comorbidity, perceived physical health, and treatment outcome in panic disorder. After 12 sessions of cognitive-behavioral treatment, 71% of patients who perceived their physical health as good met recovery criteria compared to only 35% of those who perceived their health as poor. Similar results were obtained at follow-up.

## Generalized Anxiety Disorder

Starcevic *et al.* (1994) compared hypochondriacal fears and beliefs—as measured by the IAS—in patients with GAD and panic disorder. Patients with GAD displayed significantly fewer hypochondriacal symptoms (except for health habits) than did patients with panic disorder. Only 18% of GAD patients could be considered hypochondriacal, and only about 30% of those who worried about their health also scored in the hypochondriacal range of the IAS. The study thus suggests that health and illness may be the object of GAD worries, but that these are not specifically linked to hypochondriasis.

## Obsessive-Compulsive Disorder

In recent years there has been an upsurge of interest in the relationship between hypochondriasis and obsessive-compulsive disorder (OCD). Hypochondriacal patients are often obsessed with fearful thoughts about having a disease, and patients with OCD are frequently afraid of illness or contamination (Starcevic, 1990). As a result, overlaps in diagnosis and treatment have been observed.

A model has been developed whereby the thought of illness in hypochondriasis is comparable to an obsessional idea that intrudes on consciousness and leads to increased anxiety (Warwick and Salkovskis, 1990). The hypochondriacal patients try to reduce their anxiety by seeking reassurance that they are not ill, but, as with the performance of compulsive rituals, after a short-lived period of relief, anxiety levels increase again and further reassurance is required (Warwick and Salkovskis, 1990).

Hollander (1993a, 1993b) proposed that hypochondriasis was one of the "obsessive-compulsive spectrum disorders." This suggestion was made on the basis of the similarities with OCD in the symptom profile and in the selective response to certain types of cognitive-behavior therapy and pharmacotherapy (serotonin reuptake inhibitors). Hollander and Benzaquen (1997) hypothesized that hyperfrontality and increased serotonergic sensitivity represented a common neurobiological substrate for illnesses in the "obsessive-compulsive spectrum disorders."

There is little empirical support, however, for an association between hypochondriasis and OCD. Lifetime prevalence of OCD was reported to be low in patients with hypochondriasis (Barsky et al., 1992; Noyes et al., 1994). The IAS scales were administered to patients with OCD and healthy control subjects, matched for sociodemographic variables (Savron et al., 1996). Scores on all IAS scales (including Health Habits) were significantly higher in patients with OCD. However, no significant differences existed between patients and controls in the number of subjects whose symptom intensity exceeded a clinical threshold for hypochondriasis and disease phobia. Furthermore, hypochondriacal fears and beliefs were poorly correlated with obsessions and compulsions. The results suggest the presence of nonspecific abnormal illness behavior in patients with OCD, as in patients with GAD.

## Clinical Implications

The studies reviewed here suggest that anxiety disorders and various hypochondriacal features frequently coexist. The question then becomes how clinically relevant these features are and whether they warrant specific treatment. Certain findings and observations may help the clinician in this regard.

The first issue is concerned with the chronology—that is, with the primary/secondary distinction (Fava, 1996a). It is important to define whether the onset of anxiety disorder preceded that of hypochondriacal symptoms (secondary hypochondriasis). In this case, treatment of the underlying disorder is likely to result in abatement of health concerns. This has been shown to occur in panic disorder, with pharmacotherapy (Noyes *et al.*, 1986) or exposure therapy without cognitive restructuring (Fava *et al.*, 1988a). It is conceivable, although yet to be tested, that similar considerations apply to treatment of secondary hypochondriasis in GAD and OCD. This is particularly important to investigate because health concerns in hypochondriasis may bear significant similarities to the corresponding worries in GAD and to obsessions in OCD.

Hypochondriacal symptoms may be defined as primary when their onset predates that of an anxiety disorder. This has been clearly described in the setting of panic disorder (Barsky *et al.*, 1994; Fava *et al.*, 1990a). Patients with a chronologically primary hypochondriacal disorder are less frequent than those with secondary hypochondriasis (Barsky *et al.*, 1994). It is conceivable that in these cases, hypochondriacal features warrant specific therapy even after treatment of the anxiety disorder has resulted in significant improvement. Without careful assessment, a need for continued and specific hypochondriasis-directed treatment could be overlooked.

The primary/secondary distinction is a first helpful step, but it may not be sufficient or easily applicable in clinical practice. For instance, hypochondriacal phenomena and disease phobia, in particular, often precede, together with agoraphobic avoidance, the onset of panic attacks (Fava *et al.*, 1988b, 1992; Perugi *et al.*, 1998), but they become much worse afterwards, in the subsequent course of panic disorder. Should they be viewed as primary or secondary?

The primary/secondary distinction needs to be integrated into a longitudinal view of illness, encompassing the prodromal, acute, and residual phases of the disorders (Fava, 1996b). Indeed, a follow-up approach should become the rule in the management of all patients with comorbidity of hypochondriasis and anxiety disorders. The "rollback phenomenon" (as the illness remits, it progressively recapitulates, even though in reverse order, the sequence of symptoms that preceded its onset) appears to be of considerable value. Translated into clinical decisions, this means that if treatment of panic disorder is regarded as the primary issue and hypochondriacal phenomena are seen as a consequence of panic disorder, attention should be directed mainly to the elimination of panic attacks. If panic attacks are indeed chronologically primary, hypochondriacal phenomena should disappear in the course of the treatment of panic attacks. Conversely, if hypochondriacal phenomena preceded the onset of panic attacks, hypochondriacal phenomena are likely to remain as residual, after successful treatment of panic disorder and disappearance of panic attacks.

The work of Schmidt and Telch (1997) suggests that the comorbidity of hypochondriacal phenomena and panic disorder may have considerable prognostic value in panic disorder because abnormal illness behavior and health perception, associated with hypochondriasis, affect negatively the outcome of treatment and hinder lasting recovery.

The *DSM-IV* conceptualization of hypochondriasis appears to be inadequate for satisfactory assessment and treatment of hypochondriacal phenomena (Fava, 1998). Research based on the IAS in anxiety disorders has clearly shown different and relatively specific associations with various aspects and dimensions of hypochondriasis. The DCPR criteria (Fava *et al.*, 1995) offer an important integration in this regard, but they need to be tested and validated. Health anxiety (worry about illness, concern about pain, bodily preoccupation) appears to be frequently observed in any type of anxiety disorder. Hypochondriasis and disease phobia, as clinical syndromes, were found to be associated with panic disorder more than with GAD and OCD. Thanatophobia was found to occur both in panic disorder and OCD, but its role has yet to be defined (Fava, 1998).

The distinction between the *DSM-IV* concept of hypochondriasis and the DCPR concept of disease phobia is likely to carry both clinical and, especially, treatment implications. The treatment approach to these syndromes should take into account their specific features, and patients should be treated according to principles outlined in other chapters of this book.


## Conclusion

The strength of association between anxiety disorders and hypochondriacal features has—not surprisingly—given rise to proposals to classify hypochondriasis among anxiety disorders. Such an association is particularly frequent in the setting of panic disorder, but occurs also in GAD and OCD. The relationship between hypochondriasis and panic disorder is exceedingly complex. Hypochondriacal phenomena are so frequently encountered as an important part of panic disorder that a multidimensional assessment of panic disorder should always include hypochondriacal tendencies. Hypochondriasis has also been considered one of the OCD-spectrum disorders. Despite much conceptual overlap and many similarities in the clinical presentation (also reviewed in Chapters 2 and 6), there is good evidence that specific anxiety disorders and hypochondriasis represent distinct clinical entities.

Anxiety appears to be conducive to health concerns, and these generally wane when anxiety decreases. However, this does not always occur, and it is important to ascertain when hypochondriacal phenomena precede and predispose to the onset of anxiety disorders, particularly panic disorder. Under such circumstances, hypochondriacal features are likely to continue to be present even after the symptoms of an anxiety disorder have abated, thus calling for specific treatment attention.

The official diagnostic (*DSM-IV*) concept of hypochondriasis is insufficient to capture all the "nuances" of the heterogeneous dimensions of hypochondriasis. It is recommended that clinical assessment of associations with various anxiety disorders take into account not only the clinical syndrome of hypochondriasis but also the hypochondriasis-related conditions: health anxiety, disease phobia, and thanatophobia.

Although much research into these relationships remains needed, findings to date indicate that, except for health anxiety, specific anxiety disorders have specific patterns of association with hypochondriacal syndrome, disease phobia, and thanatophobia. The clinical syndromes of hypochondriasis and disease phobia are particularly worthy of clinical attention when they occur with anxiety disorders, as they may warrant specific treatment.

## Acknowledgments

This work was supported in part by a grant from the Mental Health Project (Istituto Superiore di Sanità, Rome, Italy). It is dedicated to the memory of Robert Kellner.

### References

American Psychiatric Association. 1980. *Diagnostic and Statistical Manual of Mental Disorders, Third Edition* (*DSM-III*). Washington, DC: American Psychiatric Association.

American Psychiatric Association. 1994. *Diagnostic and Statistical Manual of Mental Disorders, Fourth Edition* (*DSM-IV*). Washington, DC: American Psychiatric Association.

Bach M., Nutzinger D.O., Harti L. 1996. Comorbidity of anxiety disorders and hypochondriasis considering different diagnostic systems. *Comprehensive Psychiatry* 37: 62–67.

Barsky A.J., Wyshak G. 1989. Hypochondriasis and related health attitudes. *Psychosomatics* 30: 412–420.

Barsky A.J., Wyshak G., Klerman G.L. 1992. Psychiatric comorbidity in DSM-III-R hypochondriasis. *Archives of General Psychiatry* 49: 101–108.

Barsky A.J., Barnett M.C., Cleary P.D. 1994. Hypochondriasis and panic disorder. *Archives of General Psychiatry* 51: 918–925.

Bartolucci G., Savron G., Fava G.A., Grandi S., Trombini G., Orlandi C. 1989. Psychological reactions to thermography and mammography. *Stress Medicine* 5: 195–199.

Benedetti A., Perugi G., Toni C., Simonetti B., Mata B., Cassano G.B. 1997. Hypochondriasis and illness phobia in panic-agoraphobic patients. *Comprehensive Psychiatry* 38: 124–131.

Bianchi G.M. 1971. Origins of disease phobia. *Australian and New Zealand Journal of Psychiatry* 5: 241–257.

Fava G.A. 1996a. The definition, diagnosis and clinical relevance of somatoform disorders. *Reviews in Contemporary Pharmacotherapy* 7: 269–277.

Fava G.A. 1996b. The concept of recovery in affective disorders. *Psychotherapy and Psychosomatics* 65: 2–13.

Fava G.A. 1998. The concept of psychosomatic disorder. In *Handbook of Psychosomatic Medicine* (eds. Fava G.A., Freyberger H.), Madison, CT: International Universities Press.

Fava G.A., Molnar G., Spinks M., Loretan A., Bartlett D. 1984. Health attitudes and psychological distress in patients attending a lithium clinic. *Acta Psychiatrica Scandinavica* 70: 591–593.

Fava G.A., Molnar G., Zielezny M. 1987. Health attitudes of psychiatric inpatients. *Psychopathology* 20: 180–186.

Fava G.A., Kellner R., Zielezny M., Grandi S. 1988a. Hypochondriacal fears and beliefs in agoraphobia. *Journal of Affective Disorders* 14: 239–244.

Fava G.A., Grandi S., Canestrari R. 1988b. Prodromal symptoms in panic disorder with agoraphobia. *American Journal of Psychiatry* 145: 1564–1567.

Fava G.A., Grandi S., Saviotti F.M., Conti S. 1990a. Hypochondriasis with panic attacks. *Psychosomatics* 31: 351–353.

Fava G.A., Grandi S., Michelacci L., Saviotti F.M., Conti S., Bovicelli L., Trombini G., Orlandi C. 1990b. Hypochondriacal fears and beliefs in pregnancy. *Acta Psychiatrica Scandinavica* 82: 70–72.

Fava G.A., Grandi S., Rafanelli C., Canestrari R. 1992. Prodromal symptoms in panic disorder: a replication study. *Journal of Affective Disorders* 25: 85–88.

Fava G.A., Freyberger H.J., Bech P., Christodoulou G., Sensky T., Theorell T., Wise T.N. 1995. Diagnostic criteria for use in psychosomatic research. *Psychotherapy and Psychosomatics* 63: 1–8.

Furer P., Walker J.R., Chartier M.J., Stein M.B. 1997. Hypochondriacal concerns and somatization in panic disorder. *Depression and Anxiety* 6: 78–85.

Hollander E. 1993a. *Obsessive-Compulsive Related Disorders*. Washington, DC: American Psychiatric Press.

Hollander E. 1993b. Obsessive-compulsive spectrum disorders: an overview. *Psychiatric Annals* 23: 355–358.

Hollander E., Benzaquen S.D. 1997. The obsessive-compulsive spectrum disorder. In *Focus on Obsessive-Compulsive Spectrum Disorders* (eds. den Boer J.A., Westenberg H.G.M.), Amsterdam: Syn-Thesis Publishers.

Kellner R. 1986. *Somatization and Hypochondriasis*. New York: Praeger.

Kellner R., Fava G.A., Lisansky J., Perini G.I., Zielezny M. 1986a. Hypochondriacal fears and beliefs in DSM-III melancholia. *Journal of Affective Disorders* 10: 21–26.

Kellner R., Wiggins R.G., Pathak D. 1986b. Hypochondriacal fears and beliefs in medical and law students. *Archives of General Psychiatry* 43: 487–489.

Kellner R., Abbott P., Winslow W.W., Pathak D. 1987. Fears, beliefs and attitudes in DSM-III hypochondriasis. *Journal of Nervous and Mental Disease* 175: 20–25.

Kellner R., Slocumb J.C., Rosenfeld R.C., Pathak D. 1988. Fears and beliefs in patients with the pelvic pain syndrome. *Journal of Psychosomatic Research* 32: 303–310.

McNally R.J., Lorenz M. 1987. Anxiety sensitivity in agoraphobics. *Journal of Behavior Therapy and Experimental Psychiatry* 18: 3–11.

Noyes R., Reich J., Clancy J., O'Gorman T.W. 1986. Reduction in hypochondriasis with treatment of panic disorder. *British Journal of Psychiatry* 149: 631–635.

Noyes R., Kathol R.G., Fisher M.M., Phillips B.M., Snelzer M.I., Woodman C.L. 1994. Psychiatric comorbidity among patients with hypochondriasis. *General Hospital Psychiatry* 16. 78–87.

Otto M.W., Pollack M.H., Sachs G.S., Rosenbaum J.F. 1992. Hypochondriacal concerns, anxiety sensitivity, and panic disorder. *Journal of Anxiety Disorders* 6: 93–104.

Otto M.W., Demopulos C.M., McLean N.E., Pollack M.H., Fava M. 1998. Additional findings on the association between anxiety sensitivity and hypochondriacalconcerns: examination of patients with major depression. *Journal of Anxiety Disorders* 12: 225–232.

Perugi G., Toni C., Benedetti A., Simonetti B., Simoncini M., Torti C., Musetti L., Akiskal H.S. 1998. Delineating a putative phobic-anxious temperament in 126 panic-agoraphobic patients. *Journal of Affective Disorders* 47: 11–23.

Pilowsky I. 1967. Dimensions of hypochondriasis. *British Journal of Psychiatry* 113: 89–93.

Pilowsky I. 1968. The response to treatment in hypochondriacal disorders. *Australian and New Zealand Journal of Psychiatry* 2: 88–94.

Reiss S., Peterson R.A., Gursky D.M., McNally R.J. 1986. Anxiety sensitivity, anxiety frequency and the prediction of fearfulness. *Behaviour Research and Therapy* 24: 1–8.

Ryle J.A. 1928. *Angor animi*, or the sense of dying. *Guy's Hospital Reports* 78: 230–235.

Ryle J.A. 1948. Nosophobia. *Journal of Mental Science* 94: 1–17.

Ryle J.A. 1949. The sense of dying. A postscript. *Guy's Hospital Reports* 99: 224–235.

Saviotti F.M., Grandi S., Savron G., Ermentini R., Bartolucci G., Conti S., Fava G.A. 1991. Characterologic traits of recovered patients with panic disorder and agoraphobia. *Journal of Affective Disorders*. 23: 113–117.

Savron G., Fava G.A., Grandi S., Rafanelli C., Raffi A.R., Belluardo P. 1996. Hypochondriacal fears and beliefs in obsessive-compulsive disorder. *Acta Psychiatrica Scandinavica* 93: 345–348.

Schmidt N.B., Telch M.J. 1997. Non-psychiatric medical comorbidity, health perceptions, and treatment outcome in patients with panic disorder. *Health Psychology* 16: 114–122.

Starcevic V. 1990. Relationship between hypochondriasis and obsessive-compulsive personality disorder: close relatives separated by nosological schemes? *American Journal of Psychotherapy* 44: 340–347.

Starcevic V., Kellner R., Uhlenhuth E.H., Pathak D. 1992. Panic disorder and hypochondriacal fears and beliefs. *Journal of Affective Disorders* 29: 73–85.

Starcevic V., Fallon S., Uhlenhuth E.H., Pathak D. 1994. Generalized anxiety disorder, worries about illness, and hypochondriacal fears and beliefs. *Psychotherapy and Psychosomatics* 61: 93–99.

Warwick H.M.C., Marks I.M. 1988. Behavioral treatment of illness phobia and hypochondriasis. *British Journal of Psychiatry* 152: 239–241.

Warwick H.M.C., Salkovskis P.M. 1990. Hypochondriasis. *Behaviour Research and Therapy* 28: 105–117.

# 5

# Hypochondriasis and Personality Disturbance

## MICHAEL HOLLIFIELD

I have sent for you, Doctor, to consult you about a distemper, of which
I am very well assured I shall never be cured.

Mandeville, 1730, p. 1

There is evidence that hypochondriasis is associated with many "attitudes," personality traits, and personality disorders. This evidence comes from descriptive and theoretical literature and from empirical findings. However, both the quality and the strength of the relationship between hypochondriasis and personality disturbance are not well understood. This is so in part because most of the data about the subject is descriptive or comes from cross-sectional research. Further, there is a debate about the classification of hypochondriasis; it has support as a mental state disorder, and there is also some support for it as a personality construct. Likewise, the debate about classification of personality disorders is ongoing. This classification confusion is further problematic because Axis I and Axis II disorders are both diagnosed on the basis of persistent symptoms and change of behavior. Moreover, differences between Axis I and Axis II disorders are not clearly separable by theory, phenomenology, or psychobiology.

This chapter reviews the theoretical, descriptive, and empirically derived relationships between hypochondriasis and personality disturbances. The first section is a brief account of how hypochondriasis and personality have been conceptualized, providing a logical backdrop for the second section about the relationship between the two. Both sections highlight how, despite much work, there remains confusion about hypochondriasis, personality, and their relationship. Finally, there is a discussion about hypochondriasis as a personality construct, which further highlights nosological difficulties, and a discussion about the relationship between hypochondriasis and traumatic experiences.

## Section I: Concepts of Hypochondriasis and Personality

Authors who have written about hypochondriasis and personality disturbance have done so from various conceptual perspectives, but without necessarily clarifying the issue. It is hoped that the reader will note that the current nosological concepts of both hypochondriasis and personality are "works in progress"; thus, the relationship between the two remains both problematic and a source for needed research.

## Concepts of Hypochondriasis

### Hypochondriasis as a Psychiatric Disorder

Pilowsky (1967) well identified the three dimensions of bodily preoccupation, disease phobia, and disease conviction with a failure to respond to reassurance that are seen in hypochondriasis, and this work has since been replicated (Barsky et al., 1986; Kellner, 1986). Hypochondriasis overlaps with, but is probably distinct from, some other psychiatric disorders (Barsky et al., 1994a). External validity has been demonstrated in hypochondriasis (Noyes et al., 1993), and the construct of hypochondriasis is stable in a population over periods of 1 to 5 years (Barsky et al., 1998; Noyes et al., 1994a).

However, some studies lead to questions about hypochondriasis as a distinct diagnosis. Discriminant validity for the diagnosis is less sound than internal and external validity (Noyes et al., 1993), and both family and twin studies have failed to yield evidence for a genetic component in hypochondriasis (Noyes et al., 1997; Torgersen, 1986). Therefore, the overall validity of the diagnosis of hypochondriasis remains unclear (see also Chapter 2).

A major epistemological problem is that hypochondriasis and somatization are frequently conceptualized together and are usually linked in empirical studies, partly due to research methodology (Barsky et al., 1992; Hollifield et al., 1999a). Hollifield and colleagues (1999b) utilized the Illness Attitude Scales (Kellner, 1987a) and the Symptom Questionnaire (Kellner, 1987b) to demonstrate that, while there is overlap between hypochondriasis and somatization, they may be distinct entities, with somatization being more associated with personality and attitudinal abnormalities than hypochondriasis. This corroborates the work of Barsky et al. (1992), which calls into question research where the two entities are not considered separately. Because hypochondriasis and somatization are often considered together, both the theoretical and empirical formulations about personality disturbance in hypochondriasis and somatization are confounded.

## Primary versus Secondary Hypochondriasis

There is support for the concept of primary hypochondriasis, with the core psychopathological feature being the conviction of an undiagnosed disease beginning early in life (Kellner, 1988)—that is, not caused by another medical or psychiatric disorder. There is also support for secondary hypochondriasis (Baker and Merskey, 1983; Pilowsky, 1970) where disease phobia and illness beliefs are induced by another illness—for example, melancholia (Kellner *et al.*, 1986), depression (Kellner *et al.*, 1987), panic disorder with or without agoraphobia (Fava *et al.*, 1988; Noyes *et al.*, 1986; Sheehan *et al.*, 1980; Starcevic *et al.*, 1992), or medical disorders (Kellner, 1986).

It is often assumed that primary and not secondary hypochondriasis is associated with personality disturbance (Bass and Murphy, 1995), but only one study to date compares personality traits in primary and secondary hypochondriasis (Pilowsky, 1970). Another study (Starcevic *et al.*, 1992) assessed personality disorder in secondary hypochondriasis. Both studies are reviewed later in this chapter.

## Other Views and Types of Hypochondriasis

In their reviews of the history of hypochondriasis, Ladee (1966) and Kellner (1985) discuss various hypochondriacal syndromes. For a long time, authors have observed the relationship between hypochondriasis and melancholia, depression, neurasthenia (Arndt, 1885; Burton, 1883; Keynes, 1962; Lewis, 1934; Tuczeck, 1883; Ziehen, 1902), and anxiety (Kenyon, 1964; Ladee, 1966; Starcevic *et al.*, 1992; Tyrer, 1976). Hypochondriasis has also been associated with paranoia (Cotard, 1880), and some authors have suggested that there is a particular way of thinking in hypochondriasis (Dubois, 1833), akin to having delusions of physical disease (Beard, 1880; Flint, 1866). Wollenberg (1904) distinguished between "incidental" and "constitutional" hypochondriasis; the latter was considered to be a form of personality disorder. Hypochondriasis has also been conceptualized as a psychological process (Barsky and Klerman, 1983), a perceptual and cognitive style (Barsky and Klerman, 1983), a style of communication and defense (Kellner, 1985; Kenyon, 1965), and as a personality disorder (Kenyon, 1965; Tyrer *et al.*, 1990).

To summarize, in writing about types of hypochondriasis, authors have communicated two basic ideas: Hypochondriasis either develops along with other illness and is thus secondary, or is constitutional and a persistent part of the individual, and thus primary. Symptoms that are "part of the self" in a persistent way are also core features of personality constructs. This diagnostic similarity between primary hypochondriasis and personality disorder has, in part, led to the nosological confusion between hypochondriasis as a mental state disorder and hypochondriasis as a personality disturbance.

## Concepts of Personality and Personality Disorders

### Diagnostic and Nosological Issues

Personality disorders as diagnoses retain utility for psychiatrists. This is reflected by their inclusion in formal illness classifications (American Psychiatric Association, 1994; World Health Organization, 1992), despite difficulties in establishing a reliable and valid classification (Tyrer, 1995; Tyrer and Alexander, 1979). Advances have been made in personality nosology, but there remain a few major problems in this field. The following comments about such problems are derived from a review of the subject by Tyrer (1995).

First, overlap among the 10 *DSM-IV* (American Psychiatric Association, 1994) personality disorders is common, and mixed personality disorders are the rule rather than the exception. Second, there is no international consensus on the criteria by which to establish a personality disorder diagnosis; ICD-10 (World Health Organization, 1992) requires subjective distress and social dysfunction to make a diagnosis, but the *DSM-IV* requires only subjective distress. (The *DSM-IV* actually requires "clinically significant distress *or* impairment" [American Psychiatric Association, 1994, p. 630].) Third, separation of Axis I and Axis II disorders is also problematic as they are both characterized by symptoms and abnormal behavior; the high "comorbidity" between Axis I and Axis II disorders may be largely a problem of construct validity in general. Fourth, the *DSM-IV* criterion of "an enduring pattern of inner experience and behavior" (American Psychiatric Association, 1994, p. 630) for making a diagnosis of personality disorder applies to many psychiatric and, for that matter, other medical disorders; again, construct validity is problematic.

Finally, the presence of Axis I disorders affects personality characteristics, and the presence of personality disorder affects the course and outcome of Axis I disorders. Illustrative of the epistemological confusion in assessing personality disturbance in hypochondriasis is a recommendation by Tyrer and colleagues (1990) that there be a diagnosis of hypochondriacal personality disorder largely because "it is possible to conceive of hypochondriasis as a personality characteristic" (p. 637) based on the criteria of the illness as enduring and pervasive. It would seem no more logical to consider persistent hypochondriasis a valid Axis II disorder than a valid Axis I disorder because of these criteria. There is currently no scientifically sound way to distinguish many Axis I state disorders from Axis II personality disorders, or between various personality disorders.

## Dimensional Conceptualization of Personality

Some experts claim that personality is best classified dimensionally rather than categorically (Widiger and Costa, 1994), although the norm has been to classify normal personality traits dimensionally and abnormal traits categorically (Livesley, 1995). Assessing personality dimensionally acknowledges that there are degrees of personality disturbance; the course of Axis I disorders can be affected when adverse conditions cause greater maladaptive expression of the personality disturbance (Tyrer, 1995).

There are a number of dimensional or "factor" models of personality. The few mentioned below have been utilized in studies of hypochondriasis. Costa and McCrae (1992) developed the NEO Five-Factor Inventory to assess neuroticism, extraversion, openness, agreeableness, and conscientiousness. The Eysenck Personality Inventory (Eysenck, 1987) posits the three dimensions of neuroticism, extraversion, and psychoticism. Tyrer and colleagues (1988) developed the Personality Assessment Schedule, which identifies thirteen personality dimensions, and is considered in detail later in this chapter.

The literature on hypochondriasis is replete with descriptions of associated "attitudes," and these attitudes were often meant to be descriptions of character traits or personality dimensions. However, the relationship of these attitudes to personality constructs is not clear.

## Section II: The Relationship Between Hypochondriasis and Personality Disturbance

The fact that there are many ways in which both hypochondriasis and personality are conceptualized and measured creates many possible interactive combinations between them. This contributes to the confusion about their relationship. Bass and Murphy (1995) delineate this confusion regarding personality and somatoform disorders in general. The variability of the constructs and the multiple potential interactions between somatoform disorders and personality have partially arisen from ideas that mental states appear in the context of developing personality, that personality shapes the clinical presentation of mental state disorders, and that personality variables affect prognosis of mental state disorders. Further, there are many models of "comorbidity" between Axis I and Axis II disorders, as highlighted by Starcevic (1992) in a paper about panic disorder and personality disturbance.

Empirical data about the relationship between hypochondriasis and personality disturbances are derived from clinical interviews and self-report questionnaires for assessing both hypochondriasis and personality disorders. Self-report questionnaires that assess hypochondriasis, such as the Illness Attitude Scales (Kellner, 1987a) and the Whiteley Index (Pilowsky, 1967), have demonstrated sensitivity to diagnosis (Barsky et al., 1992; Kellner et al., 1987). Self-report questionnaires that assess personality disorders are not reliable and have not demonstrated validity, whereas the diagnostic performance of interviews has been inconsistent; the psychometric properties of these instruments are discussed elsewhere (Ferguson and Tyrer, 1988; Perry, 1992).

Because personality, as discussed in the literature, is most often constructed in one of three ways, the following section will consider the relationships between hypochondriasis and the following: (1) attitudes, (2) personality traits and dimensions, and (3) personality disorders. These are often forced distinctions; however, they best reflect the current state of the art in the field. "Attitudes" are more heterogeneous than traits and dimensions; in turn, the latter are broader than disorders. Each of these sections is further divided into (1) Theoretical and clinical observations and (2) Research observations.

## Attitudes

### Theoretical and Clinical Observations

Bernard de Mandeville (1730) was the first to write about the "attitudes" of disease phobia and disease conviction seen in hypochondriasis. Romberg (1851) first noted the phenomenon of bodily preoccupation and amplification in hypochondriasis when he attributed the disorder to a "sensitivity of the nerves" and stated, "The disease arises only when . . . mental intention creates new sensations" (quoted from Kellner, 1986, p. 3). These three "attitudes" (disease phobia, disease conviction, and bodily preoccupation) were initially seen as personality characteristics associated with hypochondriasis as a physical disorder, but were included many years later in the diagnostic criteria of Axis I hypochondriasis, after its conceptualization had shifted from a physical disorder with constitutional "attitudes," to a mental disorder.

The dominant trend of viewing hypochondriasis as a psychopathological condition in the early twentieth century is also reflected in Emil Kraepelin's consideration of hypochondriasis as part of depression, dementia praecox, and paranoia (Kraepelin, 1921), not unlike Freud's conceptualization (Freud, 1911).

The twentieth century has seen an explosion of literature about "attitudes" in hypochondriasis. Whether these attitudes are etiologic to, part of, or personality characteristics associated with hypochondriasis is not always clear. The most common attitudes, besides those that are now constructed as the diagnostic criteria for hypochondriasis, pertain to defense and conflict resolution, communication style, hostility and anger, and a cognitive style related to a heightened awareness of bodily sensations.

**Defense and resolution of conflict.** Defense and conflict resolution are variably operative in different personality styles associated with hypochondriasis. For example, several authors (Busse, 1956; Maslow and Mittlemann, 1951; Sullivan, 1953) considered hypochondriasis a defense, a distraction from stressful interpersonal situations. Sullivan (1953) postulated that the hypochondriacal person was not capable of securely engaging in the interpersonal field except via his bodily symptoms. Likewise, Maslow and Mittlemann (1951) believed that the hypochondriacal person solved his (interpersonal) problems by increasing social detachment and focusing on the self, using his symptoms for social engagement, a view similarly taken by Busse (1956). Most views about hypochondriasis as defense and means of conflict resolution focus on bodily preoccupation and symptoms as ways to withdraw into the self because of a sense of inadequacy in coping with interpersonal and social situations (Vaillant, 1977; Wahl, 1964).

**Communication style, hostility, and anger.** Hypochondriasis has been considered a communication style for defensive and repressive purposes (Brown and Vaillant, 1981; Busse, 1956; Kellner, 1988; Maslow and Mittlemann, 1951; Sullivan, 1953; Vaillant, 1977; Wahl, 1964). Views about the association between hostility/anger and hypochondriasis have been reviewed by Kellner (1988), and they center around the ideas that hostility and anger are either etiologically linked to hypochondriasis, or that hypochondriasis is utilized as a defense against hostility and anger. In essence, it was speculated that the hypochondriacal person could not or would not communicate verbally because of a fear of hostility, a sense of inadequacy, or a need to connect interpersonally and socially while lacking skills to do so.

Hypochondriasis has also been viewed as a learned social behavior, an aspect of the "sick role" as defined by Parsons (1964), as well as a nonverbal interpersonal communication style (Barsky and Klerman, 1983). The sick role has in fact been associated with characterological features such as inhibited affect and denial, as reflected in the constructs of the Illness Behavior Questionnaire (IBQ) of Pilowsky and Spence (1975). Moreover, patients with abnormal illness behavior do have interpersonal friction and difficulty in conveying feelings to others (Pilowsky and Katsikitis, 1994).

**Cognitive style.** The concept of cognitive style has been related to that of personality (Kellner, 1988). Hypochondriasis has been associated with the cognitive styles of abnormal self-observation (Brautigam, 1956; Feldmann, 1977), selective perception of somatic sensations (Feldmann, 1977; Kellner, 1985), amplification of physical sensations (Barsky, 1979), and a belief that the physical sensations mean that there is an illness in one's body (Kellner, 1987c). Additionally, hypochondriasis has been often associated with excessive perception of bodily vulnerability and overestimation of the likelihood of being ill and at risk of death, with a consequently heightened fear of death (Barsky and Wyshak, 1989; Hollifield *et al.*, 1999b; Kellner *et al.*, 1987c; Schäfer, 1982; Starcevic, 1989a; Starcevic *et al.*, 1992; Stolorow, 1979).

## Research Observations

A substantial literature empirically links "attitudes" to hypochondriasis. Investigators have found lower self-esteem in patients with hypochondriasis compared to control subjects using structured interviews (Bianchi, 1971) and self-report questionnaires (Hollifield *et al.*, 1999b). Inhibition of anger was found to be a component of hypochondriasis in one study (Bianchi, 1973). Pilowsky and Katsikitis (1994) reported that a large number of patients with chronic pain had abnormal illness behavior (as assessed by the IBQ), and that hypochondriasis was highly associated with abnormal illness behavior. They also found that while one subset of patients with abnormal illness behavior viewed their pain within a psychological framework, another subset rejected a psychological perspective with regard to chronic pain. Such findings lend credence to the notion that hypochondriasis is in part a defense against inadequacy, anger, and having to cope with interpersonal situations in daily life.

Although many studies inferred abnormal communication in hypochondriasis, no studies directly investigated how people with hypochondriasis differ from controls in their communication style.

Anger and aggression have been associated with the tendency to somatize (Harris, 1951) and with disease fears (Bianchi, 1971). Tanabe (1973) conducted an uncontrolled psychoanalytic study of hypochondriacal patients using interviews; it was determined that these patients harbor anger and distrust toward other people and are likely to hold grudges. Utilizing the Illness Attitude Scales, Kellner and colleagues (1985) did not find a relationship between hypochondriacal fears and beliefs and hostility; they did find associations between somatization and hostility.

Several studies demonstrate that perceptual set and cognitive styles are associated with hypochondriasis. Hypochondriacal people have an inherent supersensitivity and a lower threshold for perception of physiological processes (Abadie, 1930; Kellner, 1986), and they amplify physical sensations (Barsky *et al.*, 1988, 1998). Rief and colleagues (1998) found that hypochondriacal persons "catastrophized" minor bodily complaints and had a self-concept of being weak and unable to tolerate stress. In comparison with subjects with low scores, those with high scores on scales measuring hypochondriasis are more accurate in distinguishing between two different flashes of light in rapid succession (Hanback and Revelle, 1978), more accurate in estimating their heart rate (Tyrer *et al.*,

1980), but less accurate in perceiving somatic sensations (Steptoe and Noll, 1997). Moreover, subjects with higher scores over-report symptoms during pulmonary function tests (Wright *et al.*, 1977) and notice symptoms more often when they read about them (Kellner *et al.*, 1987). Experimental evidence suggests that hypochondriacal patients differ from normal subjects and anxious patients in both their perception and their misinterpretation of normal bodily sensations (Salkovskis and Clark, 1993). This may be due to affective fluctuations in hypochondriacal patients (Steptoe and Noll, 1997) (see also Chapter 10).

In a recent report, Hollifield and colleagues (1999b) found that subjects who scored above the cutoff for hypochondriasis on the Illness Attitude Scales (Kellner, 1987a) were more negative in their self-appraisal on the Attitudes to Self Scale (Kellner, 1992) than were controls, but they did not exhibit more loneliness or emotional inhibition. When an analysis of variance (ANOVA) was conducted, the negative self-appraisal was mostly accounted for by somatization, as assessed by the Symptom Questionnaire (Kellner, 1987b), and not by hypochondriasis. This highlights how investigators may find spurious relationships between personality features and hypochondriasis if somatization is not controlled for.

## Personality Traits and Dimensions

### Theoretical and Clinical Observations

Prior to the twentieth century, hypochondriasis was most associated with the concept of hysteria. Personality features that have been associated with hypochondriasis in the twentieth-century literature include egocentricity, pride of a defiant nature, miserliness, reliability, conscientiousness in performing petty duties, obstinacy, irascibility, vindictiveness (Gillespie, 1928), orderliness and parsimoniousness (Freud, 1922), neuroticism (Hollifield *et al.*, 1999b; Noyes *et al.*, 1993; Tyrer *et al.*, 1990), narcissism (Freud, 1914; Kernberg, 1975; Kohut, 1971; Nemiah, 1980; Starcevic, 1989b), avoidance, and histrionic and borderline traits (Starcevic *et al.*, 1992).

The concept of neuroticism has become prominent in theory and research related to hypochondriasis (Hollifield *et al.*, 1999b; Nemiah, 1980; Noyes *et al.*, 1994b). There are six facets of the neuroticism scale on the NEO Five-Factor Inventory: anxiety, hostility, depression, self-consciousness, impulsivity, and vulnerability, most of which are associated with hypochondriasis. It is thus not surprising that the relationship between hypochondriasis and neuroticism is so strong.

In addition to obsessive personality traits (Pilowsky, 1970; Starcevic, 1990), narcissism has been the personality trait most closely linked with hypochondriasis (Christensen, 1978; Dorfman, 1968; Freud, 1914; Grosch, 1957–58; Kernberg, 1975; Kohut, 1971; Laughlin, 1967; Nemiah, 1980). Both classical (Klein, 1958) and contemporary (Starcevic, 1989b) authors have emphasized how hypochondriasis develops from or is part of a defective ego structure (possibly as a consequence of poor object relations), and how narcissistic injury results in a defensive focus on the body-self. A defensive concern with perfect health results in amplified and selective somatic perception, cognitive distortions about the meaning of symptoms, and fear of illness and death because of the belief that "inner badness" may cause the body to suddenly and perhaps fatally betray the individual at any time.

## Research Observations

Although there are suggestions of abnormal personality development or abnormal personality traits in hypochondriasis, other studies do not demonstrate characteristic traits (Kellner, 1985). In his review of the empirical literature until the mid-1980s, Kellner (1986) concluded that studies varied widely regarding the percentage of hypochondriacal individuals with abnormal personality traits, and he suggested that the conflicting data were largely a function of the different populations studied and the methods used. Kellner also noted a problem of the different methods and criteria to assess abnormal personality traits associated with hypochondriasis.

Pisztora (1967) conducted psychological testing of 135 hypochondriacal patients and reported that 34 demonstrated psychotic personalities, 21 had hypochondriacal personalities, 42 exhibited psychopathic and other personalities, and 79 were considered to suffer from neuroses. Twenty-two subjects lacked conspicuous personality traits before the onset of hypochondriasis. Pisztora concluded that it is the basic personality of the individual that will determine how the illness will manifest itself.

Based on his work among 225 hypochondriacal patients, Ladee (1966) believed that there was a subgroup of patients who were "constitutionally nervous with a vegetative-dystonic substratum." He wrote that others had character neuroses, with subtypes of "organ hypochondriacal development, paranoid hypochondria, the hystero-psychopathic form acting out type, and chronic hypochondriacal depersonalization" (quoted from Kellner, 1986, p. 160).

Hollifield and colleagues (1999b) recently investigated the relationship between hypochondriasis and personality dimensions using the NEO Five-Factor Inventory (Costa and McCrae, 1985). Subjects identified as hypochondriacal using the Illness Attitude Scales were more neurotic and less extroverted than were control subjects, but they did not differ from controls in openness, conscientiousness, or agreeableness. The study sample also had somatizers, and an

ANOVA demonstrated that the abnormalities in personality dimensions were accounted for by somatization and not by hypochondriasis, although interaction was observed between the two regarding extroversion. This again demonstrates the importance of distinguishing between hypochondriasis and somatization in research studies. Further, this corroborated the finding of Noyes and colleagues (1994b) of high levels of neuroticism in hypochondriacal individuals.

Scant data exist about the relationship of gender to hypochondriasis and personality traits. Katzenelbogen (1942) reviewed charts of 26 women and 25 men from the Phipps Psychiatric Clinic in Baltimore to determine symptoms, personality, and environmental influences in hypochondriacal patients without other mental disorders. The most prevalent personality features in men, of thirteen listed, were conscientiousness (40%), rigidity (40%), stubbornness (40%), being opinionated (40%), seclusiveness (36%), and sensitivity (32%). The most prevalent personality features in women, of seventeen listed, were conscientiousness (35%), sociability (35%), stubbornness (27%), and sensitivity (27%).

A few workers have attempted to tease out the temporal relationship between hypochondriasis and personality traits. Sarkisov (1972) studied personality development in 72 hypochondriacal patients without a premorbid personality disorder. He believed there were three stages in this development, the last of which was characterological disturbances. These disturbances were of three types: the hysterohypochondriacal, the obsessional hypochondriacal, or the asthenohypochondriacal. Bobrov (1976) conducted structured examinations in 51 hypochondriacal patients in whom a personality disorder had seemed to appear prior to the onset of hypochondriasis. He found a high prevalence of psychopathic traits, inadequacy, and poor social adaptation, including diminished work performance. These patients appeared more ill than subjects in other studies.

## Personality Disorders

### Theoretical and Clinical Observations

Tyrer (1995) notes that Emil Kraepelin may have been the first to write about persistent hypochondriasis as a personality characteristic. Wollenberg (1904) postulated that hypochondriasis may be "constitutional," or a form of personality disorder. Freud (1914) discussed the psychopathology of hypochondriasis in a paper on narcissism, which was the first description of hypochondriasis related to what would later be defined as a specific personality disorder. Narcissistic traits have been well described in association with hypochondriasis, as discussed above, but the link to narcissistic personality disorder has received little attention.

Starcevic (1990) reviewed a relationship between hypochondriasis and obsessive-compulsive personality disorder, and noted their four common characteristics: (*1*) excessive experience of personal vulnerability and insecurity, (*2*) excessive need for control, (*3*) poor tolerance of uncertainty, and (*4*) peculiar cognitive style with marked attention to detail, diminished ability to withdraw attention from undesirable signals, and overall cognitive constriction and rigidity.

## Research Observations

Kellner's review of the literature (Kellner, 1986) concluded that studies varied widely regarding the reported percentage of hypochondriacal individuals with associated personality disorders, and noted that different methods had been used for assessment.

A substantial number of patients with hypochondriasis do not have an established personality disorder upon clinical assessment (Kellner, 1983; Ladee, 1966). Kellner (1983) studied 36 patients with hypochondriacal neurosis in England and found 12 with a personality disorder. Eight of these patients had no evidence of a personality disorder before the onset of hypochondriasis.

Pilowsky (1970) evaluated premorbid personalities in patients with both primary and secondary hypochondriasis utilizing a clinical examination and the current British nosology. In men, the most prevalent personalities in primary hypochondriasis were obsessional (84%), hypochondriacal (65%), anxiety prone (60%), and sensitive (43%); in women, the most common personalities were obsessional (79%), anxiety prone (79%), sensitive (51%), and hypochondriacal (41%). In secondary hypochondriasis, both men and women were anxiety prone (86%), obsessional (75%), and hypochondriacal (69%) prior to the onset of hypochondriasis.

Starcevic and colleagues (1992) utilized the Structured Clinical Interview for *DSM-III-R* Personality Disorders (SCID-II) (Spitzer *et al.*, 1987) and found an increased prevalence of avoidant, histrionic, and borderline personality disorders in panic disorder patients with secondary hypochondriasis in comparison with panic disorder patients without hypochondriasis. However, personality disorder in general was not associated with secondary hypochondriasis in panic patients, and the increased prevalence of the three specific personality disorders may be due to an association of panic disorder itself with these types of character pathology (Mavissakalian, 1990; Starcevic, 1992).

Barsky and colleagues (1992) utilized a 5-item subscale of the Personality Diagnostic Questionnaire (Hyler *et al.*, 1988) in an outpatient medical clinic in Boston and found that the 42 hypochondriacal individuals were more likely than the 76 nonhypochondriacal individuals to have a probable personality disorder (63% vs. 17%). Further, 8 (19%) hypochondriacal subjects were diagnosed with antisocial personality disorder compared with 4 (5.3%) nonhypochondriacal subjects. Noyes *et al.* (1994b) also used the Personality Diagnostic Questionnaire and found a higher likelihood of personality pathology in hypochondriacal than in nonhypochondriacal subjects.

## Hypochondriacal Personality

Katzenelbogen (1942) surveyed charts of 51 patients who were preoccupied "with their bodily health, either physical or mental, or both, without any apparently reasonable foundation" or who exhibited "excessive preoccupation with existing physical or mental disorders that is disproportionate to their seriousness" (Katzenelbogen, 1942, p. 818). In this uncontrolled study, Katzenelbogen concluded that rather than having a distinct personality type, the only common characteristic shared by hypochondriacal patients is their unusual and peculiar attitude toward health and sickness.

Other work supports the concept of hypochondriacal personality. Bianchi (1971) utilized structured interviews and Pisztora (1967) conducted personality testing to demonstrate the presence of a hypochondriacal personality. However, it is not clear what criteria were used to support concepts of hypochondriacal personality.

Tyrer and colleagues (1990) argued that hypochondriasis should be considered separately in the personality disorder domain, perhaps in addition to the Axis I domain. Hypochondriacal personality disorder (HCPD) has received support from cluster analyses of the Personality Assessment Schedule (PAS; Tyrer and Alexander, 1988), with hypochondriasis being the most marked feature of the disorder in addition to prominent anxiousness, conscientiousness, and dependence. The PAS was developed from clinical experience and literature review of personality disorders, and included hypochondriasis as one of the original items. The PAS was also developed on the assumption that a personality disorder is an entity in which "certain traits dominate behaviour adversely and are persistent" (Tyrer *et al.*, 1990, p. 638). A cluster analysis initially identified four "abnormal personalities," with subsequent data creating nine others, one of which was HCPD. It was considered part of the anankastic (obsessive-compulsive) group (Tyrer *et al.*, 1990).

Tyrer and colleagues (1999) recently reported on a sample of 181 patients with neurotic disorders, 17 (9%) of whom met criteria for HCPD. In comparison with patients with other personality disorders or no personality disorder, patients with HCPD had a worse outcome at 2 and 5 years, as measured by the Comprehensive Psychopathological Rating Scale (Asberg *et al.*, 1978). However, the 5-year outcome was determined from chart review. The lack of improvement was associated with somatization in HCPD. This study provides some evidence for the validity of HCPD.

**Table 5.1.** Side-by-side comparison of the *DSM-IV* criteria for hypochondriasis and criteria for hypochondriacal personality disorder

| *DSM-IV* Hypochondriasis* | Hypochondriacal Personality Disorder[†] |
|---|---|
| A. *Preoccupation* with fears of having, or the idea that one has, a serious disease based on the person's *misinterpretation of bodily symptoms* | *Excessive preoccupation* with maintenance of health with associated behavior<br>The *perception* of minor ailments and physical symptoms *is distorted and magnified* into major and life-threatening disorder |
| B. The *preoccupation persists* despite appropriate medical evaluation and reassurance | *Rigidity of beliefs* about health and lifestyle ensures their persistence |
| C. The belief in Criterion A is not of delusional intensity and is not restricted to a circumscribed concern about appearance | |
| D. The preoccupation causes *clinically significant distress or impairment* in social, occupational, or other important areas of functioning | *Repeated recourse to consultation* with medical and associated disciplines for reassurance, investigation, and treatment |
| E. The *duration* of the disturbance is *at least 6 months* | |

*Adapted from American Psychiatric Association, 1994.
[†]Adapted from Tyrer *et al.*, 1990.

The features of HCPD are very similar to those of hypochondriasis as a state disorder. These features are compared in Table 5.1. Hypochondriasis and HCPD are both defined by persistent and rigid preoccupation with amplified bodily symptoms, the belief that these symptoms equal illness, and behaviors designed to refute these frightening beliefs but which reinforce them because of the rigidity of the conviction. Hypochondriasis and HCPD are different in some of the language used to describe each criterion; in hypochondriasis, the emphasis is on disease fears and beliefs and on misinterpretation of bodily symptoms that are all presumed to be ego-dystonic; in HCPD the emphasis is on preoccupation with health maintenance and help-seeking behaviors that are presumed to be ego-syntonic. Both the shared and the unshared features of hypochondriasis and HCPD have empirical support as part of the broader concept of hypochondriasis (Barsky *et al.*, 1986; Kellner, 1986; Noyes *et al.*, 1993; Pilowsky, 1967; Warwick and Salkovskis, 1989). Furthermore, all of the phenomena for both constructs can be viewed as the result of abnormal cognitive processing that includes amplification and misinterpretation of bodily symptoms and the behavioral outcomes of help-seeking coupled with resistance to reassurance.

The problem of hypochondriasis versus HCPD is an epistemological one: Why should there be two diagnoses when both are referring to a similar construct? If it is a question of early onset and persistence of traits that dominate behavior, evidence already exists that these characterize a primary form of hypochondriasis. However, it appears that chronicity and pervasiveness are easily attributed to or identified with a personality disturbance. The trend of transforming chronic Axis I disorders into personality disorders because of their duration and, to a certain extent, their pervasiveness is already evident with other disorders: Thus, social phobia is often constructed as an avoidant personality disorder, and dysthymia is considered a depressive personality disorder.

Alternatively, if HCPD receives further empirical support, then "primary" hypochondriasis should no longer be thought of as valid, and Axis I hypochondriasis should be diagnosed when it is associated with other medical and psychiatric disorders. Even in this case, hypochondriasis may be a manifestation of personality traits becoming maladaptive under adverse conditions. Thus, it may be just as logical to suggest that this "secondary" form of hypochondriasis is the "personality form" of the disorder. Various medical conditions, including asthma, diabetes, and seizure disorders, have early- and late-onset forms. Even where there are personality traits associated with these illnesses, an important research goal has been to understand the mechanisms of each form. Likewise, it is this author's view that it is important to understand the mechanisms of the primary and secondary forms of hypochondriasis and incorporate personality as either a risk factor or a consequence of hypochondriasis.

If further research weakens support for hypochondriasis as a mental state disorder, then the alternative will be to consider hypochondriasis purely in the personality domain. Bass and Murphy (1995) and Tyrer (1995) discuss an alternative to the current descriptive and taxonomic approach to psychopathology with regard to somatoform disorders. This approach utilizes developmental and life-span perspectives to demonstrate that somatoform disorders develop in the context of developmental tasks and processes, and are thus more similar than dissimilar to personality disorders. For support, Bass and Murphy note the work of Craig and colleagues (1993), who speculate that early childhood illness and lack of parental care are two separate factors during development that come together in adulthood as somatization. This work is similar to the multiprocess view of Millon (1990) regarding the formation of personality disorder and provides another important paradigm for understanding hypochondriasis as a "developmental disorder." However, there are two difficulties with this view.

First, research into pathogenesis is difficult to conduct because of the longitudinal and prospective design of the studies. Second, and perhaps more importantly, other psychiatric disorders such as schizophrenia and childhood obsessive-compulsive disorder also arise in the context of development, but they are not considered personality constructs, even though they easily meet the *DSM-IV* criteria for personality disorder. Perhaps it should be emphasized that there is a hierarchical relationship between "developmental" disorders and more pervasive mental disorders that also appear during development (e.g., schizophrenia), so that the diagnosis of the latter precludes that of the former.

## Hypochondriasis, Personality Disorders, and Trauma

Given that personality disorder and hypochondriasis are both linked to vulnerability in development, it is surprising that there is very little research into a relationship of trauma to hypochondriasis, especially when associated with personality disturbance. Although there are numerous reports on somatization and somatoform disorders in specific traumatized populations (Bryer *et al.*, 1987; Drossman *et al.*, 1990; Morrison, 1989), there is only one study about trauma related to hypochondriasis. Barsky and colleagues (1994b) utilized the Childhood Traumatic Events Scale (Pennebaker, 1993; Pennebaker and Susman, 1988) in 60 outpatients with hypochondriasis and 60 nonhypochondriacal patients from the same clinic. Significantly more hypochondriacal patients than nonhypochondriacal patients reported traumatic sexual contact (29% vs. 7%), physical violence (32% vs. 7%), and major parental upheaval before age 17 (29% vs. 9%). The hypochondriacal patients reported being sick more often as children and missing school for health reasons, but did not differ on six other measures of childhood health.

The relationship between trauma as a risk factor for hypochondriasis and personality disorder in the context of hypochondriasis warrants further investigation. Given the known relationship between childhood trauma and personality disorders (Modestin *et al.*, 1998), the conflicting data on the relationship between childhood trauma and adult somatization (Figueroa *et al.*, 1997), and the evidence for abnormal personality traits in hypochondriasis, it can be speculated that a significant relationship exists between trauma and early-onset hypochondriasis, which is associated with personality disturbance.

## Conclusion

There is no pathognomonic personality disturbance in hypochondriasis. The relationship between hypochondriasis and personality disorders or abnormal personality traits is unclear and warrants further investigation. Traits most reliably associated with hypochondriasis are narcissism, obsessive-compulsivity, neuroticism, introversion, and negative self-appraisal. By definition, all hypochondriacal people have bodily preoccupation and disease fears, and some are convinced they have a disease. Concepts derived from these diagnostic features have been considered personality attributes by some investigators, giving rise to a call for hypochondriasis to be conceptualized as a personality disorder or dimension.

A lack of epistemological precision and of knowledge of psychobiological factors involved in pathogenesis have greatly hampered understanding of the relationship between hypochondriasis and personality.

First, from a phenomenological viewpoint, hypochondriasis and personality disorders as distinct diagnoses cannot be considered truly valid. The nosological separation between somatoform disorders and personality disorders, and between Axis I and Axis II disorders in general, is not clear. Second, the good intentions to provide better or more accurate understanding of hypochondriasis and personality through various conceptualizations and measurements have not clarified the relationship between the two. However, because the psychobiological patho genesis of both hypochondriasis and personality disturbance may never be fully known, the relationship between them may always be shrouded under incomplete data. For the future, better understanding of phenomenology and psychobiology, and better understanding of developmental risk factors for hypochondriasis, including temperament and personality, will be of paramount importance.

The presence of personality disturbance may have implications for the treatment of hypochondriasis. It is known that personality disorders can complicate the treatment of mental state disorders, but the possible extent of this interference is unknown regarding hypochondriasis. When hypochondriasis is secondary, has been present for a brief time, and is without personality disturbance, reassurance and education are likely to be effective. Primary hypochondriasis with or without personality disturbance, notwithstanding the nosological issue, is more refractory and requires a more comprehensive assessment and more elaborate treatment planning.

Understanding the relationship between hypochondriasis and personality will likely be advanced if research is informed first by theory and second by hypothesis testing. Epistemology must also be attended to. First, further validation of hypochondriasis as a diagnosis will be important, thus distinguishing it from somatization, and understanding whether it is a developmental trait, exacerbated by stressors, or a mental state disorder. Second, the theoretical construction of personality and the most appropriate ways to assess its deviance likely will be always at issue. Relevant to the relationship to hypochondriasis, this field will benefit from information about personality as a risk for or a manifestation of hypochondriasis, assuming the latter to be a state disorder. Third, construct validity must be established if there are to be disorders with relationships between them. A nosological separation between somatoform disorders and personality states must be accomplished from a theoretical position that will allow phenomenological and psychobiological research to actually find construct distinctions. The current overlap of diagnostic criteria in these constructs defeats good attempts to distinguish them and find relationships between them. Finally, standardization of assessment between studies is important, and will only be accomplished after the constructs are better defined and validated.

### References

Abadie J. 1930. L'Hypocondrie et la constitution hypocondrique. *Journal de Médecine de Bordeaux* 107: 783–791.

American Psychiatric Association. 1994. *Diagnostic and Statistical Manual of Mental Disorders, Fourth Edition (DSM–IV)*. Washington, DC: American Psychiatric Association.

Arndt R. 1885. *Die Neurasthenie, ihr Wesen, ihre Bedeutung und Behandlung vom anatomischphysiologischen Standpunkt*. Wien: Urban und Schwarzenberg.

Asberg M., Montgomery S.A., Perris C., Schalling D., Sedvall G. 1978. A Comprehensive Psychopathological Rating Scale. *Acta Psychiatrica Scandinavica* 58 (Suppl. 271): 5–29.

Baker B., Merskey H. 1983. Classification and associations of hypochondriasis in patients from a psychiatric hospital. *Canadian Journal of Psychiatry* 28: 629–634.

Barsky A.J. 1979. Patients who amplify bodily symptoms. *Annals of Internal Medicine* 91: 63–70.

Barsky A.J., Klerman G.L. 1983. Overview: hypochondriasis, bodily complaints, and somatic styles. *American Journal of Psychiatry* 140: 273–283.

Barsky A.J., Wyshak G. 1989. Hypochondriasis and related health attitudes. *Psychosomatics* 30: 412–420.

Barsky A.J., Wyshak G., Klerman G.L. 1986. Hypochondriasis: an evaluation of the DSM-III criteria in medical outpatients. *Archives of General Psychiatry* 43: 493–500.

Barsky A.J., Geringer E., Wool C.A. 1988. A cognitive-educational treatment for hypochondriasis. *General Hospital Psychiatry* 10: 322–327.

Barsky A.J., Wyshak G., Klerman G.L. 1992. Psychiatric comorbidity in DSM-III-R hypochondriasis. *Archives of General Psychiatry* 49: 101–108.

Barsky A.J., Barnett M.D., Cleary P.D. 1994a. Hypochondriasis and panic disorder: boundary and overlap. *Archives of General Psychiatry* 51: 918–925.

Barsky A.J., Wool C., Barnett M.C., Cleary P.D. 1994b. Histories of childhood trauma in adult hypochondriacal patients. *American Journal of Psychiatry* 151: 397–401.

Barsky A.J., Fama J.M., Bailey E.D., Ahern D.K. 1998. A prospective 4- to 5-year study of DSM-III-R hypochondriasis. *Archives of General Psychiatry* 55: 737–744.

Bass C., Murphy M. 1995. Somatoform and personality disorders: syndromal comorbidity and overlapping developmental pathways. *Journal of Psychosomatic Research* 39: 403–427.

Beard G.M. 1880. *American Nervousness. A Practical Treatise on Nervous Exhaustion (Neurasthenia): Its Symptoms, Nature, Sequences, Treatment.* New York: William Wood.

Bianchi G.N. 1971. Origins of disease phobia. *Australian and New Zealand Journal of Psychiatry* 5: 241–257.

Bianchi G.N. 1973. Patterns of hypochondriasis: a principal components analysis. *British Journal of Psychiatry* 122: 541–548.

Bobrov A.S. 1976. Pathological hypochondriacal personality development. *Zhurnal Nevropatologii i Psikhiatrii* 76: 1347–1352.

Brautigam V.W. 1956. Analyse der hypochondrischen Selbstbeobachtung. *Nervenarzt* 27: 409–418.

Brown H.N., Vaillant G.E. 1981. Hypochondriasis. *Archives of Internal Medicine* 141: 723–726.

Bryer J.B., Nelson B.A., Miller J.B., Krol P.A. 1987. Childhood sexual and physical abuse as factors in adult psychiatric illness. *American Journal of Psychiatry* 144: 1426–1430.

Burton R. 1883. *The Anatomy of Melancholy.* London: Oxford University Press (Original work published 1611).

Busse E.W. 1956. The treatment of the chronic complainer. *Medical Record Annals* 50: 196–200.

Christensen C.W. 1978. The hypochondriacal syndrome. *Comprehensive Therapy* 4: 22–25.

Costa P.T., Jr., McCrae R.R. (eds). 1985. *The NEO Personality Inventory Manual, Form S and Form R.* Odessa, FL: Psychological Assessment Resources.

Costa P.T., Jr., McCrae R.R. 1992. The five-factor model of personality and its relevance to personality disorders. *Journal of Personality Disorders* 6: 343–359.

Cotard J. 1880. Du délire hypochondriaque dans une forme grave de la mélancholie anxieuse. *Annales Médico-Psychologiques* 38: 168–174.

Craig T.K.J., Boardman A.P., Mills K., Daly-Jones O., Drake H. 1993. The South London somatisation study: I. Longitudinal course and the influence of early life experiences. *British Journal of Psychiatry* 163: 579–588.

Dorfman W. 1968. Hypochondriasis as a defense against depression. *Psychosomatics* 9: 248–251.

Drossman D.A., Leserman J., Nachman G., Li Z.M., Gluck H., Toomey T.C., Mitchell C.M. 1990. Sexual and physical abuse in women with functional or organic gastrointestinal disorders. *Annals of Internal Medicine* 113: 828–833.

Dubois E.F. (d'Amiens) 1833. *Historie philosophique de l'hypocondrie et de l'hystérie.* Paris: Cavelin, Librairie de Deville.

Eysenck H. 1987. The definition of personality disorders and the criteria appropriate for their description. *Journal of Personality Disorders* 1: 211–219.

Fava G.A., Kellner R., Zielezny M.A., Grandi S. 1988. Hypochondriacal fears and beliefs in agoraphobia. *Journal of Affective Disorders* 14: 239–244.

Feldmann H. 1977. Symptomwahrnehmung und Uberbewertung bei der Hypochondrie. *Archiv für Psychiatrie und Nervenkrankheiten* 224: 235–245.

Ferguson B.G., Tyrer P. 1988. Classifying personality disorder. In *Personality Disorders: Diagnosis, Management and Course* (ed. Tyrer P.), London: Wright.

Figueroa E.F., Silk K.R., Huth A., Lohr N.E. 1997. History of childhood sexual abuse and general psychopathology. *Comprehensive Psychiatry* 38: 23–30.

Flint A. 1866. *A Treatise on the Principles and Practice of Medicine.* Philadelphia: Henry C. Lea.

Freud S. 1911. *Psycho-analytic Notes on an Autobiographical Account of a Case of Paranoia (Dementia Paranoides), Standard Edition* 12: 3–86. London: Hogarth Press, 1955.

Freud S. 1914. *On Narcissism: An Introduction, Standard Edition* 14: 69–102. London: Hogarth Press, 1955.

Freud S. 1922. *Introductory Lectures.* London: Allen and Unvia.

Gillespie R.D. 1928. Hypochondria: its definition, nosology and psychopathology. *Guy's Hospital Report* 78: 408–460.

Grosch M. 1957–58. Über Hypochondrie. *Zeitschrift für Psychosomatische Medizin und Psychoanalyse* 4: 195–205.

Hanback J.W., Revelle W. 1978. Arousal and perceptual sensitivity in hypochondriacs. *Journal of Abnormal Psychology* 32: 50–55.

Harris I.D. 1951. Mood, anger and somatic dysfunction. *Journal of Nervous and Mental Disease* 113: 152–158.

Hollifield M., Paine S., Tuttle L., Kellner R. 1999a. Hypochondriasis, somatization, and perceived health and utilization of health care services. *Psychosomatics* 40: 380–386.

Hollifield M., Tuttle L., Paine S., Kellner R. 1999b. Hypochondriasis and somatization related to personality and attitudes toward self. *Psychosomatics* 40: 387–395.

Hyler S.E., Rieder R.O., Williams J.B.W., Spitzer R.L., Hendler J., Lyons M. 1988. The Personality Diagnostic Questionnaire: development and preliminary results. *Journal of Personality Disorders* 2: 229–238.

Katzenelbogen S. 1942. Hypochondriacal complaints with special reference to personality and environment. *American Journal of Psychiatry* 98: 815–822.

Kellner R. 1983. Prognosis of treated hypochondriasis: a clinical study. *Acta Psychiatrica Scandinavia* 67: 69–79.

Kellner R. 1985. Functional somatic symptoms and hypochondriasis: a survey of empirical studies. *Archives of General Psychiatry* 42: 821–833.

Kellner R. 1986. *Somatization and Hypochondriasis.* New York: Praeger.

Kellner R. 1987a. *Abridged Manual of the Illness Attitude Scales.* Albuquerque, NM: Department of Psychiatry, University of New Mexico School of Medicine.

Kellner R. 1987b. *Manual of the Symptom Questionnaire.* Albuquerque, NM: Department of Psychiatry, University of New Mexico School of Medicine.

Kellner R. 1987c. Hypochondriasis and somatization. *Journal of the American Medical Association* 258: 2718–2722.

Kellner R. 1988. *Theories and Research in Hypochondriasis. The 1988 C. Charles Burlingame, M.D. Award Lecture.* Hartford, CT: The Institute of Living.

Kellner R. 1992. *Scoring of the Attitude to Self Scale.* Albuquerque, NM: Department of Psychiatry, University of New Mexico School of Medicine.

Kellner R., Slocumb J., Wiggins R.G., Abbott P.J., Winslow W.W., Pathak D. 1985. Hostility, somatic symptoms, and hypochondriacal fears and beliefs. *Journal of Nervous and Mental Disease* 173: 554–560.

Kellner R., Fava G.A., Lisansky J., Perini G.I., Zielezny M. 1986. Hypochondriacal fears and beliefs in DSM-III melancholia: changes with amitriptyline. *Journal of Affective Disorders* 10: 21–26.

Kellner R., Abbott P., Winslow W.W., Pathak D. 1987. Fears, beliefs, and attitudes in DSM-III hypochondriasis. *Journal of Nervous and Mental Disease* 175: 20–25.

Kenyon F.E. 1964. Hypochondriasis: a clinical study. *British Journal of Psychiatry* 110: 478–488.

Kenyon F.E. 1965. Hypochondriasis: a survey of some historical, clinical and social aspects. *British Journal of Medical Psychology* 38: 117–133.

Kernberg O.F. 1975. *Borderline Conditions and Pathological Narcissism*. New York: Jason Aronson.

Keynes G. 1962. *Timothie Bright (1550–1615): A Survey of His Life with a Bibliography of His Writings*. London: Wellcome Historical Medical Library.

Klein M. 1958. On the development of mental functions, In *Contributions to Psycho–Analysis, 1921–1945* (ed. Klein M.), London: Hogarth Press.

Kohut H. 1971. *The Analysis of the Self*. New York: International Universities Press.

Kraepelin E. 1921. *Dementia Praecox and Paraphrenia* (ed. Robertson G.M.), Chicago: Chicago Medical Book Co.

Ladee G.A. 1966. *Hypochondriacal Syndromes*. Amsterdam: North-Holland Publishing.

Laughlin H.P. 1967. *The Neuroses*. Washington, DC: Butterworths.

Lewis A.J. 1934. Melancholia: clinical survey of depressive states. *Journal of Mental Science* 80: 277–378.

Livesley W.J. (ed.). 1995. *The DSM-IV Personality Disorders*. New York: Guilford Press.

Mandeville B. 1730. *A Treatise of the Hypochondriack and Hysterick Passions, Second Edition*. London: J. Tonson.

Maslow A.H., Mittlemann B. 1951. *Principles of Abnormal Psychology: The Dynamics of Psychic Illness*. New York: Harper & Row.

Mavissakalian M. 1990. The relationship between panic disorder/agoraphobia and personality disorders. *Psychiatric Clinics of North America* 13: 661–684.

Millon T. 1990. *Towards a New Personology: An Evolutionary Model*. New York: John Wiley.

Modestin J., Oberson B., Erni T. 1998. Possible antecedents of DSM-III-R personality disorders. *Acta Psychiatrica Scandinavia* 97: 260–266.

Morrison J. 1989. Childhood sexual histories of women with somatization disorder. *American Journal of Psychiatry* 146: 239–241.

Nemiah J.C. 1980. Somatoform disorders. In *Comprehensive Textbook of Psychiatry, Third Edition* (eds. Kaplan H.I., Freedman A.M., Sadock B.J.), Baltimore: Williams & Wilkins.

Noyes R., Jr., Reich J., Clancy J., O'Gorman T.W. 1986. Reduction of hypochondriasis with treatment of panic disorder. *British Journal of Psychiatry* 149: 631–635.

Noyes R., Jr., Kathol R.G., Fisher M.M., Phillips B.M., Suelzer M.T., Holt C.S. 1993. The validity of DSM-III-R hypochondriasis. *Archives of General Psychiatry* 51: 961–970.

Noyes R., Jr., Kathol R.G., Fisher M.M., Phillips B.M., Suelzer M.T., Woodman C.L. 1994a. A one-year follow-up of medical outpatients with hypochondriasis. *Psychosomatics* 35: 533–545.

Noyes R., Jr., Kathol R.G., Fisher M.M., Phillips B.M., Suelzer M.T., Woodman C.L. 1994b. Psychiatric comorbidity among patients with hypochondriasis. *General Hospital Psychiatry* 16: 78–87.

Noyes R., Jr., Holt C.S., Happel R.L., Kathol R.G., Yagla S.J. 1997. A family study of hypochondriasis. *Journal of Nervous and Mental Disease* 185: 223–232.

Parsons T. 1951. *The Social System.* New York: The Free Press.

Parsons T. 1964. *Social Structure and Personality.* London: Collier-Macmillan.

Pennebaker J.W. 1993. Social mechanisms of constraint. In *Handbook of Mental Control* (eds. Wegner D.M., Pennebaker J.W.), Englewood Cliffs, NJ: Prentice Hall.

Pennebaker J.W., Susman J.R. 1988. Disclosure of traumas and psychosomatic processes. *Social Science and Medicine* 26: 327–332.

Perry J.C. 1992. Problems and considerations in the valid assessment of personality disorders. *American Journal of Psychiatry* 149: 1645–1653.

Pilowsky I. 1967. Dimensions of hypochondriasis. *British Journal of Psychiatry* 113: 89–93.

Pilowsky I. 1970. Primary and secondary hypochondriasis. *Acta Psychiatrica Scandinavia* 46: 273–285.

Pilowsky I. 1978. Pain as abnormal illness behavior. *Journal of Human Stress* 4: 22–27.

Pilowsky I., Spence N.D. 1975. Patterns of illness behaviour in patients with intractable pain. *Journal of Psychosomatic Research* 19: 279–287.

Pilowsky I., Katsikitis M. 1994. A classification of illness behaviour in pain clinic patients. *Pain* 57: 91–94.

Pisztora F. 1967. A szemelyseg meghatarozo szerepe a coenasethesias-hipochondrias korkepek patogeneziseben. *Pszichologiai Tanulmanyok* 10: 575–579.

Rief W., Hiller W., Margraf J. 1998. Cognitive aspects of hypochondriasis and the somatization syndrome. *Journal of Abnormal Psychology* 107: 587–595.

Romberg M.H. 1851. *Lehrbuch der Nervenkrankheiten des Menschen, Second Edition.* Berlin: Duncker.

Salkovskis P.M., Clark D.M. 1993. Panic disorder and hypochondriasis. *Advances in Behaviour Research and Therapy* 15: 23–48.

Sarkisov S.A. 1972. The clinical picture of hypochondriac development. *Zhurnal Nevropatologii i Psikhiatrii* 72: 446–450.

Schäfer M.L. 1982. Phenomenology and hypochondria. In *Phenomenology and Psychiatry* (eds. de Koning A.J., Jenner F.A.), New York: Grune & Stratton.

Sheehan D.V., Ballenger J., Jacobsen G. 1980. Treatment of endogenous anxiety with phobic, hysterical, and hypochondriacal symptoms. *Archives of General Psychiatry* 37: 51–59.

Spitzer R.L., Williams J.B.W, Gibbon M. 1987. *Structured Clinical Interview for DSM-III-R Personality Disorders (SCID-II).* New York: New York State Psychiatric Institute.

Starcevic V. 1989a. Pathological fear of death, panic attacks, and hypochondriasis. *American Journal of Psychoanalysis* 49: 347–361.

Starcevic V. 1989b. Contrasting patterns in the relationship between hypochondriasis and narcissism. *British Journal of Medical Psychology* 62: 311–323.

Starcevic V. 1990. Relationship between hypochondriasis and obsessive-compulsive personality disorder: close relatives separated by nosological schemes? *American Journal of Psychotherapy* 44: 340–347.

Starcevic V. 1992. Comorbidity models of panic disorder/agoraphobia and personality disturbance. *Journal of Personality Disorders* 6: 213–225.

Starcevic V., Kellner R., Uhlenhuth E.H., Pathak D. 1992. Panic disorder and hypochondriacal fears and beliefs. *Journal of Affective Disorders* 24: 73–85.

Steptoe A., Noll A. 1997. The perception of bodily sensations, with special reference to hypochondriasis. *Behaviour Research and Therapy* 35: 901–910.

Stolorow R.D. 1979. Defensive and arrested developmental aspects of death anxiety, hypochondriasis and depersonalization. *International Journal of Psychoanalysis* 60: 201–213.

Sullivan H S. 1953. *The Interpersonal Theory of Psychiatry*. New York: WW Norton & Co.

Tanabe K. 1973. A clinical study on hypochondriasis. *Kyashu Neuro-Psychiatry* 19: 73–109.

Torgersen S. 1986. Genetics of somatoform disorders. *Archives of General Psychiatry* 43: 502–505.

Tuczeck J. 1883. Zur Lehre von der Hypochondrie. *Zeitschrift der Psychiatrie* 39: 653–663.

Tyrer P. 1976. *The Role of Bodily Feelings in Anxiety*. London: Oxford University Press.

Tyrer P. 1995. Somatoform and personality disorders: personality and the soma. *Journal of Psychosomatic Research* 39: 395–397.

Tyrer P., Alexander J. 1979. The classification of personality disorder. *British Journal of Psychiatry* 135: 163–167.

Tyrer P., Alexander J. 1988. Personality Assessment Schedule. In *Personality Disorders: Diagnosis, Management and Course* (ed. Tyrer P.), London: Wright.

Tyrer P., Lee I., Alexander J. 1980. Awareness of cardiac function in anxious, phobic and hypochondriacal patients. *Psychological Medicine* 10: 171–174.

Tyrer P., Fowler-Dixon R., Ferguson B., Kelemen A. 1990. A plea for the diagnosis of hypochondriacal personality disorder. *Journal of Psychosomatic Research* 34: 637–642.

Tyrer P., Seivewright N., Seivewright H. 1999. Long-term outcome of hypochondriacal personality disorder. *Journal of Psychosomatic Research* 46: 177–185.

Vaillant G. 1977. *Adaptation to Life*. Boston: Little, Brown.

Wahl C.W. 1964. Psychodynamics of the hypochondriacal patient. In *New Dimensions in Psychosomatic Medicine* (ed. Wahl C.W.), Boston: Little, Brown.

Warwick H.M.C., Salkovskis P.M. 1989. Hypochondriasis. In *Cognitive Therapy and Clinical Practice* (eds. Scott J., Williams J.M.G., Beck A.T.), London: Gower.

Widiger T.A., Costa P.T. 1994. Personality and personality disorders. *Journal of Abnormal Psychology* 103: 78–91.

Wollenberg R. 1904. *Die Hypochondrie.* Wien: Alfred Holder.

World Health Organization. 1992. *The ICD-10 Classification of Mental and Behavioural Disorders. Clinical Descriptions and Diagnostic Guidelines.* Geneva, Switzerland: World Health Organization.

Wright D.D., Kane R.L., Olsen D.M., Smith T.J. 1977. The effects of selected psychosocial factors on the self-reporting of pulmonary symptoms. *Journal of Chronic Diseases* 30: 195–206.

Ziehen T. 1902. *Psychiatrie für Arzte und Studierende, 2nd Edition.* Leipzig: S. Hirzel.

# 6

# Epidemiology of Hypochondriasis

## RUSSELL NOYES, JR.

Relatively little is known about the epidemiology of hypochondriasis. The reasons for this are several, but, importantly, no surveys of the general population have been completed. Consequently, data from the community concerning prevalence, risk factors, morbidity, and so on, are not available, and information from clinical samples may be influenced by selection bias. The Epidemiologic Catchment Area Study and the National Comorbidity Survey failed to include hypochondriasis. Authors of these and other large epidemiologic surveys may have regarded it as a less important disorder or one that might not be diagnosed reliably in those whose health status is unknown. Regardless of the reason, large gaps exist in our knowledge of how the disorder is distributed and factors that influence its distribution.

Most information about the occurrence of hypochondriasis comes from medical populations where hypochondriacal patients manifest their persistent care-seeking behavior. Even there, however, the disorder is rarely diagnosed, so that investigators have had to rely upon a variety of screening methods. Many have used scales, such as the Whiteley Index (Pilowsky, 1967), for the measurement of hypochondriacal symptoms and have examined correlations with the level of such symptoms throughout the population (Pilowsky and Spence, 1983). Such dimensional assessment assumes that hypochondriasis is distributed along a continuum of severity. However, few studies using this approach have taken medical morbidity, an important determinant of health worry, into account. Others have taken a categorical approach and employed two-step case-identification procedures, so that following a measure of hypochondriacal symptoms a structured interview is administered to those scoring above a particular cutoff. Such procedures tend to increase sensitivity and yield higher rates than might be obtained when the entire range of psychiatric disorders is studied. Rates are also influenced by the criteria for diagnosis. The *Diagnostic and Statistical Manual of Mental Disorders* (3rd ed. revised) (*DSM-III-R*) criteria excluded patients whose symptoms were simply those of panic attacks (American Psychiatric Association, 1987). However, the fourth edition of the *DSM* (*DSM-IV*) criteria exclude patients whose hypochondriacal symptoms are better accounted for by most other anxiety, depressive, and somatoform disorders (American Psychiatric Association, 1994). Because the rate of coexisting disorders is high, such hierarchical rules can be expected to reduce rates considerably. Also, hypochondriasis has been studied in populations ranging from student volunteers to psychiatric inpatients, and findings vary from one setting to the next (Mabe *et al.*, 1996).

Epidemiologic data are important for establishing the existence of a disorder and formulating the criteria by which it is defined. Investigations in psychiatric populations have shown hypochondriacal patients to have anxious or phobic symptoms, a focus on bodily sensations, and a particular cognitive set about disease. For example, in his original research, Pilowsky (1967) demonstrated dimensions of disease phobia, bodily preoccupation, and disease conviction. And, others have reported similar findings (Bianchi, 1973; Hanback and Revelle, 1978; Kellner *et al.*, 1987a; Pilowsky and Spence, 1975, 1976; Pilowsky *et al.*, 1977). More recently, Barsky *et al.* (1986a) demonstrated the presence of a hypochondriacal syndrome in medical outpatients. Among these patients, they showed that disease conviction, disease fear, bodily preoccupation, and somatic symptoms were significantly intercorrelated. Thus, there appears to be considerable internal consistency for *DSM-III* hypochondriasis. Increased health care utilization and disability among patients with these characteristics provided external validation of the syndrome (Barsky *et al.*, 1986a).

Barsky *et al.* (1992a) extended this work by developing a structured diagnostic interview for hypochondriasis. Using that interview, these investigators and Noyes *et al.* (1993) examined the validity of the *DSM-III-R* hypochondriasis. Noyes *et al.* (1993) compared 50 patients who met *DSM-III-R* criteria for hypochondriasis with 50 age- and sex-matched controls from the same general medicine clinic. Clinic physicians rated the hypochondriacal patients as having more unrealistic fear of illness and diagnosed psychiatric and functional somatic syndromes (e.g., fibromyalgia) more frequently in these patients than in controls. Their hypochondriacal patients viewed their health as worse, had more health worries, and exhibited more severe psychiatric symptoms than did controls. These patients also reported poorer physical functioning and work performance, greater health care utilization, poorer response to medical treatment, and less satisfaction with the care they received than did controls. The results provided several indicators of internal and external validity for this diagnostic category (see also Chapter 2).

Hypochondriasis appears to be distinct from other forms of somatization in primary care. For example, Kirmayer and Robbins (1991) identified three forms of somatization—one of them hypochondriacal worry—that were separate from one another and were associated with different sociodemographic and illness behavior characteristics. Most studies show some overlap between hypochondriasis and subsyndromal somatization disorder (variously defined), yet most show the former to have fewer unexplained somatic symptoms (Barsky *et al.*, 1992b; Escobar *et al.*, 1998; Noyes *et al.*, 1994a). Also, while patients with subsyndromal somatization disorder are predominantly women, unmarried, and from lower socioeconomic status, those with hypochondriasis appear not to differ from non-hypochondriacal patients with respect to most demographic characteristics (Escobar *et al.*, 1998). Such findings support the view that these somatoform disorders are separable.

Epidemiologic studies are dependent upon reliable and valid measures of hypochondriasis. Where two-step case-identification procedures are employed for the sake of efficiency, the Whiteley Index has been used, and in one study it showed a sensitivity of 87% and specificity of 72% (Speckens *et al.*, 1996a). Also, a modified Whiteley Index used in combination with the Somatic Symptom Inventory (the Minnesota Multiphasic Personality Inventory [MMPI; Greene, 1991] hypochondriasis scale plus Symptom Checklist-90 [Lipman *et al.*, 1979] somatization scale) showed a sensitivity of 90% and specificity of 67% (Barsky *et al.*, 1992a; Noyes *et al.*, 1993). However, some items on the Whiteley Index may be influenced by symptoms of physical illness, prompting Robbins *et al.* (1990) to develop a modification, the Illness Worry Scale. On this scale they suggested a cutoff of four out of nine items for case identification (Robbins and Kirmayer, 1996).

The Illness Attitude Scales are also available (Kellner, 1981, 1986; Kellner *et al.*, 1983–84). A principal components analysis of this instrument yielded two dimensions, Health Anxiety and Illness Behavior (Speckens *et al.*, 1996b). In one study, the Illness Attitude Scales showed a sensitivity of 79% and specificity of 74% (Speckens *et al.*, 1996a). As indicated, a second-stage structured interview has been developed by Barsky *et al.* (1992a). This is a module of the Structured Clinical Interview for *DSM-III-R* (Spitzer *et al.*, 1990) that begins with a series of probe questions. The interview has been shown to have adequate psychometric properties. The instruments for assessing hypochondriasis and assessment issues are discussed in more detail in Chapter 3.

## Prevalence

### General Population

In addition to one community survey of somatoform disorders that included hypochondriasis, there are several sources of information. Agras *et al.* (1969) reported that 16.5% of people in Burlington, Vermont, had some fear of illness (excluding fear of injury) and 3.1% had phobia of actual illness or injury. According to Marks (1987), illness phobia may be a subtype of hypochondriasis in which one or more specific illnesses are the focus of concern. Illness phobia appears to be distinct from blood-needle phobia, although this issue, like that of illness phobia itself, has received little study (Marks, 1988). Phobias of illness in this survey had a peak onset in the fifth decade and were associated with anxious personality traits. Recently, Noyes et al. (2000) found that 4%–5% of individuals in the general population had fears of illness or injury that interfered with their medical care.

Early researchers found between 4% and 25% of the general population to be hypochondriacal (Langner and Michael, 1963; Leighton, 1959). Later, Kellner and colleagues obtained estimates using the Illness Attitude Scales from a variety of nonclinical study samples (Kellner, 1986). For instance, they found that 2% of employees, when told by a doctor that they had no physical illness, refused to believe it, compared to 9% of family practice patients (Kellner et al., 1983–84). They also found that 9% and 13% of people in England and New Mexico, respectively, were worried they might have a serious disease (Kellner and Sheffield, 1973), and 3% of employees were worried they might get serious illness in the future (Kellner et al., 1983). In addition, Kellner et al. (1986a) observed that 8% of medical and law students scored 3 or more on the subscales of the Illness Attitude Scales, which indicate hypochondriasis. They found few differences between medical and law students, and because of the small numbers they had little opportunity to identify factors associated with hypochondriacal concerns.

Faravelli et al. (1997) completed a community survey of somatoform disorders in Florence, Italy, based upon interviews with 673 randomly selected residents of that city who were interviewed by their general practitioners. Four such practitioners with training in psychiatry conducted interviews. One-year prevalence rates were 0.3% for conversion disorder, 0.6% for somatoform pain disorder, 0.7% for somatization disorder, 4.5% for hypochondriasis, and 13.8% for undifferentiated somatoform disorder. Individuals who met criteria for hypochondriasis were at increased relative risk for an associated depressive disorder (3.8 for dysthymia and 4.2 for major depression) but not an anxiety disorder. Also, one study of people aged 65 and over found rates of hypochondriasis of 1.1% in Liverpool, England, and 1.8% in Zaragoza, Spain (Saz et al., 1995).

Recently, Noyes et al. (1997) completed a preliminary family study of hypochondriasis. The probands consisted of general medical patients with hypochondriasis and nonhypochondriacal controls from the same clinic. All available first-degree relatives were interviewed using the Structured Clinical Interview for DSM-IV (SCID-I; First et al., 1997). Because the frequency of hypochondriasis was comparable in the two groups of relatives, they were combined for a comparison of hypochondriacal and nonhypochondriacal individuals. Hypochondriasis was diagnosed in 7.7% of these relatives, and when subthreshold cases were added, the proportion rose to 10.7% (Noyes *et al.*,1999). Although hypochondriasis was not strongly associated with demographic variables, it was related to psychiatric comorbidity, functional impairment, and utilization of health care. These hypochondriacal relatives showed most of the same characteristics that have been identified among hypochondriacal patients from clinical populations (Noyes *et al.*, 1999).

## General Medical Patients

A number of investigators have examined the occurrence of hypochondriasis among general medical patients. As shown in Table 6.1, the current prevalence in these studies has ranged from 0.8 to 10.3%. The authors of a cross-national survey, Gureje *et al.* (1997), noted that, if the criterion of failure to respond to reassurance were dropped, 2.2% of their primary care patients qualified for the diagnosis and were just as impaired as those who met this criterion. Taking that into consideration and limiting prevalence estimates to those obtained using diagnostic criteria, the range narrows in seven studies to 2.2% to 6.9%. Several factors appeared to influence estimates in these studies. Higher rates were obtained when scales were used to assess hypochondriasis than when diagnostic criteria were employed. In addition, studies that focused upon a single diagnosis—in this case hypochondriasis—yielded higher rates than those that assessed all psychiatric diagnoses.

Hypochondriacal concerns appear to be higher in medical patients than in the general population, and higher still among psychiatric patients (Kellner *et al.*, 1983–84; Speckens *et al.*, 1996a). Seeking treatment on the part of hypochondriacal persons likely contributes to these differences, but experience with illness and interaction with physicians may also contribute (Barsky *et al.*, 1986b). Also, among psychiatric patients, hypochondriasis frequently accompanies anxiety and depressive syndromes, which may contribute to its occurrence.

Hypochondriasis may be especially prevalent among medical specialty populations where large proportions of patients have functional disturbances. For instance, one survey identified hypochondriasis among 13% of otolaryngology clinic patients (Schmidt *et al.*, 1993). These patients made frequent use of medical services and took large amounts of medicine. They also had a more negative view of their health despite being less ill than nonhypochondriacal patients. Furthermore, when the level of hypochondriasis is compared in patients with functional and organic conditions, it has tended to be higher in the former. For example, Gomborone *et al.* (1995) observed higher hypochondriasis scores in irritable bowel patients than in patients with organic gastrointestinal disease or in

**Table 6.1.** Studies examining the prevalence of hypochondriasis in primary care populations

| | N | Population | Criteria* | Percent | Comment |
|---|---|---|---|---|---|
| Kellner *et al.* (1983–84) | 44 | Family practice | Illness Attitude Scales | 9.3 | 2.0% of employees hypochondriacal |
| Beaber and Rodney (1984) | 109 | Family practice | Whiteley Index ≥10 | 5.5 | |
| Palsson (1988) | 78 | General practice (Sweden) | Whiteley Index ≥6 | 10.3 | Subtypes of hypochondriasis identified |
| Barsky *et al.* (1990a) | 1,389 | General medical | SCID | 6.3 | Estimate based on structured interview and diagnostic criteria |
| Kirmayer and Robbins (1991) | 685 | Family practice | Illness Worry Scale ≥4 | 7.7 | Patients with hypochondriacal worry distinguished from other forms of somatization |
| van Hemert *et al.* (1993) | 191 | General medical | Present State Examination, *DSM-II-R* | 4.7 | Hypochondriasis more frequent among patients with unexplained symptoms |
| El-Rufaie and Absood (1993) | 217 | Primary care | Clinical Interview Schedule, ICD-9 | 2.3 | Represents less than 10% of minor psychiatric disorders |
| Noyes *et al.* (1994a) | 1,182 | General medical | SCID | 6.9 | |
| Spitzer *et al.* (1994) | 1,000 | Primary care | PRIME-MD, *DSM-IV* | 2.2 | |
| Preveler *et al.* (1997) | 175 | Primary care | Whiteley Index ≥6 | 9.0 | |
| Gureje *et al.* (1997) | 5,447 | Primary care (cross-national) | CIDI, ICD-10 | 0.8 | 2.2% if failure of reassurance criterion set aside |
| Escoar *et al.* (1998) | 1,456 | Primary care | CIDI, *DSM-IV* | 3.4 | |

*SCID = Structured Clinical Interview for *DSM-II-R*; CIDI = Composite International Diagnostic Interview.

healthy volunteers. Similarly, dyspeptic patients without evidence of *Helicobacter pylori* infection achieved higher hypochondriasis scores than did those with infection (Andersson *et al.*, 1994). In contrast, the level of hypochondriasis was not higher in patients with fibromyalgia compared to those with rheumatoid arthritis (Robbins *et al.*, 1990).

As might be expected, hypochondriasis appears to be especially high among medical inpatients. Using a cutoff on the Whiteley Index of 8, Mabe *et al.* (1988) identified a third of hospitalized patients on various medical wards as having hypochondriasis. Likewise, Pilowsky and Spence (1983) reported higher mean scores on this measure among medical inpatients than among outpatients. And, Fava *et al.* (1982) found hypochondriacal concerns related to depression among inpatients.

## Psychiatric Patients

The prevalence of hypochondriasis in psychiatric populations appears especially high, but estimates are quite variable and difficult to evaluate. Definitions have ranged from unexplained somatic symptoms to unfounded fear of disease. Population studies have included inpatients as well as outpatients, and among the former, delusional as well as nondelusional cases. In addition, most interest has focused on particular diagnostic groups, especially depressive and anxiety disorders, which were themselves variously selected. Few studies used recently developed diagnostic criteria.

Among unselected outpatients, Ray and Advani (1962) identified 13% as having hypochondriasis, and Kellner *et al.* (1983–84) found 12% to 22% to be hypochondriacal based on responses to the Illness Attitude Scales. In a study of unselected inpatients, Brown (1936) identified 45% as hypochondriacal, and Stenback and Rimon (1964) assigned this label to 30% based on clinical assessment. They reported higher rates among neurotic (49%) than among psychotic (22%) patients.

Not many psychiatric patients are given the diagnosis of hypochondriasis. Kenyon (1964), for example, reported that only 0.9% of outpatients and 1.0% of inpatients had received hypochondriasis as a primary diagnosis. Similarly, among patients with medically unexplained symptoms seen on a psychiatric consultation service, only 3% were diagnosed as having hypochondriasis (Slavney and Teitelbaum, 1985).

## Risk Factors

Risk factors for unexplained somatic symptoms include female gender, younger age, nonwhite race, less education, and lower income (Escobar *et al.*, 1991). However, relatively few of these factors appear important for hypochondriasis. As reviewed by Barsky *et al.* (1990a) and Hernandez and Kellner (1992), findings with respect to gender and age have been inconsistent. Although Noyes *et al.* (1993) found that hypochondriacal subjects were more often women (80% vs. 58%, $P <$ 0.002) and younger (40 years vs. 48 years, $P < 0.0001$) than new patients attending the clinic in which their study was conducted, Barsky *et al.* (1990a) and Gureje *et al.* (1997) reported that gender and age distributions reflected the clinical populations from which they drew their samples. Also, Barsky *et al.* (1991a) found no relationship between age and hypochondriasis. In their study, hypochondriacal patients were not older than comparison patients. In addition, hypochondriacal patients over age 65 did not differ from those who were younger with respect to hypochondriacal attitudes, somatization, tendency to amplify bodily sensations, or global assessment of health.

With respect to other demographic variables, Kirmayer and Robbins (1991) reported that their hypochondriacal somatizers had fewer years of education and lower income than did nonsomatizing patients. Furthermore, Gerdes *et al.* (1996) observed a negative correlation ($r = -0.27$) between level of education and Whiteley Index scores. Otherwise, few relationships with educational attainment or occupational level have been observed (Barsky *et al.*, 1990a; Noyes *et al.*, 1993). Barsky *et al.* (1990a) reported that hypochondriacal patients were more likely to be black, even after socioeconomic status had been taken into account.

Studies have shown that patients with multiple somatic symptoms, even somatization disorder, have no more physical disease than do other patients of comparable age (Coryell, 1981; Smith *et al.*, 1986). The same situation appears to apply to those with hypochondriasis. In primary care samples, no relationship between severity of documented physical disease and hypochondriasis has been found (Barsky *et al.*, 1992a; Noyes *et al.*, 1993). Gureje *et al.* (1997) reported that more hypochondriacal patients were rated by examining physicians as having moderate to severe physical illness (29% vs. 17%, $P < 0.001$). However, more of these patients were referred for further diagnostic investigation, reflecting physicians' uncertainty. Also, when physician ratings of overall health were controlled for physical illness, no differences remained. Barsky *et al.* (1991b) were unable to find any relationship between physical illness and hypochondriasis. In their sample of medical outpatients, they observed no difference in aggregate medical morbidity between hypochondriacal and comparison patients. Within the comparison sample, higher levels of morbidity were associated with higher levels of hypochondriasis. This was because the most serious illnesses were associated with bodily preoccupation, disease conviction, and somatization. However, within the hypochondriacal sample, no significant correlation existed between medical morbidity and level of hypochondriasis. Noyes *et al.* (1993) replicated these findings. This lack of relationship to medical illness is consistent with the lack of association with age (Costa and McCrae, 1985a). Acute experience with illness may give rise to transient, but not persistent, hypochondriasis (Barsky *et al.*, 1993).

Beyond demographic and illness (coexisting physical and psychiatric) variables, not very much is known about risk factors that may be important in the development of hypochondriasis (Barsky and Klerman, 1983). Most studies have involved patients with somatization, not hypochondriasis specifically (Robbins and Kirmayer, 1991; Stuart and Noyes, 1999). Also, most studies have examined highly selected samples and have compared cases and controls. These studies provide clues for future epidemiological inquiry, however.

For instance, childhood environment may prove important in the development of adult hypochondriasis (Bianchi, 1971). Factors might include childhood illness, parental illness, parental attitudes (e.g., lack of care, overprotection), and childhood trauma (e.g., sexual, physical). In their study of primary care outpatients, Craig *et al.* (1993) obtained reports of severe physical illness in childhood and adverse early environment, including physical and sexual abuse, more often from adult somatizers than from medical patients. Barsky *et al.* (1994a) examined childhood variables in hypochondriacal medical outpatients and found reports of childhood illness and abuse more frequent in hypochondriacal than in control patients. Also, Mabe *et al.* (1988) found a history of serious childhood illness correlated with hypochondriacal symptoms in medical inpatients.

Likewise, not much is known about physiologic vulnerability or personality predisposition to hypochondriasis (Kirmayer *et al.*, 1994). Using a screening instrument, Barsky *et al.* (1992b) identified almost two-thirds of hypochondriacal medical patients as having high likelihood of a personality disorder, compared to 17% of nonhypochondriacal patients. Various personality traits have been described, including anxious, obsessional, narcissistic, and so on, but no systematic studies of personality have been undertaken in hypochondriacal patients. Neuroticism has been observed to correlate with hypochondriasis, but it is difficult to determine whether this is a premorbid characteristic, the result of hypochondriasis, or even of coexisting anxiety and depressive disorders (Hollifield *et al.*, 1999; Noyes *et al.*, 1993). Neuroticism and negative affectivity are related to symptom reporting, and it has been hypothesized that such traits interact with stressful events to produce somatization and hypochondriasis (Pennebaker and Watson, 1991).

Stressful life events may contribute to the development of hypochondriasis, and illness events may be rather specific in this regard. An example is that of "cardiac neurosis" following myocardial infarction. Kellner *et al.* (1983) showed that, among employees of a retail firm, life events were associated with hypochondriacal concerns as well as with other psychological and somatic symptoms. Barsky *et al.* (1990b) observed a group of general medical patients whose elevation in hypochondriacal symptoms had subsided in 3 weeks. Compared to non-hypochondriacal patients they had more lifetime psychiatric disorders, more personality disorders, and more medical disorders. Robbins and Kirmayer (1996) reported similar characteristics in a group of family medicine patients who became hypochondriacal during a year follow-up interval. At initial assessment they had higher levels of illness worry, were more likely to see their health as poor, and displayed more unexplained symptoms. The authors hypothesized that these patients may have been predisposed to hypochondriasis by high levels of illness worry and a learned schema of physical vulnerability.

## Morbidity

Despite the lack of difference in physical disease, patients with hypochondriasis have been shown to be more impaired in physical functioning and work performance than patients who are not hypochondriacal (Barsky et al., 1992a; Noyes et al., 1993). They view their health as worse, are more physically disabled, and are more impaired in their occupational roles than are nonhypochondriacal patients (Gureje et al., 1997). They also use more medical services and are less satisfied with the care they receive. This increased utilization includes the number of physicians seen as well as the number of visits, laboratory tests, medications taken, hospitalizations, and so on (Noyes et al., 1993). According to Gureje et al. (1997), hypochondriacal patients more often disagreed with physicians about their health status. And, according to Noyes et al. (1993), they were more likely than nonhypochondriacal patients to feel that their health problems had not been thoroughly evaluated or explained. Also, Beaber and Rodney (1984) reported that hypochondriacal patients were less likely to keep scheduled appointments. These findings are consistent with those reported by other researchers (Barsky and Wyshak, 1989; Kellner, 1990; Pilowsky et al., 1987).

Hypochondriasis appears to be related to impairment in both functional and organic disease. For example, hypochondriacal scores were related to quality of life and disability in patients with chronic fatigue (Manu et al., 1996), irritable bowel syndrome (Gomborone et al., 1995), and fibromyalgia (Robbins et al., 1990). Lichtenberg et al. (1986) reported that hypochondriasis was the strongest predictor of pain due to osteoarthritis. Likewise, hypochondriasis was among the predictors of angina and disability in patients with coronary artery disease (Hlatky et al., 1986; Williams et al., 1986). Similarly, both impairment and disability among patients with chronic lung disease are related to fear of illness and hypochondriasis arising from anxiety-provoking breathlessness and asthmatic attacks (Noyes and Hoehn-Saric, 1998). Of course, distressing symptoms and disability may provoke hypochondriacal concerns, and hypochondriacal worry may, in turn, increase symptoms and lead to disproportionate impairment, thus creating a vicious circle (Kellner, 1990).

As is true of patients with other psychiatric disorders, hypochondriacal patients tend not to be recognized by primary care physicians. In fact, studies have shown that the diagnosis is almost never made (Beaber and Rodney, 1984; Noyes *et al.*, 1993; Palsson, 1988). However, physician recognition apart from diagnosis may be somewhat higher. For instance, Gureje *et al.* (1997) found that more hypochondriacal patients satisfying abridged criteria were identified as psychiatric cases than nonhypochondriacal patients (57.4% vs. 23.5%, $P < 0.0001$). Also, Noyes *et al.* (1993) reported that medical clinic physicians rated hypochondriacal patients higher on unrealistic fear of illness (hypochondriasis) and lower on the extent to which disease explains symptoms. However, Gerdes *et al.* (1996) observed that the basis for this recognition was largely unexplained symptoms. Conversely, Kirmayer *et al.* (1993) showed that hypochondriasis increased the recognition of anxiety disorders among primary care physicians.

## Comorbidity

Hypochondriacal primary care patients have high levels of psychiatric distress, including anxiety, depressive, and somatoform symptoms (Kellner *et al.*, 1987b). A number of studies have shown strong positive correlations between depressive ($r = 0.58$), anxiety ($r = 0.55$), and somatic symptoms ($r = 0.52$) and hypochondriacal concerns among medical outpatients (Barsky *et al.*, 1986a; Noyes *et al.*, 1993). For instance, Gureje *et al.* (1997) observed higher mean General Health Questionnaire (Goldberg and Williams, 1988) scores among their patients with abridged hypochondriasis than among patients without. Scores on the subscales measuring depression, anxiety, and somatization were all significantly higher in their hypochondriacal patients ($P < 0.0001$). They also observed ICD-10 major depression and generalized anxiety disorder in a greater proportion of hypochondriacal patients (36.9% vs. 9.8% and 21.5% vs. 7.5%, respectively). Two studies that examined psychiatric comorbidity among primary care hypochondriacal patients in some detail found greater proportions of hypochondriacal patients with anxiety, depressive, and somatoform disorders (Barsky *et al.*, 1992b; Noyes *et al.*, 1994a).

In both instances, general medical patients with *DSM-III-R* hypochondriasis were compared with a random sample of nonhypochondriacal patients from the same clinic. Findings from these studies are shown in Table 6.2. The proportion of hypochondriacal and control patients having one or more comorbid Axis I disorder was 88% versus 51% in one study and 62% versus 30% in the other. Anxiety and depressive disorders both contributed to the excess among the

**Table 6.2.** Comorbidity identified in patients with *DSM-III-R* hypochondriasis

| | Barsky *et al.* (1992b) | | | Noyes *et al.* (1994a) | | |
|---|---|---|---|---|---|---|
| | Hypochon-driasis subjects (*n* = 42) % | Control subjects (*n* = 76) % | *P* | Hypochon-driasis subjects (*n* = 50) % | Control subjects (*n* = 50) % | *P* |
| Major depressive disorder | 43 | 18 | 0.004 | 28 | 6 | 0.005 |
| Dysthymic disorder | 45 | 9 | 0.0001 | 8 | 2 | *ns* |
| Panic disorder | 17 | 3 | 0.006 | 16 | 6 | *ns* |
| Generalized anxiety disorder | 71 | 28 | 0.0001 | 0 | 0 | *ns* |
| Phobic disorders | 43 | 21 | 0.013 | 6 | 2 | *ns* |
| Obsessive-compulsive disorder | 10 | 3 | 0.04 | 0 | 0 | *ns* |
| Alcohol abuse/ dependence | 10 | 18 | *ns* | 14 | 12 | *ns* |
| Other drug abuse/ dependence | 12 | 4 | *ns* | 8 | 10 | *ns* |
| Somatization disorder | 21 | 0 | 0.0001 | | | |
| Any depressive disorder | 55 | 20 | 0.0001 | 44 | 18 | 0.005 |
| Any anxiety disorder | 86 | 36 | 0.01 | 22 | 6 | 0.02 |
| Any substance abuse/dependence | 17 | 20 | *ns* | 20 | 18 | *ns* |

*ns* = nonsignificant.

hypochondriacal group. Odds ratios for any lifetime anxiety disorder (5.9) and any depressive disorder (4.9) were significant, as were odds ratios for most individual disorders. Findings from these studies are quite similar except for generalized anxiety disorder and dysthymia, diagnoses that may be less reliable in medical patients.

Several studies have shown that only a small proportion of hypochondriacal patients qualify for a diagnosis of somatization disorder, but that a much higher proportion meet criteria for the subsyndromal disorder. Rates for somatization disorder (requiring 14 symptoms for women and 12 for men) ranged from 7% to 21%, but for the subsyndromal disorder (requiring 6 and 4 symptoms, respectively) they ranged from 32% to 83% (Barsky *et al.*, 1992b; Escobar *et al.*, 1998; Kirmayer and Robbins, 1991; Noyes *et al.*, 1994a). Barsky *et al.* (1992b) found that the symptoms of somatization disorder were not correlated with hypochondriasis but that other functional somatic symptoms were. They suggested that these disorders might be distinguishable on the basis of type of somatic symptoms.

## Relationship to Depression

Hypochondriasis has been viewed by some as a manifestation of depression. Kenyon (1964), for example, reported that, among inpatients, hypochondriasis was almost always secondary to another disorder, usually depression. This view prompted surveys of its prevalence among depressed psychiatric patients and examination of the relationship between these disorders. Demopulos *et al.* (1996) found hypochondriacal symptoms prominent among depressed outpatients although few met *DSM-III-R* criteria for hypochondriasis. Among depressed inpatients, however, estimates based on clinical assessment have ranged from 18% to 69% (Bianchi, 1973; El-Islam *et al.*, 1988; Kellner *et al.*, 1986b; Lewis, 1934; Stenback and Jalava, 1961). Two studies reported rates of 60% and 64% among elderly depressed inpatients (de Alarcon, 1964; Kramer-Ginsberg *et al.*, 1989).

Various authors have examined the temporal relationship between hypochondriasis and depression to see which might be primary. De Alarcon (1964) found that hypochondriacal symptoms usually develop during the course of a depressive syndrome. According to this author, only 19.5% of patients had lifelong hypochondriacal concerns. Also, Burns and Nichols (1972) reported that many depressed patients with chest symptoms had fear or conviction of disease (sometimes of delusional proportions) that remitted after treatment with antidepressants or electrotherapy. Similarly, Kellner *et al.* (1986b) observed that, while over a third of their melancholic patients were hypochondriacal, only 5% remained so after treatment. However, both Kramer-Ginsberg *et al.* (1989) and Demopulos *et al.* (1996) observed some persistence of hypochondriacal concerns after antidepressant treatment and concluded that such features are a mixture of state and trait phenomena.

Few differences have been found between hypochondriacal and nonhypochondriacal depressed patients to explain the relationship. Neither Kramer-Ginsberg *et al.* (1989) nor Demopulos *et al.* (1996) found any relationship between hypochondriacal features and severity of depression, but both found associations with anxiety and somatic symptoms. Likewise, few variables contributing to hypochondriasis in depressed patients have been identified. A high frequency of hypochondriasis among elderly depressives suggests that age might be a factor. In fact, Brown *et al.* (1984) observed that depressed patients over age 50 had more hypochondriasis as well as agitation and initial insomnia than did those under age 50. However, within a population age 60 and older, Kramer-Ginsberg *et al.* (1989) found no relationship to age. According to Ball and Clare (1990), cultural factors may be important. These authors found hypochondriasis more common in Jewish compared to non-Jewish depressive patients, confirming earlier observations.

## Relationship to Anxiety

Just as some have viewed hypochondriasis as a manifestation of depression, others have seen it as a feature of anxiety (Noyes, 1999). Although relationships between several anxiety disorders have been considered, most interest has focused on panic disorder. Noyes *et al.* (1986) and Fava *et al.* (1988) reported that patients with panic disorder and agoraphobia scored nearly as high on measures of hypochondriasis as hypochondriacal psychiatric patients. Also, Starcevic *et al.* (1992) found that half of their panic patients scored in the hypochondriacal range on the Illness Attitude Scales, and Bach *et al.* (1996), Benedetti *et al.* (1997), and Furer *et al.* (1997) found that between 45% and 51% of their patients with panic disorder and agoraphobia met *DSM-III-R* criteria for hypochondriasis. Furer *et al.* (1997) found hypochondriasis in a greater proportion of patients with panic disorder (48%) than in patients with social phobia (17%) or controls (14%).

To explore the relationship further, several authors sought to determine what features of panic disorder might be most closely associated with hypochondriasis. Starcevic *et al.* (1992) found a strong relationship between hypochondriacal concerns and agoraphobia in a series of panic patients. They speculated that hypochondriacal features might be attributed to greater severity of panic disorder or that hypochondriasis might be associated with agoraphobia. However, other investigators failed to find such an association (Bach *et al.*, 1996; Benedetti *et al.*, 1997; Otto *et al.*, 1992). Instead, Otto *et al.* (1992) found hypochondriacal concerns most strongly associated with anxiety sensitivity. Anxiety sensitivity, a fear of anxiety symptoms, and a tendency to respond anxiously to arousal, appears common to both panic disorder and hypochondriasis and may have explanatory significance for both.

Several studies have examined the temporal relationship of panic disorder and hypochondriasis in an effort to understand further the relationship between them. In three of these, Fava *et al.* (1988, 1992) and Benedetti *et al.* (1997) found hypochondriacal concerns or illness phobia in a substantial proportion of panic patients prior to their first attacks. The researchers speculated that these early symptoms might represent predisposing factors, prodromes, or early manifestations of panic disorder; they further speculated that they might also constitute separate disorders (Fava and Kellner, 1993). For instance, Fava *et al.* (1990) identified a series of cases in which not only did hypochondriasis precede the onset of panic disorder but attacks arose from hypochondriacal concerns. Attacks were prompted in these patients by fearful hypochondriacal cognitions; pharmacological treatment, while reducing panic, had little effect on hypochondriasis.

The studies cited involved psychiatric populations, and only the most recent study employed diagnostic criteria. When this was done, findings were somewhat different. Barsky *et al.* (1994b) examined the relationship of *DSM-III-R* panic disorder and hypochondriasis in a general medicine clinic. They found that 25% of panic patients had current hypochondriasis and 13% of hypochondriacal patients had current panic disorder. Although the disorders co-existed more often than expected by chance, patients more often had them separately than concurrently. Also, they differed demographically; patients with hypochondriasis were older and more often women than were those with panic disorder. In addition, patients with the two disorders had somewhat different patterns of comorbidity. Barsky *et al.* (1994b) concluded that, despite the overlap between them, hypochondriasis and panic disorder are independent disorders.

Other anxiety disorders with definitional or phenomenological resemblance to hypochondriasis include specific phobia, generalized anxiety disorder, and obsessive-compulsive disorders (Noyes, 1999). Specific phobia of illness, although prevalent in the general population, has received little study (Agras *et al.*, 1969). Worry about health or illness may also occur as a part of generalized anxiety disorder, but according to Starcevic *et al.* (1994) such worries are infrequent. In their series, 31% of patients worried about health, but only 18% had hypochondriasis. Others have reported similar findings (Borkovec *et al.*, 1991; Craske *et al.*, 1989; Sanderson and Barlow, 1990). Obsessions may involve fears of illness, injury or contamination, and compulsions may involve checking the body for signs of illness and cleaning to prevent infection or toxic exposure. In one series of patients with obsessive-compulsive disorder (OCD), 33% had somatic obsessions and 50% had obsessions involving contamination (Rasmussen and Eisen, 1992). There is, however, only one estimate of the prevalence of hypochondriasis in such patients. Using the Illness Attitude Scales, Savron *et al.* (1996) identified only 10% of patients with OCD as hypochondriacal.

## Family and Twin Data

Often, family and twin studies not only provide evidence for the validity of diagnostic categories but also yield information about the contribution of genetic and environmental factors to the development of psychiatric disorders. For example, a series of family studies of somatization disorder and its forerunner, Briquet's syndrome, showed that not only is this disturbance prevalent among female family members but also that it is associated with antisocial personality disorder among male relatives (Guze *et al.*, 1986). These findings of family aggregation were supportive of validity and suggested that genetic factors might have a role in transmission (Coryell, 1980). However, few such studies have been undertaken for other somatoform disorders such as hypochondriasis.

Recently, Noyes *et al.* (1997) completed a preliminary family study of hypochondriasis. Nineteen probands meeting *DSM-III-R* criteria for hypochondriasis were identified in a general medicine clinic, and 24 nonhypochondriacal control probands were obtained from the same clinic. Available first-degree relatives of these probands were interviewed blindly using the Structured Diagnostic Interview for *DSM-IV* (First *et al.*, 1997). As shown in Table 6.3, no significant differences existed in the frequency of lifetime or current psychiatric diagnoses except that somatization disorder was more frequent among relatives of hypochondriasis probands. There was a trend toward greater frequency of anxiety disorders among the hypochondriasis relatives as well. Also, no differences were observed between hypochondriasis and control relatives on measures of hypochondriasis, including the Whiteley Index, Illness Attitude Scales, MMPI hypochondriasis scale, and Somatosensory Amplification Scale (Barsky *et al.*, 1990c).

**Table 6.3.** Frequency of lifetime and current psychiatric diagnoses in interviewed first-degree relatives of probands with hypochondriasis and control probands

|  | Lifetime diagnoses | | Current diagnoses | |
|---|---|---|---|---|
|  | Hypochon-driasis relatives $n = 72$ % | Control relatives $n = 97$ % | Hypochon-driasis relatives $n = 72$ % | Control relatives $n = 97$ % |
| Major depressive disorder | 31.9 | 34.0 | 11.3 | 8.2 |
| Dysthymia[†] | 4.2 | 1.0 | 4.2 | 1.0 |
| Alcohol abuse or dependence | 30.6 | 29.9 | 4.2 | 6.2 |
| Drug abuse or dependence | 9.7 | 8.2 | 0.0 | 2.1 |
| Panic disorder | 9.7 | 10.3 | 5.6 | 7.2 |
| Agoraphobia | 4.2 | 4.1 | 4.2 | 3.1 |
| Social phobia | 11.1 | 6.2 | 5.6 | 2.1 |
| Specific phobia | 8.3 | 9.3 | 8.5 | 5.2 |
| Generalized anxiety disorder[†] | 9.7 | 3.1 | 9.7 | 3.1 |
| Posttraumatic stress disorder | 11.1 | 8.2 | 2.8 | 1.0 |
| Obsessive-compulsive disorder | 1.4 | 1.0 | 1.4 | 1.0 |
| Somatization disorder | 12.5 | 3.1** | 12.5 | 3.1** |
| Hypochondriasis | 6.9 | 8.2 | 6.9 | 8.2 |
| Other somatoform disorders | 2.8 | 2.0 | 2.8 | 2.0 |

[†]Current diagnoses only.

**P < 0.05.

Although the relatives of hypochondriasis probands did not differ from relatives of control probands with respect to hypochondriasis, they did differ on several measures of somatic and psychological symptoms, attitude toward health care, and personality traits. Hypochondriasis relatives scored significantly higher on the somatization, obsessive-compulsive, hostility, paranoid ideation, and psychoticism subscales of the Brief Symptom Inventory (Derogatis and Spencer, 1983). They also rated themselves as having poorer social adjustment on the Functional Status Questionnaire (Jette *et al.*, 1986). With respect to health care, hypochondriasis relatives had a less favorable attitude toward doctors, responded less well to treatment, and were less satisfied with the care they received than were control relatives. Concerning personality, hypochondriasis relatives scored lower on the dimensions of agreeableness and conscientiousness (NEO Personality Inventory; Costa and McCrae, 1985b) and higher on the alexithymic dimension of inability to express feelings.

The findings from this study suggest that hypochondriasis is not familial. They indicate that this may not be an independent disorder but a variable feature of other psychiatric disorders, involving other dimensions of psychopathology (e.g., symptoms, personality, and so on). In this study, an association between hypochondriasis and somatization disorder was observed. As indicated earlier, a number of studies have found that these somatoform disorders coexist. Both are characterized by multiple unexplained somatic symptoms, and the boundary between them seems far from clear. Hypochondriacal relatives did differ from control relatives on a number of interrelated symptoms, traits, and attitudes often associated with somatization. Perhaps the most consistent finding from the study by Noyes and associates was that these relatives scored higher on measures of mistrust and antagonism in interpersonal relationships. Such traits and attitudes, often seen in patients with somatization disorder and hypochondriasis, may confer a vulnerability to somatoform disorders.

Findings from the family study suggest that hypochondriasis and somatization disorder, as defined in *DSM-IV*, are closely related. The question concerns how they are related and how future studies might address this relationship. It may simply be one of definitional overlap (Schmidt, 1994). For instance, few studies have compared the somatic symptoms of hypochondriasis (once located in the hypochondriac region below the costal cartilages) and somatization disorder, and while attitudinal differences have been proposed, few studies have examined them. According to ICD-10, hypochondriacal patients are concerned with the possible presence of serious disease and its consequences, whereas patients with multiform somatization disorder are preoccupied with individual symptoms (World Health Organization, 1993). In addition, hypochondriacal patients are believed to seek reassurance, whereas those with somatization disorder seek sanction for the sick role (Murphy, 1990). But, as indicated earlier, important demographic differences exist despite extensive overlap (see also Chapter 2).

The Swedish adoption study of somatoform disorders conducted by Cloninger, Sigvardsson and colleagues is relevant to the classification of hypochondriasis (Bohman et al., 1984; Cloninger et al., 1984, 1986; Sigvardsson et al., 1984, 1986). Based upon information available on individuals adopted at an early age, these investigators identified two distinct groups of somatizers. Adoptees consisted of nearly 1800 men and women born in Stockholm prior to 1949. "Asthenic somatizers" had a lower frequency and diversity of complaints but were more often disabled by fatigue, weakness or common minor illnesses. "Diversiform somatizers" had higher frequency of brief sickness with a wide diversity of complaints, especially pain in the head, joints, and abdomen. Asthenic somatizers, who more closely resembled hypochondriacal patients, were more often men, whereas diversiform somatizers were more often women. Men with asthenic somatization were characterized by high cognitive anxiety, high anticipatory anxiety, slow recuperation from stress, and low sociability. The separation of two discrete clinical disorders was supported by a finding of lower criminality among the biological parents of asthenic somatizers than among the parents of nonsomatizers. The investigators concluded that genetic factors are important in men with asthenic somatization. This investigation relied upon limited registry data, and it is not clear to what extent the disorders that were identified resemble those found in current classifications.

Data concerning twins with hypochondriasis are likewise sparse (Shields, 1962). An early twin study by Gottesman (1962) found no correlation between adolescent monozygotic twins on the hypochondriasis scale of the MMPI. However, in a later study, the same group found a modest correlation ($r = 0.30$) on the scale between twins reared apart (Gottesman et al., 1984). These results are difficult to interpret because physical illness was not controlled for and the hypochondriasis scale measures only physical symptoms. Based on a twin study of somatoform disorders, Torgersen (1986) concluded that these disorders are familial. However, he found little evidence of genetic transmission for hypochondriasis. Six of his probands, who had been psychiatric inpatients, had hypochondriasis but none of their co-twins (two monozygotic and four dizygotic) had the same disorder. One had major depression and the remainder had no psychiatric disorder. In addition, two co-twins had hypochondriasis. The proband for one (monozygotic) had conversion disorder and the other (dizygotic) had pain disorder. Torgersen (1986) found an increase in generalized anxiety disorder among the co-twins of probands with somatoform disorders, supporting findings from family and adoption studies.

Recently, a population-based twin study of blood-injury fears and phobias was reported (Neale et al., 1994). Because the relationship between fears of blood, needles, hospitals, and illness—which were examined as a group in this study—is uncertain, it is not clear how the findings may apply to hypochondriasis. However, 11 of the 124 female probands who reported fear of illness alone were examined separately. The tetrachoric correlations for fear of illness were 0.26 for monozygotic and 0.32 for dizygotic twins. Fear of illness appeared to aggregate within families, based more on shared environmental than on genetic factors. This fear appeared separate from blood-injury fear, which was strongly influenced by genetic factors. The results suggest that blood-injury phobia with or without illness phobia develops in response to traumatic events (classical conditioning) and some social learning (modeling). However, susceptibility to classical conditioning may be influenced by genetic factors (Neale *et al.*, 1994).

## Natural History

Follow-up of representative samples may not only provide evidence of diagnostic stability, as mentioned earlier, but also indicate what factors influence the course and outcome of a disorder, in this case hypochondriasis. Four studies examined the course of representative primary care patients with hypochondriasis or hypochondriacal worry (Barsky *et al.*, 1990b, 1998; Noyes *et al.*, 1994b; Robbins and Kirmayer, 1996). Barsky *et al.* (1990b) identified a group of patients with transient hypochondriasis. These were patients who scored high on measures of hypochondriasis but failed to meet *DSM-III-R* criteria for the disorder. When reassessed 3 weeks after their visit to the medical clinic, their hypochondriacal symptoms had decreased substantially. Compared with hypochondriacal patients, the transiently hypochondriacal patients had fewer psychiatric disorders and more medical morbidity, but compared to nonhypochondriacal patients they had more psychiatric disorders, more personality pathology, greater somatosensory amplification, and more medical disorders. Barsky *et al.* (1990b) concluded that, when confronted with physical illness, patients with psychiatric symptoms, personality pathology, and sensitivity to somatic sensations are more likely to develop transient hypochondriasis.

Noyes *et al.* (1994b) and Robbins and Kirmayer (1996) followed patients for a year and examined predictors of remission or reduction in Illness Worry Scale scores. Noyes *et al.* (1994b) found that two-thirds of their subjects with *DSM-III-R* hypochondriasis continued to meet criteria for the disorder after a year, and the remaining third had persisting hypochondriacal symptoms. The hypochondriacal subjects as a whole were improved on most measures but still differed from control subjects with regard to attitudes, perceptions, and behaviors that had distinguished them initially. More severe symptoms, longer duration of hypochondriasis, and coexisting psychiatric illness were all predictive of a worse outcome. Neuroticism, a measure of personality psychopathology, was also associated with sustained hypochondriasis. Robbins and Kirmayer (1996) reported similar findings for their patients with hypochondriacal worry, about half of whom showed persisting symptoms and the other half, transient symptoms. In addition to psychiatric comorbidity, they found fears of emotional instability, pathological symptom attribution, and interpersonal vulnerability among those who had continuing hypochondriasis.

Barsky *et al.* (1998) reported similar findings from a long-term follow-up study of hypochondriacal outpatients. After 5 years, these patients showed considerable decline in symptoms and improvement in role functioning, but two-thirds still met criteria for hypochondriasis. At follow-up, the hypochondriacal patients remained substantially more hypochondriacal, had more somatization and somatosensory amplification, were more functionally impaired, and more psychiatrically disordered than were nonhypochondriacal patients. The researchers concluded that hypochondriasis carries a substantial long-term burden of morbidity, functional impairment, and personal distress.

## Conclusion

Community surveys of hypochondriasis are needed to address critical questions related to this syndrome. Such surveys are important because clinical populations are influenced by treatment-seeking, a bias that appears especially important in the case of hypochondriasis. Two-step screening procedures, using a modified Whiteley Index followed by the hypochondriasis module of the Structured Clinical Interview for *DSM-III-R*, have shown satisfactory reliability and validity. One problem for community surveys, as for studies of hypochondriasis in general, is accurate assessment of physical health status, which often requires physical examination and testing. Of course, one important issue has to do with the relationship of hypochondriasis to physical illness, both acute and chronic. Another has to do with its relationship to psychiatric illness. Studies examining comorbidity must attempt to determine the temporal relationship as well as predominance of one disturbance or the other.

There appears to be considerable heterogeneity within the category of hypochondriasis as well as overlap with other somatoform disorders. Some patients appear to have primary hypochondriasis, whereas others have hypochondriacal syndromes that are secondary, meaning that hypochondriasis is limited to an episode of a more pervasive disorder (e.g., major depression). Also, there may be subtypes of hypochondriasis. Some patients may be more disease phobic, whereas others may have more disease conviction; the former tend to have anxious features and the latter may be closer to depression (Barsky, 1992). The relationship of hypochondriasis to illness phobia, which may be prevalent in the population, remains unexplored as does the relationship of both to blood-injury phobia. Part of the importance of these disorders is the impact they may have on medical care, an aspect that takes on increasing importance in an age of preventive services and efforts to control the costs of care (Barsky and Borus, 1995). Both persistent treatment-seeking and avoidance of health care are likely to have a major impact on outcomes.

Information concerning risk factors for hypochondriasis is very limited at present. There is little evidence that demographic variables are important, and this lack of relationship may distinguish hypochondriacal patients from those with somatization or somatization disorder. Still, we should remember that gender has been related historically to hypochondriasis, and there is evidence from an adoption study for gender-specific somatoform syndromes (Cloninger *et al.*, 1984). A model for the development of hypochondriasis might assume some genetically determined traits such as neuroticism or negative affectivity. Developmental factors might encompass adverse early environment, including negative parental attitudes and childhood experience of illness. Adult vulnerability that is increased by general psychopathology might include an amplifying perceptual style and cognitive schema of serious illness.

Finally, stressful life events might, in susceptible individuals, produce hypochondriacal symptoms that are reinforced by interpersonal and social factors, including gains of illness. A model of this kind, based on clinical studies, awaits verification through epidemiologic investigation.

## References

Agras S., Sylvester D., Oliveau D. 1969. The epidemiology of common fears and phobia. *Comprehensive Psychiatry* 10: 151 156.

American Psychiatric Association. 1987. *Diagnostic and Statistical Manual of Mental Disorders, Third Edition, Revised* (*DSM-III-R*), Washington, DC: American Psychiatric Association.

American Psychiatric Association. 1994. *Diagnostic and Statistical Manual of Mental Disorders, Fourth Edition* (*DSM-IV*), Washington, DC: American Psychiatric Association.

Andersson S.I., Hovelius B., Molstad S., Wadstrom T. 1994. Dyspepsia in general practice: psychological findings in relation to *Helicobacter pylori* serum antibodies. *Journal of Psychosomatic Research* 38: 241–247.

Bach M., Nutzinger D.O., Hartl L. 1996. Comorbidity of anxiety disorders and hypochondriasis considering different diagnostic systems. *Comprehensive Psychiatry* 37: 62–67.

Ball R.A., Clare A.W. 1990. Symptoms and social adjustment in Jewish depressives. *British Journal of Psychiatry* 156: 379-383.

Barsky A.J. 1992. Hypochondriasis and obsessive-compulsive disorder. *Psychiatric Clinics of North America* 15: 791–801.

Barsky A.J., Klerman G.L. 1983. Overview: hypochondriasis, bodily complaints and somatic styles. *American Journal of Psychiatry* 140: 273–282.

Barsky A.J., Wyshak G. 1989. Hypochondriasis and related health attitudes. *Psychosomatics* 30: 412–420.

Barsky A.J., Borus J.F. 1995. Somatization and medicalization in the era of managed care. *Journal of the American Medical Association* 274: 1931–1934.

Barsky A.J., Wyshak G., Klerman G.L. 1986a. Hypochondriasis: an evaluation of the *DSM-III* criteria in medical outpatients. *Archives of General Psychiatry* 43: 493–500.

Barsky A.J., Wyshak G., Klerman G.L. 1986b. Medical and psychiatric determinants of outpatient medical utilization. *Medical Care* 24: 548–560.

Barsky A.J., Klerman G.L., Wyshak G., Latham K.S. 1990a. The prevalence of hypochondriasis in medical outpatients. *Social Psychiatry and Psychiatric Epidemiology* 14: 89–94.

Barsky A.J., Wyshak G., Klerman G.L. 1990b. Transient hypochondriasis. *Archives of General Psychiatry* 47: 746–752.

Barsky A.J., Wyshak G., Klerman G.L. 1990c. The Somatosensory Amplification Scale and its relationship to hypochondriasis. *Journal of Psychiatric Research* 24: 323–334.

Barsky A.J., Frank C.B., Cleary P.D., Wyshak G., Klerman G.L. 1991a. The relation between hypochondriasis and age. *American Journal of Psychiatry* 148: 923–928.

Barsky A.J., Wyshak G., Klerman G.L. 1991b. The relationship between hypochondriasis and medical illness. *Archives of Internal Medicine* 151: 84–88.

Barsky A.J., Cleary P.D., Wyshak G., Spitzer R.L., Williams J.B.W., Klerman G.L. 1992a. A structured diagnostic interview for hypochondriasis: a proposed criterion standard. *Journal of Nervous and Mental Disease* 180: 20-27.

Barsky A.J., Wyshak G., Klerman G.L. 1992b. Psychiatric comorbidity in *DSM-III-R* hypochondriasis. *Archives of General Psychiatry* 49: 101–108.

Barsky A.J., Cleary P.D., Sarnie M.K., Klerman G.L. 1993. The course of transient hypochondriasis. *American Journal of Psychiatry* 150: 484–488.

Barsky A.J., Wool C., Barnett M.C., Cleary P.D. 1994a. Histories of childhood trauma in adult hypochondriacal patients. *American Journal of Psychiatry* 151: 397–401.

Barsky A.J., Barnett M.C., Cleary P.D. 1994b. Hypochondriasis and panic disorder: boundary and overlap. *Archives of General Psychiatry* 51: 918-925.

Barsky A.J., Fama J.M., Bailey E.D., Ahern D.K. 1998. A prospective 4- to 5-year study of DSM-III-R hypochondriasis. *Archives of General Psychiatry* 55: 737–744.

Beaber R.J., Rodney W.M. 1984. Underdiagnosis of hypochondriasis in family practice. *Psychosomatics* 25: 39–45.

Benedetti A., Perugi G., Toni C., Simonetti B., Mata B., Cassano G.B. 1997. Hypochondriasis and illness phobia in panic-agoraphobic patients. *Comprehensive Psychiatry* 38: 124–131.

Bianchi G.N. 1971. The origins of disease phobia. *Australian and New Zealand Journal of Psychiatry* 5: 241–257.

Bianchi G.N. 1973. Patterns of hypochondriasis: a principal components analysis. *British Journal of Psychiatry* 122: 541–548.

Bohman M., Cloninger C.R., von Knorring A-L., Sigvardsson S. 1984. An adoption study of somatoform disorders: III. Cross-fostering analysis and genetic relationship to alcoholism and criminality. *Archives of General Psychiatry* 41: 872–878.

Borkovec T.D., Shadick R.N., Hopkins M. 1991. The nature of normal and pathological worry. In *Chronic Anxiety: Generalized Anxiety Disorder and Mixed Anxiety-Depression* (eds. Rapee R.M., Barlow D.H.), New York: Guilford Press.

Brown F. 1936. The body complaint: a study of hypochondriasis *Journal of Mental Science* 82: 295–359.

Brown R.P., Soveeney J., Loutsch E., Kocsis J., Frances A. 1984. Involutional melancholia revisited. *American Journal of Psychiatry* 141: 24–28.

Burns B.H., Nichols M.A. 1972. Factors related to the localization of symptoms to the chest in depression. *British Journal of Psychiatry* 121: 405–409.

Cloninger C.R., Sigvardsson S., von Knorring A-L., Bohman M. 1984. An adoption study of somatoform disorders: II. Identification of two discrete disorders. *Archives of General Psychiatry* 41: 863–871.

Cloninger C.R., von Knorring A-L., Sigvardsson S., Bohman M. 1986. Symptom patterns and causes of somatization in men: II. Genetic and environmental independence from somatization in women. *Genetic Epidemiology* 3: 171–185.

Coryell W. 1980. A blind family history study of Briquet's syndrome: further validation of the diagnosis. *Archives of General Psychiatry* 37: 1266–1269.

Coryell W. 1981. Diagnosis-specific mortality: primary unipolar depression and Briquet's syndrome (somatization disorder). *Archives of General Psychiatry* 38: 939–942.

Costa P.T., McCrae R.R. 1985a. Hypochondriasis, neuroticism and aging: when are somatic complaints unfounded? *American Psychologist* 40: 19–28.

Costa P.T., McCrae R.R. 1985b. *The NEO Personality Inventory Manual*. Odessa, FL: Psychological Assessment Resources.

Craig T.K.J., Broadman A.P., Mills K., Daly-Jones O., Drake H. 1993. The South London Somatization Study: I. Longitudinal course and the influence of early life experiences. *British Journal of Psychiatry* 163: 579–588.

Craske M.G., Rapee R.M., Jackel L., Barlow D.H. 1989. Qualitative dimensions of worry in DSM-III-R generalized anxiety disorder subjects and non-anxious controls. *Behaviour Research and Therapy* 27: 397–402.

de Alarcon R. 1964. Hypochondriasis and depression in the aged. *Gerontology Clinics* 6: 266–277.

Demopulos C., Fava M., McLean N.E., Alpert J.E., Nierenberg A.A., Rosenbaum J.F. 1996. Hypochondriacal concerns in depressed outpatients. *Psychosomatic Medicine* 58: 314–320.

Derogatis L.R., Spencer P.M. 1983. *The Brief Symptom Inventory: Administration, Scoring, and Procedures Manual*. Baltimore: Clinical Psychometric Research.

El-Islam M.F., Malasi T.A., Suleiman M.A., Mirza I.A. 1988. The correlates of hypochondriasis in depressed patients. *International Journal of Psychiatry in Medicine* 18: 253–261.

El-Rufaie O.E.F., Absood G.H. 1993. Minor psychiatric morbidity in primary health care: prevalence, nature and severity. *International Journal of Social Psychiatry* 39: 159–166.

Escobar J.I., Swartz M., Rubio-Stipec M., Manu P. 1991. Medically unexplained symptoms: distribution, risk factors and comorbidity. In: *Current Concepts of Somatization: Research and Clinical Perspectives* (eds. Kirmayer L.J., Robbins J.M.), Washington DC: American Psychiatric Press.

Escobar J.I., Gara M., Waitzkin H., Silver R.C., Holman A., Compton W. 1998. DSM-IV hypochondriasis in primary care. *General Hospital Psychiatry* 20: 155–159.

Faravelli C., Salvatori S., Galassi F., Aiazzi L., Drei C., Cabras P. 1997. Epidemiology of somatoform disorders: a community survey in Florence. *Social Psychiatry and Psychiatric Epidemiology* 32: 24–29.

Fava G.A., Pilowsky I., Fierfederici A., Bernardi M., Pathak D. 1982. Depression and illness behavior in a general hospital: a prevalence study. *Psychotherapy and Psychosomatics* 38: 141–153.

Fava G.A., Kellner R., Zielezny M., Grandi S. 1988. Hypochondriacal fears and beliefs in agoraphobia. *Journal of Affective Disorders* 14: 239–244.

Fava G.A., Grandi S., Saviotti F.M., Conti S. 1990. Hypochondriasis with panic attacks. *Psychosomatics* 31: 351–353.

Fava G.A., Grandi S., Rafanelli C., Canestrari R. 1992. Prodromal symptoms in panic disorder with agoraphobia: a replication study. *Journal of Affective Disorders* 26: 85–88.

Fava G.A., Kellner R. 1993. Staging: a neglected dimension in psychiatric classification. *Acta Psychiatrica Scandinavica* 87: 225–230.

First M.B., Spitzer R.L., Gibbon M., Williams J.B.W. 1997. *User's Guide for the Structured Clinical Interview for DSM-IV Axis I Disorders (SCID-I)—Clinician Version.* Washington, DC: American Psychiatric Press.

Furer P., Walker J.R., Chartier M.J., Stein M.B. 1997. Hypochondriacal concerns and somatization in panic disorder. *Depression and Anxiety* 6: 78–85.

Gerdes T.T., Noyes R., Kathol R.G., Phillips B.M., Fisher M.M., Morcuende M.A., Yagla S.J. 1996. Physician recognition of hypochondriacal patients. *General Hospital Psychiatry* 18: 106–112.

Goldberg D.P., Williams P. 1988. *A User's Guide to the General Health Questionnaire.* Windsor, England: NFER-Nelson.

Gomborone J., Dewsnap P., Libby G., Farthing M. 1995. Abnormal illness attitudes in patients with irritable bowel syndrome. *Journal of Psychosomatic Research* 39: 227–230.

Gottesman I.I. 1962. Differential inheritance of the psychoneuroses. *Eugenics Quarterly* 9: 223–227.

Gottesman I.I., Bouchard T.J., Carey G. 1984. MMPI findings in the Minnesota study of twins reared apart. Bloomington, Indiana University: *Proceedings of the Fourth Annual Meeting of the Behavior Genetics Association.*

Greene R.L. 1991. *The MMPI-2/MMPI: An Interpretive Manual.* Boston: Allyn & Bacon.

Gureje O., Üstün T.B., Simon G.E. 1997. The syndrome of hypochondriasis: a cross-national study in primary care. *Psychological Medicine* 27: 1001–1010.

Guze S.B., Cloninger C.R., Martin R.L., Clayton P.J. 1986. A follow-up and family study of Briquet's syndrome. *British Journal of Psychiatry* 149: 18–23.

Hanback J.W., Revelle W. 1978. Arousal and perceptual sensitivity in hypochondriacs. *Journal of Abnormal Psychology* 87: 523–530.

Hernandez J., Kellner R. 1992. Hypochondriacal concerns and attitudes toward illness in males and females. *International Journal of Psychiatry in Medicine* 22: 251–263.

Hlatky M.A., Haney T., Barefoot J.C., Califf R.M., Mark D.B., Pryor D.B., Williams R.B. 1986. Medical, psychological and social correlates of work disability among men with coronary artery disease. *American Journal of Cardiology* 58: 911–915.

Hollifield M., Tuttle L., Paine S., Kellner R. 1999. Hypochondriasis and somatization related to personality and attitudes toward self. *Psychosomatics* 40: 387–395.

Jette A.M., Davies A.R., Cleary P.D., Calkins D.R., Rubenstein L.V., Fink A., Kosecott J., Young R.T., Brook R.H., Delbanco T.L. 1986. The Functional Status Questionnaire: reliability and validity when used in primary care. *Journal of General Internal Medicine* 1: 143–149.

Kellner R. 1981. *Abridged Manual for the Illness Attitude Scales.* Albuquerque, NM: University of New Mexico.

Kellner R. 1986. *Somatization and Hypochondriasis.* New York: Praeger.

Kellner R. 1990. Somatization: theories and research. *Journal of Nervous and Mental Disorder* 178: 150–160.

Kellner R., Sheffield B.F. 1973. The one-week prevalence of symptoms in neurotic patients and normals. *American Journal of Psychiatry* 130: 102–105.

Kellner R., Pathak D., Romanik R., Winslow W.W. 1983. Life events and hypochondriacal concerns. *Psychiatric Medicine* 1: 133–141.

Kellner R., Abbot H.P., Pathak D., Winslow W.W., Umland B.E. 1983–84. Hypochondriacal beliefs and attitudes in family practice and psychiatric patients. *International Journal of Psychiatry in Medicine* 13: 127–139.

Kellner R., Wiggins R.G., Pathak D. 1986a. Hypochondriacal fears and beliefs in medical and law students. *Archives of General Psychiatry* 43: 487–489.

Kellner R., Fava G.A., Lisansky J., Perini G.I., Zielezny M. 1986b. Hypochondriacal fears and beliefs in DSM-III melancholia: changes with amitriptyline. *Journal of Affective Disorders* 10: 21–26.

Kellner R., Abbot P.J., Winslow W.W., Pathak D. 1987a. Fears, beliefs and attitudes in DSM-III hypochondriasis. *Journal of Nervous and Mental Disease* 175: 2–25.

Kellner R., Slocumb J.C., Wiggins R.J. 1987b. The relationship of hypochondriacal fears and beliefs to anxiety and depression. *Psychiatric Medicine* 4: 15–24.

Kenyon F.E. 1964. Hypochondriasis: a clinical study. *British Journal of Psychiatry* 110: 478–488.

Kirmayer L.J., Robbins J.M. 1991. Three forms of somatization in primary care: prevalence, co-occurrence and sociodemographic characteristics. *Journal of Nervous and Mental Disease* 179: 647–655.

Kirmayer L.J., Robbins J.M., Dworkind M., Yaffe M.J. 1993. Somatization and the recognition of depression and anxiety in primary care. *American Journal of Psychiatry* 150: 734–741.

Kirmayer L.J., Robbins J.M., Paris J. 1994. Somatoform disorders: personality and the social matrix of social distress. *Journal of Abnormal Psychology* 103: 125–135.

Kramer-Ginsberg E., Greenwald B.S., Aisen P.S., Brod-Miller C. 1989. Hypochondriasis in the elderly depressed. *Journal of the American Geriatric Society* 37: 507–510.

Langner T.S., Michael S.T. 1963. *Life Stress and Mental Health.* New York: Free Press.

Leighton A.H. 1959. *My Name Is Legion.* New York: Basic Books.

Lewis A. 1934. Melancholia: a clinical survey of depressive states. *Journal of Mental Science* 80: 277–378.

Lichtenberg P.A., Swenson C.H., Skehan M.N. 1986. Further investigation of the role of personality, lifestyle and arthritic severity in predicting pain. *Journal of Psychosomatic Research* 30: 327–337.

Lipman R.S., Covi L., Shapiro A.K. 1979. The Hopkins Symptom Checklist (HSCL): factors derived from the HSCL-90. *Journal of Affective Disorders* 1: 9–24.

Mabe P.A., Hobson D.P., Jones L.R., Jarvis R.G. 1988. Hypochondriacal traits in medical patients. *General Hospital Psychiatry* 10: 236–244.

Mabe P.A., Riley W.T., Jones L.R., Hobson D.P. 1996. The medical context of hypochondriacal traits. *International Journal of Psychiatry in Medicine* 26: 443–459.

Manu P., Affleck G., Tennen H., Morse P.A., Escobar J.T. 1996. Hypochondriasis influences quality-of-life-outcomes in patients with chronic fatigue. *Psychotherapy and Psychosomatics* 65: 76–81.

Marks I.M. 1987. *Fears, Phobias, and Rituals*. New York: Oxford University Press.

Marks I.M. 1988. Blood-injury phobia: a review. *American Journal of Psychiatry* 145: 1207–1213.

Murphy M.R. 1990. Classification of the somatoform disorders. In *Somatization: Physical Symptoms and Psychological Illness* (ed. Bass C.M.), London: Blackwell Scientific.

Neale M.C., Walters E.E., Eaves L.J., Kessler R.C., Heath A.C., Kendler K.S. 1994. Genetics of blood-injury fears and phobias: a population-based twin study. *American Journal of Medical Genetics* 54: 326–334.

Noyes R. 1999. Relationship of hypochondriasis to anxiety disorders. *General Hospital Psychiatry* 21: 8–17.

Noyes R., Hoehn-Saric R. 1998. *The Anxiety Disorders*. New York: Cambridge University Press.

Noyes R., Reich J., Clancy J., O'Gorman T.W. 1986. Reduction in hypochondriasis with treatment of panic disorder. *British Journal of Psychiatry* 149: 631–635.

Noyes R., Kathol R.G., Fisher M., Phillips B., Suelzer M., Holt C. 1993. The validity of DSM-III-R hypochondriasis. *Archives of General Psychiatry* 50: 961–970.

Noyes R., Kathol R.G., Fisher M., Phillips B., Suelzer M., Woodman C. 1994a. Psychiatric comorbidity among patients with hypochondriasis. *General Hospital Psychiatry* 15: 78–87.

Noyes R., Kathol R.G., Fisher M.M., Phillips B.M., Suelzer M.T., Woodman C.L. 1994b. One-year follow-up of medical outpatients with hypochondriasis. *Psychosomatics* 35: 533–545.

Noyes R., Holt C.S., Happel R.L., Kathol R.G., Yagla S.J. 1997. A family study of hypochondriasis. *Journal of Nervous and Mental Disease* 185: 223–232.

Noyes R., Happel R.L., Yagla S.J. 1999. Correlates of hypochondriasis in a nonclinical population. *Psychosomatics* 40: 461–478.

Noyes R., Hartz A.J., Doebbeling C.C., Malis R.W., Happel R.L., Werner L.A., Yagla S.J. (2000). Illness fears in the general population. *Psychosomatic Medicine* 62:318–325.

Otto M.W., Pollack M.H., Sachs G.S., Rosenbaum J.F. 1992. Hypochondriacal concerns, anxiety sensitivity, and panic disorder. *Journal of Anxiety Disorders* 6: 93–104.

Palsson N. 1988. Functional somatic symptoms and hypochondriasis among general practice patients: a pilot study. *Acta Psychiatrica Scandinavica* 78: 191–197.

Pennebaker J.W., Watson D. 1991. The psychology of somatic symptoms. In *Current Concepts of Somatization: Research and Clinical Perspectives* (eds. Kirmayer L.J., Robbins J.M.), Washington DC: American Psychiatric Press.

Peveler R., Kilkennu L., Kinmonth A-L. 1997. Medically unexplained physical symptoms in primary care: a comparison of self-reporting screening questionnaire and clinical opinion. *Journal of Psychosomatic Research* 42: 245–252.

Pilowsky I. 1967. Dimensions of hypochondriasis. *British Journal of Psychiatry* 131: 89–93.

Pilowsky I., Spence N.D. 1975. Patterns of illness behavior in patients with intractable pain. *Journal of Psychosomatic Research* 19: 279–287.

Pilowsky I., Spence N.D. 1976. Illness behavior syndromes associated with intractable pain. *Pain* 2: 61–71.

Pilowsky I., Spence N.D. 1983. *Manual for the Illness Behaviour Questionnaire (IBQ), Second Edition*. Adelaide, Australia: Department of Psychiatry, University of Adelaide.

Pilowsky I., Chapman C.R., Bonica J.J. 1977. Pain, depression, and illness behavior in a pain clinic population. *Pain* 4: 183–192.

Pilowsky I., Smith Q.P., Katsikitis M. 1987. Illness behavior and general practice utilization: a prospective study. *Journal of Psychosomatic Research* 31: 177–183.

Rasmussen S.A., Eisen J.L. 1992. The epidemiology and clinical features of obsessive-compulsive disorder. *Psychiatric Clinics of North America* 15: 743–758.

Ray S.D., Advani M.T. 1962. A survey of 200 cases of hypochondriasis. *Journal of the Indian Medical Association* 39: 419–421.

Robbins J.M., Kirmayer L.J. 1991. Cognitive and social factors in somatization. In *Current Concepts of Somatization: Research and Clinical Perspectives* (eds. Kirmayer L.J., Robbins J.M.), Washington, DC: American Psychiatric Press.

Robbins J.M., Kirmayer L.J. 1996. Transient and persistent hypochondriacal worry in primary care. *Psychological Medicine* 26: 575–589.

Robbins J.M., Kirmayer L.J., Kapusta M.A. 1990. Illness worry and disability in fibromyalgia syndrome. *International Journal of Psychiatry in Medicine* 20: 49–63.

Sanderson W.C., Barlow D.H. 1990. A description of patients diagnosed with *DSM-III-R* generalized anxiety disorder. *Journal of Nervous and Mental Disease* 178: 588–591.

Savron G., Fava G.A., Grandi S., Rafanelli C., Raffi A.R., Belluardo P. 1996. Hypochondriacal fears and beliefs in obsessive-compulsive disorder. *Acta Psychiatrica Scandinavica* 93: 345–348.

Saz P., Copeland J.R.M., de la Camara C., Lobo A., Dewey M.E. 1995. Cross-national comparison of prevalence of symptoms of neurotic disorders in older people in two community samples. *Acta Psychiatrica Scandinavica* 91: 18–22.

Schmidt A.J.M. 1994. Bottlenecks in the diagnosis of hypochondriasis. *Comprehensive Psychiatry* 35: 306–315.

Schmidt A.J.M., Van Roosmalen R., Van Der Beek J.M.H., Lousberg R. 1993. Hypochondriasis in ENT practice. *Clinical Otolaryngology* 18: 508–511.

Shields J. 1962. *Monozygotic Twins Brought Up Apart and Brought Up Together*. New York: Oxford University Press.

Sigvardsson S., von Knorring A-L., Bohman M., Cloninger C.R. 1984. An adoption study of somatoform disorders. I. The relationship of somatization to psychiatric disability. *Archives of General Psychiatry* 41: 853–859.

Sigvardsson S., Bohman M., von Knorring A-L., Cloninger C.R. 1986. Symptom patterns and causes of somatization in men. I. Differentiation of two discrete disorders. *Genetic Epidemiology* 3: 153–169.

Slavney P.R., Teitelbaum M.L. 1985. Patients with medically unexplained symptoms: *DSM-III* diagnosis and demographic characteristics. *General Hospital Psychiatry* 7: 21–25.

Smith G.R., Monson R.A., Ray D.C. 1986. Patients with multiple unexplained symptoms: their characteristics, functional health, and health care utilization. *Archives of Internal Medicine* 146: 69–72.

Speckens A.E.M., van Hermert A.M., Spinhoven P., Bolk J.H. 1996a. The diagnostic and prognostic significance of the Whiteley Index, the Illness Attitude Scales and the Somatosensory Amplification Scale. *Psychological Medicine* 26: 1085–1090.

Speckens A.E.M., Spinhoven P., Sloekers P.P.A., Bolk J.H., van Hermert A.M. 1996b. A validation study of the Whiteley Index, the Illness Attitude Scales, and the Somatosensory Amplification Scale in general medicine and general practice patients. *Journal of Psychosomatic Research* 40: 95–104.

Spitzer R.L., Williams J.B.W., Gibbon M., First M.B. 1990. *Structured Clinical Interview for DSM-III-R (SCID)*. Washington, DC: American Psychiatric Press.

Spitzer R.L., Williams J.B.W., Kroenke K., Linzer M., deGruy F.V. 3rd, Hahn S.R., Brody D., Johnson J.G. 1994. Utility of a new procedure for diagnosing mental disorders in primary care: the PRIME-MD 1000 study. *Journal of the American Medical Association* 272: 1749–1756.

Starcevic V., Kellner R., Uhlenhuth E.H., Pathak D. 1992. Panic disorder and hypochondriacal fears and beliefs. *Journal of Affective Disorders* 24: 73–85.

Starcevic V., Fallon S., Uhlenhuth E.H., Pathak D. 1994 Generalized anxiety disorder, worries about illness, and hypochondriacal fears and beliefs. *Psychotherapy and Psychosomatics* 61: 93–99.

Stenback A., Jalava V. 1961. Hypochondria and depression. *Acta Psychiatrica Scandinavica 37* (Suppl. 162): 240–246.

Stenback A., Rimon R. 1964. Hypochondria and paranoia. *Acta Psychiatrica Scandinavica* 40: 379–385.

Stuart S., Noyes R. 1999. Attachment and interpersonal relationships in somatization. *Psychosomatics* 40: 34–43.

Torgersen S. 1986. Genetics of somatoform disorders. *Archives of General Psychiatry* 43: 502–505.

van Hemert A.M., Hengeveld M.W., Bolk J.H., Rooijmans H.G.M., Vandenbroucke J.P. 1993. Psychiatric disorders in relation to medical illness among patients of a general medical out-patient clinic. *Psychological Medicine* 23: 167–173.

Williams R.B., Haney T.L., McKinnis R.A., Harrell F.E., Lee K.L., Pryor D.B., Calif R., Kong Y.-Y., Rosati R.A., Blumenthal J.A. 1986. Psycho-social and physical predictors of anginal pain relief with medical management. *Psychosomatic Medicine* 48: 20–210.

World Health Organization. 1993. *The ICD-10 Classification of Mental and Behavioural Disorders: Diagnostic Criteria for Research*. Geneva: World Health Organization.

# 7

# Hypochondriasis in Primary Care

LAURENCE J. KIRMAYER
KARL J. LOOPER

---

**Case 1**

Ms. A, a 46-year-old single clerical worker who lives with and cares for her disabled mother, presented to a community walk-in clinic with concern about a 2 cm bruise on her left hand. She did not know how she had received the bruise. The clinic physician told her that it would resolve spontaneously and she was offered no follow-up. She returned 2 days later, however, with the complaint that "my left arm is not right." She explained that in the past week she had had the feeling that her left arm felt different than usual, and was slightly swollen. Six months earlier she had had an episode of chest pain. The pain was of moderate severity, radiated down her left arm, but was not associated with shortness of breath, palpitations or diaphoresis, and was relieved by rest. She did not seek help at that time but feared that she had suffered a heart attack. She now believes that the swollen arm, bruise on her hand, and the episode of chest pain indicate that she has had a myocardial infarction and that she risks imminent death.

Ms. A. acknowledged that she was under significant stress caring for her disabled mother. On the day of her chest pain she had had a heated argument with her mother and brother. However, she did not believe that the chest pain could have been a manifestation of stress alone and stated emphatically: "I know everything seems fine but, doctor, I *know* something is not right." Apart from her physical symptoms and concern about having a cardiac condition she denied other symptoms including insomnia, anorexia, difficulty concentrating, and low mood. She did report a loss of enjoyment of life and guilt over her mother's illness. She denied alcohol and drug use. She did not appear sad but remained anxious and was only partially satisfied with the reassurance that her symptoms were not likely to be related to cardiac illness. She was reassured somewhat after an electrocardiogram showed no abnormality, and felt relieved that she would have a cardiac stress test in a few weeks.

---

## Case 2

Mr. B. is a 28-year-old university student who lives with his brother. He presented to the student health clinic 6 months earlier with dizziness, chest pain, and anxiety since breaking up with his girlfriend two months prior. Since then he has been seen by his family physician several times for gastrointestinal complaints and was referred to a gastroenterologist who performed a colonoscopy to confirm that he did not have inflammatory bowel disease. He also visited three emergency rooms for chest pain and anxiety (on one occasion following marijuana consumption) where he had consistently normal physical exams and electrocardiograms.

His medical history includes a period of treatment for various unexplained somatic complaints 3 years ago after the death of his father from gastric cancer. When his father was diagnosed, the patient presented with a history of rectal pain, loose bowel movements with mucus, and weight loss. He was investigated for inflammatory bowel disease, although no physical illness was detected. Despite this, he returned to the clinic eleven times over the course of 6 months with a variety of urogenital and gastrointestinal symptoms. He had blood tests, screening for sexually transmitted diseases, stool cultures; he was referred to urology and gastroenterology specialists and treated with antibiotics for prostatitis. He finally stopped coming to the clinic when he dropped out of his program at the university, and was not seen again until this recent presentation.

The physical examination was unremarkable and the family doctor tried to reassure him that he was not physically ill but had anxiety related to the breakup of his relationship. He was prescribed a low-dose benzodiazepine. A complete blood count and thyroid function tests were ordered to rule out infection and hyperthyroidism.

The patient phoned the clinic several times over the next week, requesting the results of the investigations and a referral to the clinic psychiatrist. When he saw the psychiatrist he reported that he had had a sexual contact with a prostitute and although he had used a condom, he believed that he had contracted HIV through a small laceration on his finger that was in contact with vaginal secretions. He was educated regarding the relatively low risk of this contact and, given the incubation period, advised to have an HIV test in 3 months.

Over the next 3 months he returned to the clinic sixteen times for various physical complaints all of which he believed were caused by HIV. These included sore throat, cough, rashes, fatigue, and palpable lymph nodes. He had three negative HIV tests, was seen by an infectious disease specialist, and had an undetectable HIV viral count. Throat cultures were positive for candida, for which he was treated with antifungal medication and was seen by a dermatologist.

---

Primary care is a major arena for the management of health anxiety, illness worry, and hypochondriasis. Family physicians, general internists, and other frontline practitioners see the whole range of hypochondriacal concerns. At one end of the spectrum are patients like Ms. A., who present with acute anxiety but whose distress quickly resolves with information, reassurance or changing life circumstances. At the other extreme are patients like Mr. B., with severe incapacitating fears and the persistent or recurrent conviction that they are seriously ill, despite the doctor's most strenuous efforts to reassure.

The portrait of hypochondriasis in the psychiatric literature has tended to represent the most severe end of this broad spectrum. Cases seen in primary care often are milder and, indeed, transient acute hypochondriasis is more common than the chronic persistent disorder (Robbins and Kirmayer, 1996). The relationship between the transient and persistent forms of hypochondriasis is of great theoretical and practical significance. Are the two forms distinct problems affecting different people or can an acute form of hypochondriacal worry progress to chronicity? If the latter, under what circumstances does hypochondriacal worry emerge in primary care and what factors make some people go on to have persistent problems that may or may not respond well to specific treatments?

In this chapter, we review what is known about the clinical presentations, prevalence, and comorbidity of hypochondriasis in primary care. Next, we consider the course of hypochondriasis, which may depend crucially on interactions with primary care clinicians. We then review studies on primary care populations that elucidate some of the individual and social processes that contribute to illness worry, disease conviction, and the failure to respond to medical reassurance. Finally, we briefly consider treatment strategies appropriate for the primary care setting.

## Clinical Presentations of Hypochondriasis in Primary Care

Hypochondriasis is characterized by bodily preoccupation, illness worry, disease conviction, and failure to be reassured by medical opinion (Pilowsky, 1967, 1997). Clinically, all of these dimensions are judged against notions of appropriate illness behavior—that is, the level of illness worry that is appropriate for the symptoms or illness that the patient is suffering from, or the reasonable degree of doubt or uncertainty that one is sick given the limitations of current medical knowledge. Patients may be perceived as hypochondriacal because of manifestly high levels of anxiety, a dramatic style of illness presentation, or high rates of health care utilization.

Patients in medical settings often present with apprehensions or concerns about new symptoms or the course of chronic conditions. It might be thought, therefore, that much worry that is labeled hypochondriacal is simply anxiety that is proportional to the severity of co-occurring disease. Figure 7.1 shows data from a study in primary care in Montreal (Robbins and Kirmayer, 1996) in which symptoms of hypochondriasis were measured with a nine-item Hypochondriasis

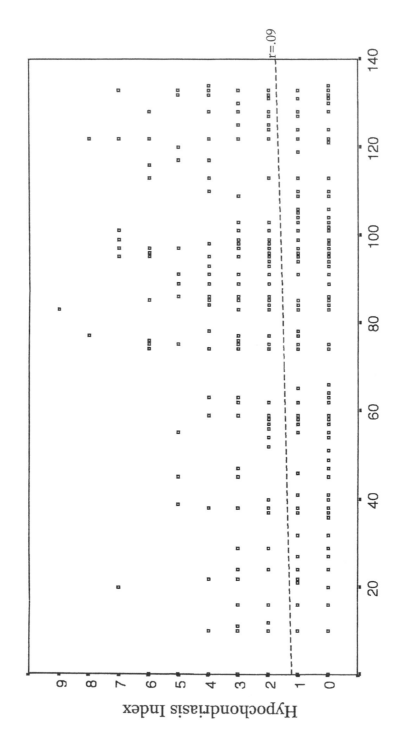

**Figure 7.1.** Distribution of level of hypochondriasis by seriousness of physical illness ($n = 683$).

Index based on the Whiteley Index (Pilowsky and Spence, 1983) and concurrent medical morbidity was rated with the Seriousness of Illness Rating Scale (Rosenberg *et al.*, 1987).[1] Clearly, the level of hypochondriasis varies widely among patients in primary care and shows only a very low correlation with disease severity ($r = 0.09$, $P = 0.02$, $N = 683$). High levels of hypochondriasis are found among patients with both mild and severe concurrent medical illness. This holds true for each of the dimensions of hypochondriasis, as shown in Figure 7.2A–C; indeed, only illness vulnerability is significantly correlated with seriousness of illness ($r = 0.12$, $P = 0.002$). The lack of correlation with seriousness of medical illness makes it evident that illness worry, illness vulnerability, and disease conviction are not simply responses to the threat posed by disease but must reflect other psychological or social processes.

While the definitions of hypochondriasis in the *DSM-IV* (American Psychiatric Association, 1994) and ICD-10 (World Health Organization, 1992) rest on the fear or idea that one has a serious disease and less on the presence of physical symptoms, studies in primary care find that patients with hypochondriasis tend to have multiple somatic symptoms. For example, in the Montreal study the mean number of current somatic complaints (on a list of twelve from the Somatization scale of the Hopkins Symptom Checklist; Lipman *et al.*, 1979) was 5.72 ($SD = 3.15$) for the hypochondriacal patients versus 3.14 ($SD = 2.73$) for the rest of the clinic sample ($t = 6.79$, $df = 683$, $P < 0.001$).

Table 7.1 displays the presenting complaints of patients with hypochondriacal worries attending primary care clinics on a self-initiated visit.[2] The most common presenting complaints were bodily pain and other somatic symptoms, which each accounted for one-third of the hypochondriacal patients' presentations. An

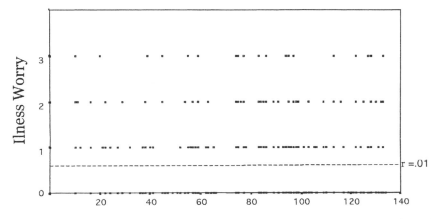

**Figure 7.2.** Distribution of illness worry, vulnerability, and disease conviction by seriousness of physical illness in primary care sample ($n = 683$).

additional 10% presented with possible somatic concomitants of anxiety and 5% with symptoms included in the vegetative symptoms of depression. Although they resembled the general clinic sample in most respects, those in the hypochondriacal group were more likely to seek help for a problem that they described in terms of a psychiatric diagnostic label (e.g.,"depressed"). Patients were also asked why they had sought help for their chief complaints and Table 7.1 presents the results. Again, hypochondriacal patients resembled the general clinic sample in that pain or discomfort and wanting a checkup or medication were the two most

**Table 7.1.** Clinical presentations of hypochondriacal patients in primary care

| | Hypochon-driacal (N = 58) | | Nonhypo-chondriacal (N = 625) | | Significance test* | |
|---|---|---|---|---|---|---|
| | N | (%) | N | (%) | $\chi^2$ | P |
| **Primary Presenting Complaint** | | | | | | |
| Pain | 19 | 32.8 | 145 | 23.2 | 2.66 | 0.10 |
| Vegetative symptoms | 3 | 5.2 | 51 | 8.2 | 0.65 | ns |
| Somatic anxiety | 6 | 10.3 | 58 | 9.3 | 0.07 | ns |
| Other somatic symptoms | 19 | 32.8 | 220 | 35.2 | 0.14 | ns |
| Psychiatric diagnosis | 5 | 8.6 | 12 | 1.9 | 9.82 | 0.01 |
| Psychosocial problem | 0 | 0 | 2 | 0.3 | 0.19 | ns |
| Health maintenance | 6 | 10.3 | 123 | 19.7 | 3.02 | 0.08 |
| Habit or substance abuse | 0 | 0 | 14 | 2.2 | 1.33 | ns |

| | Hypochon-driacal (N = 57) | | Nonhypo-chondriacal (N = 613) | | Significance test* | |
|---|---|---|---|---|---|---|
| | N | % | N | % | $\chi^2$ | P |
| **Reasons for Seeking Help for Presenting Complaint** | | | | | | |
| Pain or discomfort | 16 | 27.6 | 125 | 20.4 | 1.85 | ns |
| Checkup or change medication | 10 | 17.2 | 155 | 25.3 | 1.68 | ns |
| Anxious or afraid | 8 | 13.8 | 37 | 6.0 | 5.33 | 0.05 |
| Symptom persisted or worsened | 5 | 8.6 | 27 | 4.4 | 2.19 | ns |
| Referred by friend or other doctor | 4 | 6.9 | 30 | 4.9 | 0.49 | ns |
| Rule out lay diagnosis/find cause | 3 | 5.3 | 64 | 10.2 | 1.55 | ns |
| Unusual symptom or sign | 2 | 3.4 | 15 | 2.4 | 0.24 | ns |
| Reached limit of tolerance | 2 | 3.4 | 16 | 2.6 | 0.16 | ns |
| Monitor symptoms | 2 | 3.4 | 41 | 6.6 | 0.88 | ns |
| Want advice or treatment | 1 | 1.7 | 9 | 1.4 | 0.03 | ns |
| Activity limitation | 1 | 1.7 | 38 | 6.2 | 1.88 | ns |
| Detracts from appearance | 1 | 1.7 | 5 | 0.8 | 6.52 | ns |
| For referral | 1 | 1.7 | 3 | 0.5 | 1.41 | ns |

*Fisher exact result reported when an expected cell value is <5.

common groups of reasons for seeking help. Not surprisingly, hypochondriacal patients were more likely than nonhypochondriacal patients to seek help because they were anxious or afraid about a symptom or problem.

Although hypochondriasis is classified as a somatoform disorder, it is characterized by anxiety, and hypochondriacal patients often have serious concerns about their own emotional state. Indeed, while 46 (79.3%) in our sample of 58 hypochondriacal patients presented with a somatic symptom and only 8 (13.8%) with psychosocial complaints, 37 (63.8%) made a psychological attribution for their primary symptoms (i.e., they related their symptoms to some worry, stress, or psychosocial problem). This is compared to 241 (46.8%) of 515 nonhypochondriacal patients who made a psychological attribution (chi square = 10.18, $df = 1$, $P = 0.001$). To examine further the association of somatic and emotional distress, we constructed the Emotion Worry scale with items parallel to the Hypochondriasis Index to assess the level of worry about one's emotional state.

We found substantial correlations between the scores on Emotion Worry and the Hypochondriasis Index in the entire clinic sample ($r = 0.43$, $P < 0.001$, $N = 685$) and among the hypochondriacal patients ($r = 0.38$, $P = 0.004$, $N = 58$). Thus, people who worry about their physical health also tend to worry about their emotional vulnerability. The prominence of emotional distress in hypochondriasis accounts for the fact that, whereas medically unexplained symptoms impede the recognition of depression and anxiety in primary care, the presence of hypochondriacal worry actually increases the ability of primary care physicians to recognize that their patients have a psychosocial problem (Kirmayer *et al.*,1993).

Although physicians are generally able to identify patients with high levels of unrealistic illness worry (Gerdes *et al.*, 1996; Noyes *et al.*, 1993), the diagnosis of hypochondriasis is rarely recorded in medical charts (Beaber and Rodney, 1984). In the Montreal study, only 50% of the patients with hypochondriacal worry were identified in their charts as having a psychiatric or psychosocial problem, and only one received a somatoform diagnosis. The diagnoses or problems recorded were depression 24.1%, anxiety 8.6%, other psychiatric disorder 6.9%, stress 5.2%, somatoform disorder 1.7%, alcohol or substance abuse 1.7%, and noncompliance 1.7%. The reluctance to formally label patients hypochondriacal likely reflects physicians' awareness of the pejorative effects of such labeling and their lack of knowledge of an effective treatment.

## Prevalence and Sociodemographic Characteristics

Early estimates of the prevalence of hypochondriasis in the community ranged from 3% to 13%, with the assumption that primary care rates would be higher (Kellner, 1985). Kellner and colleagues (1983) found that 9% of a sample of patients in family medicine did not accept their physicians' reassurances that they were not seriously ill. A study of two university teaching hospital family medicine clinics found a prevalence of 7.7% of patients with high levels of illness worry (on a modified version of the Whiteley Index) in the absence of serious illness (Kirmayer and Robbins, 1991). Using a similar screening scale in a general-medicine clinic sample, Noyes and colleagues (1993) found 13.8% of patients with high levels of hypochondriacal symptoms, of whom 61.4% met *DSM-III-R* criteria for hypochondriasis for a prevalence of 8.5%. Based on clinical diagnosis, Barsky and colleagues (1990a) found a 6-month prevalence of *DSM-III-R* hypochondriasis in a general medicine clinic of 4.2% to 6.3%.

In a study of 1456 new patients seeking primary care services at a university-affiliated outpatient clinic in Southern California, Escobar and colleagues (1998) found a prevalence of *DSM-IV* hypochondriasis of 3.4% with the Composite International Diagnostic Interview (CIDI; Robins *et al.*, 1989). Hypochondriacal patients did not differ from others in gender, immigrant status, or ethnicity. The study had a low response rate (50%) and the diagnosis was based on a structured interview given by trained lay interviewers without consistent use of medical records or other secondary sources.

The WHO Collaborative Study on Psychological Problems in General Health Care examined the prevalence of hypochondriasis as measured by the CIDI at fifteen primary care sites in fourteen countries (Gureje *et al.*, 1997). A total of 25,916 patients were screened across the sites, and 5447 patients completed a second-stage evaluation; the overall response rate was 60%. The 12-month prevalence of ICD-10 hypochondriasis varied from 0% to 3.8% across sites, with an average of 0.8%. Similar rates were obtained with *DSM-III-R* criteria, with an overall prevalence of 0.7%. The relative rarity of hypochondriasis appeared to be related to the criterion requiring that patients refuse to accept medical reassurance that their symptoms had no physical cause. Disease conviction or preoccupation with a presumed deformity (the latter corresponding to body dysmorphic disorder in *DSM-IV*) had a prevalence of 6.7%. The authors concluded that the criterion of "persistent refusal to accept medical reassurance" (World Health Organization, 1992) was a bottleneck in the diagnosis of hypochondriasis in primary care. They proposed a concept of "abridged hypochondriasis," which required the triad of disease conviction, distress, or interference with functioning, and medical help-seeking. This syndrome had a prevalence of 2.2% in their sample. In support of the validity of the construct, patients meeting criteria for abridged hypochondriasis were perceived by physicians to have poorer health, were more likely to be referred for additional physical investigations, had higher rates of clinic attendance, more frequent and more severe physical disability and sick days, and were more likely to rate their own health as worse than the physician judged it to be. Compared to those with full ICD-10 criteria for hypochondriasis, the patients with abridged hypochondriasis tended to be older and were more likely to receive a diagnosis of generalized anxiety disorder (GAD); the two groups were alike in other sociodemographic and diagnostic characteristics.

Many studies have shown that hypochondriasis is not associated with age, gender, or marital status (Barsky *et al.*, 1990a; Escobar *et al.*, 1998; Gureje *et al.*, 1997; Robbins and Kirmayer, 1996). This is in contrast to somatization disorder, which is much more commonly found in women in most North American studies, although cultural variations exist in the gender ratio. Several studies in primary care have found an association of hypochondriasis with less education (Robbins and Kirmayer, 1991a; 1996).

## Comorbidity

Hypochondriasis in primary care is distinct from but often comorbid with mood and anxiety disorders as well as other somatoform disorders. Levels of comorbidity in primary care are usually higher than in the general population owing to the fact that coexisting disorders increase help-seeking.

Data on comorbidity for the Montreal study, as assessed by the Diagnostic Interview Schedule (DIS, version III-A; Robins *et al.*, 1981) are presented in Table 7.2. Patients with high levels of hypochondriacal worry were more likely than nonhypochondriacal patients to have current and lifetime major depression and abridged somatization disorder. There was a trend for them to report a lifetime history of panic disorder and somatization disorder more frequently as well.

**Table 7.2.** Comorbidity of hypochondriacal patients in primary care ($N = 685$)

| | Hypochondriacal (N = 58) | | Nonhypochondriacal (N = 627) | | Significance test* | |
|---|---|---|---|---|---|---|
| | N | (%) | N | (%) | $\chi^2$ | P |
| Major depression (lifetime) | 22 | 37.9 | 101 | 16.1 | 17.16 | <0.001 |
| Major depression (in last month) | 11 | 19 | 57 | 9.1 | 5.78 | 0.016 |
| Dysthymic disorder | 5 | 8.6 | 35 | 5.6 | 0.89 | NS |
| Generalized anxiety disorder (lifetime) | 5 | 8.6 | 39 | 6.2 | 0.51 | NS |
| Panic disorder (lifetime) | 2 | 3.4 | 5 | 0.8 | 3.69 | 0.055 |
| Obsessive-compulsive disorder (lifetime) | 3 | 5.2 | 17 | 2.7 | 1.13 | NS |
| Simple phobia (lifetime) | 3 | 5.2 | 34 | 5.4 | 0.01 | NS |
| Somatization disorder | 2 | 3.4 | 5 | 0.8 | 3.69 | 0.055 |
| Abridged somatization disorder (SSI 4.6) | 17 | 29.3 | 97 | 15.5 | 7.3 | 0.007 |

*Fisher exact result reported when an expected cell value is <5.

Barsky and colleagues (1992) compared 42 general medical patients with *DSM-III-R* hypochondriasis to 76 nonhypochondriacal patients from the same setting. On the DIS, 33% of the hypochondriacal patients had current major depression, 24% met *DSM-III* criteria for GAD, and 21% received a diagnosis of somatization disorder. There was also a threefold increase of personality disorder caseness (63.4% compared to 17.3%) among the hypochondriacal group based on the Personality Diagnostic Questionnaire (Hyler *et al.*, 1983). Noyes and colleagues (1994a) compared 50 hypochondriacal patients to 50 nonhypochondriacal controls from a general medical clinic and found that nearly 40% had subsyndromal somatization disorder; however, they found no overlap with GAD.

The study by Escobar and colleagues (1998) found significant overlap with *DSM-IV* somatization disorder (8.2% of patients with hypochondriasis vs. 1.1% of those without hypochondriasis) and abridged somatization (Escobar *et al.*, 1989) (49% of patients with hypochondriasis vs. 21% of those without hypochondriasis). Of patients with abridged somatization only 15% had hypochondriasis. These results confirm previous findings of the independence of hypochondriasis, somatization, and somatized presentations of depression and anxiety in primary care (Garcia-Campayo *et al.*, 1998; Kirmayer and Robbins, 1991).

In the WHO Collaborative Study on Psychological Problems in General Health Care (Gureje *et al.*, 1997), abridged hypochondriasis was associated with ICD-10 diagnoses of GAD (22%) and depression (37%). Again, somatization disorder was uncommon among hypochondriacal patients, although many had multiple medically unexplained symptoms and one-fifth met criteria for abridged somatization disorder.

Thus, across diverse primary care settings, roughly one-third of hypochondriacal patients have current major depression, one-quarter have GAD, and from one-fifth to one-half meet criteria for abridged somatization disorder. When GAD, panic disorder, obsessive-compulsive disorder, and phobias are considered together, 50%–75% of hypochondriacal patients have a lifetime history of some anxiety disorder. A range of personality disorders is common among patients with the most severe and persistent forms of hypochondriasis and likely contribute in many ways to their problematical relationships with clinicians (Kirmayer *et al.*, 1994). A family aggregation study found no tendency for hypochondriasis to occur in the families of probands but did find some association with somatization disorder and problematical personality traits (Noyes *et al.*, 1997).

The high rate of comorbidity of hypochondriasis with other disorders suggests that, like many other psychiatric diagnoses, it is best thought of not as a discrete entity but as a dimension of illness experience and behavior that cuts across diagnoses and complicates or precedes other disorders. Its location within the broad category of somatoform disorders reflects the dualistic organization of biomedical health care services more than any evidence of specific pathology. In a nosology organized around cognitive and physiological mechanisms, hypochondriasis might be reclassified with other anxiety disorders or used as a qualification for other major diagnoses (e.g., major depression, GAD, panic disorder, or personality disorder with hypochondriacal features).

## The Course of Hypochondriasis in Primary Care

Hypochondriasis has had the reputation of being chronic and relatively refractory to treatment (Adler, 1981; Strain, 1986). This may apply to the severe end of the spectrum but is not true as a general rule (Kellner, 1986). The most common presentation to the primary care physician is the patient with transient illness worry who does not meet full criteria for hypochondriasis, and the outcome for these patients is relatively good (Barsky *et al.*, 1990b).

Barsky and colleagues (1993a) followed 24 patients with subthreshold hypochondriasis and 22 control patients recruited from a general medicine clinic for approximately 2 years. They found illness worry was stable, with hypochondriacal patients continuing to have elevated symptom scores and physician visits on follow-up as compared to control patients. Despite this, only one patient eventually met the full *DSM-III-R* criteria for hypochondriasis. Robbins and Kirmayer (1996) followed 546 patients from a family-medicine clinic for 12 months. They compared three groups of hypochondriacal patients: 31 with persistent hypochondriacal worry ("stable"); 34 with initial worry, which had resolved by the 12-month follow-up ("transient"); and 21 who had developed worry at the second assessment ("emergent"). Both the transient and the persistent hypochondriacal patients showed improvement in depressive and somatic symptoms over the follow-up year. However, only the transient group showed lower health care utilization over the period of the study compared to the previous 12 months.

Few sociodemographic differences existed between the groups, although the transient and persistent groups had slightly less education than the nonhypochondriacal patients. Persistent hypochondriacal patients had a more serious medical history than did nonhypochondriacal patients, and both the persistent and emergent groups had more severe current medical illness than did the transient and nonhypochondriacal groups. There was more current and past psychiatric illness (major depression and anxiety disorder) in the persistently hypochondriacal group. These results suggest that both current and past medical and psychiatric diagnoses are risk factors for enduring hypochondriacal concerns.

Noyes and colleagues (1994b) conducted a 1-year follow-up study of 50 patients with *DSM-III-R* hypochondriasis and 50 control subjects, omitting the duration criterion in order to use it as a dependent variable in the outcome analysis.

No sociodemographic differences between the groups (although age and sex were controlled) were found, and no difference was seen in aggregate physical disease. Thirty percent of patients with hypochondriasis had comorbid depressive disorder, and 22% had an anxiety disorder. At 12 months, approximately 30% reduction in the measure of hypochondriasis was observed, and 16 (33%) patients in the original hypochondriacal group no longer met the criteria for diagnosis. Subjects with more severe hypochondriasis and longer duration of illness at the initial assessment had a worse outcome. Coexisting depression, anxiety, and neuroticism were also associated with more severe hypochondriacal symptoms and impairment at follow-up.

Similar results were found by Barsky and colleagues (1998) in a 4- to 5-year prospective study of 120 *DSM-III-R* hypochondriasis patients and 133 controls. On follow-up there was a significant overall improvement in symptoms, with 31 of 85 (36.5%) patients no longer meeting diagnostic criteria for hypochondriasis. Greater severity of initial symptoms predicted persistence of hypochondriasis at follow-up. Those who lost the diagnosis had developed a greater number of major medical illnesses during the intervening period than did those who retained the diagnosis. However, a review of these cases identified few situations in which the initial hypochondriacal presentation could be interpreted as accurate disease conviction or justifiable concern due to an emerging medical condition.

The response of others in the patient's social milieu may also influence the course of hypochondriasis. Clinical experience suggests that reinforcement of hypochondriacal concerns through overly solicitous behavior may contribute to chronicity. In their longitudinal study, Robbins and Kirmayer (1996) examined patients' perceptions of the response of significant others. The persistent hypochondriacal group tended to view their significant others as making fewer normalizing responses but offering less encouragement to seek medical attention. This presents a dilemma in which partners are perceived as not offering reassuring explanations for symptoms, yet not sanctioning medical help-seeking. If this perception is accurate, it may mean that others have come to doubt or ignore the hypochondriacal patient's medical concerns. However, these findings are based on patients' own perceptions of their partners' illness behavior and may reflect the same cognitive biases that give rise to hypochondriacal concerns in the first place. There is a need for studies that examine family and social interactional variables in hypochondriasis more directly.

Taken together, the available data suggest that the prognosis of the hypochondriacal patient in primary care is generally optimistic. The most common form is transient hypochondriacal worry, which has a low rate of conversion to the persistent form and a good prognosis for recovery. Patients who are at risk of a more protracted course of illness have a greater number of medical and psychiatric conditions both in the past and at the time of presentation. Although patients meeting the full *DSM* criteria for hypochondriasis tend to have substantial long-term impairment, they do show some improvement over time.

## Models of Hypochondriasis in Primary Care

Here we consider studies on primary care populations that explore some psychological and social interactional mechanisms that may underlie hypochondriasis. Many of these studies consider hypochondriasis to arise from dimensions of personality, affect, and cognition that can contribute to elevated symptom reporting and illness worry in any patient. Hypochondriasis, in turn, would then be best approached as a multidimensional construct rather than a discrete diagnostic category (Kirmayer and Taillefer, 1997; Robbins and Kirmayer, 1991b).

### Individual Factors

Pennebaker and Watson (1991) reviewed studies linking *neuroticism* and the analogous construct *negative affectivity* to somatic symptom reporting (Watson and Pennebaker, 1989). This personality trait reflects negative mood and self-concept, general pessimism, as well as a tendency to introspection, focusing on negative aspects of oneself. This results in consistently higher levels of distress and dissatisfaction over time and across situations. Neuroticism is correlated with increased reporting of all types of sensations and physical symptoms in the absence of differences in objective health markers (Costa and McCrae, 1985). Other personality traits may contribute to the rigidity with which some hypochondriacal patients hold their beliefs and to their difficulty in trusting and accepting medical reassurance (Kirmayer *et al.*, 1994; see also Starcevic, Chapter 13).

Barsky and Klerman (1983) hypothesized that the elevated symptom reporting and bodily concern of patients with hypochondriasis could be due to a general tendency to experience somatic sensation as intense, noxious, and disturbing. To test this hypothesis, Barsky and colleagues (1990c) developed the Somatosensory Amplification Scale (SSAS) in which respondents report their sensitivity to common somatic and sensory stimuli. In studies of medical outpatients, somatosensory amplification was significantly higher among patients with *DSM-III-R* hypochondriasis than among controls (Barsky *et al.*, 1990c), and they accounted for 31% of the variance in hypochondriasis as measured by the Whiteley Index (Barsky and Wyshak, 1990). Somatosensory amplification was also a significant independent predictor of symptoms, discomfort, and disability in a study of 115 patients with upper respiratory tract infections, even after controlling for medical morbidity (Barsky *et al.*, 1988a).

Kellner and colleagues (1992) examined the association of hypochondriacal concerns with anxiety, depressive and somatic symptoms in a sample of 100 general practice and 100 psychiatric outpatients. Disease conviction correlated with somatic symptoms, while the fear of having a disease was more closely associated with general anxiety. This suggests an important distinction between the processes underlying the two dimensions of hypochondriasis, namely disease conviction and fear of having a disease.

Barsky and colleagues (1993b) examined the tendency of hypochondriacal patients to have an unrealistic view of health as a symptom-free state. Using the Health Norms Sorting Task, they found that primary care patients with hypochondriasis were more likely than nonhypochondriacal patients to interpret ambiguous somatic symptoms as incompatible with good health. This narrow definition of health was more closely associated with the disease conviction and bodily preoccupation dimensions of hypochondriasis.

A related cognitive process that may contribute to hypochondriasis is the attribution of somatic symptoms to pathological causes. Robbins and Kirmayer (1991a) developed the Symptom Interpretation Questionnaire (SIQ) to measure the tendency to attribute common somatic symptoms to three types of hypothetical explanations: somatic, psychological, or normalizing. For example: "If I got dizzy all of a sudden, I would probably think that it is because: (a) there is something wrong with my heart or blood pressure [somatic explanation]; (b) I must be under a lot of stress [psychological]; or (c) I am not eating enough or I got up too quickly [normalizing]."

In a 6-month follow-up study of 100 family medicine patients, Robbins and Kirmayer (1991a) found that the number of past physical illnesses correlated positively with the somatic attribution on the SIQ, while the number of previous psychiatric illnesses correlated with a psychological attribution of somatic symptoms on the SIQ. This suggests that the experience of past illnesses affects the attribution of current somatic symptoms. After controlling for past history of medical and psychiatric illness, the score on the somatic attribution scale was a predictor of the number of presentations for somatic symptoms with and without definite medical diagnosis in the subsequent 6 months. The score on the psychological attribution scale was a predictor of the number of presentations for psychosocial symptoms over that period of time, but was not associated with the number of somatic symptoms that received no definite medical diagnosis. The score on the normalizing attribution scale was inversely related to the number of somatic and psychosocial presentations. A somatic attributional style may increase concern about unexplained somatic symptoms with subsequent high levels of health care utilization, whereas a normalizing style allows individuals to reassure themselves and reduce help-seeking.

This finding is supported by a study that compared frequent general practice attenders (more than 12 visits in the past year), who were considered by their physicians to be excessively worried about their health, to infrequent attenders (mean time to last visit, 2 years) (Sensky *et al.*, 1996). When presented with somatic symptoms from the SIQ scale and asked to write down as many potential explanations for each symptom as they could think of in one minute, the frequent attenders generated significantly fewer normalizing explanations for common bodily sensations and were less able to state reasons why a somatic attribution might be untrue. Given that most people experience frequent somatic symptoms in the ordinary course of events, this suggests that high utilizers of medical services (including transiently and persistently hypochondriacal individuals) are less able to explain away symptoms and so reassure themselves. Using a similar methodology, MacLeod and colleagues (1998) found that anxious patients made more psychological and fewer normalizing attributions, but patients with hypochondriacal concerns consistently made more somatic attributions and were more likely to provide a somatic attribution as their first explanation.

In a reanalysis of data from the Montreal study, we examined some determinants of hypochondriacal concerns in our sample of family medicine patients. The dependent variable was the Hypochondriasis Index drawn from the Whiteley Index; this scale, which has nine items, includes illness worry, perceived vulnerability to illness, and disease conviction, but eliminates items directly related to somatic symptomatology. As shown in Table 7.3, at the bivariate level,

**Table 7.3.** Multiple regression models of determinants of hypochondriasis in primary medical care ($N = 679$)

| | Bivariate $r$ | Model I $\beta$ | Model I SE | Model II $\beta$ | Model II SE |
|---|---|---|---|---|---|
| Age | −0.02 | −0.01 | 0.004 | −0.01* | 0.004 |
| Sex (female) | −0.01 | −0.07 | 0.13 | −0.11 | 0.12 |
| Education (years) | −0.19*** | −0.06*** | 0.02 | −0.05** | 0.02 |
| Married | −0.06* | −0.12 | 0.13 | −0.02 | 0.13 |
| Unemployed | 0.08* | 0.22 | 0.19 | 0.12 | 0.18 |
| Seriousness of illness | 0.09* | 0.004* | 0.002 | 0.004** | 0.001 |
| Private body-consciousness | 0.28*** | 0.15*** | 0.04 | 0.15*** | 0.04 |
| Private self-consciousness | 0.25*** | 0.14*** | 0.04 | 0.07* | 0.03 |
| Normalizing attributions | −0.24*** | −0.10*** | 0.03 | −0.02 | 0.03 |
| Somatic attributions | 0.10** | 0.03 | 0.03 | 0.06† | 0.03 |
| CES-D depressive symptoms | 0.43*** | | | 0.06*** | 0.01 |
| Constant | | 1.68 | 0.47 | 0.44 | 0.46 |
| $R^2$ | | 0.17*** | | 0.26*** | |

*$P < 0.05$.
**$P < 0.01$.
***$P < 0.001$.
†$P = 0.07$.

hypochondriacal concerns were associated with less education, unmarried and unemployed status, and greater seriousness of physical illness.

The original study measured three dimensions of illness cognition: private self-consciousness (the tendency to be introspective or to scrutinize one's own thoughts and feelings; Fenigstein et al., 1975), private body-consciousness (the tendency to be aware of one's own bodily sensations; Miller et al., 1981), and symptom attributional style (the tendency to attribute common somatic symptoms to either external, environmental causes [normalizing] or pathological somatic causes [somatic], as measured with the SIQ; Robbins and Kirmayer, 1991a).[3] All of the illness cognition measures were significantly related to hypochondriasis at the bivariate level. In a multivariate model, normalizing attributions were negatively related to hypochondriacal concerns, while somatic attributions were unrelated.

This inconsistency with the findings of MacLeod and colleagues (1998) is likely due to the limitations of the SIQ. To score high on the SIQ somatic scale, the patient must endorse attributions to many different types of somatic causes, so that this scale is less sensitive to hypochondriacal concerns than the more naturalistic measure of self-generated explanations used by Sensky and MacLeod. When depressive symptomatology was controlled in a second model, however, the effect of normalizing attributions was eliminated while the coefficient for somatic attributions increased to near significance. Body- and self-consciousness were associated with hypochondriasis in both models.

To examine these relationships further, we broke the Hypochondriasis Index into three components: illness worry, vulnerability to disease, and disease conviction. All three subscales had modest internal reliabilities (Cronbach's alpha of 0.54, 0.50, and 0.51, respectively). Illness worry was related to younger age, male gender, less schooling, greater body- and self-consciousness, and fewer normalizing attributions ($R^2 = 0.14$, $P < 0.001$). Vulnerability to illness was related to female gender, greater severity of physical illness, body-consciousness, and fewer normalizing attributions ($R^2 = 0.06$, $P < 0.001$). Disease conviction was related only to less education and greater body-consciousness ($R^2 = 0.14$, $P < 0.001$). All three dimensions were related to depressive symptomatology, which again eliminated the effect of normalizing attributions.

These results suggest that attentional, attitudinal, and attribution processes all contribute to hypochondriasis, but that the effects of attribution style are limited to the dimensions of illness worry and vulnerability to illness. The difficulty in generating normalizing attributions characteristic of hypochondriasis may be accounted for by the level of dysphoric mood or depression.

## Social and Interactional Factors

The reasons why medical opinion fails to reassure and why anxiety persists in the face of counterevidence can be sought in the personality and psychopathology of the individual. But they may also reside in the social context: in prevailing ideas about illness, and in important interactions with health care providers, family members, employers, the compensation system, and wider social circles (Kirmayer, 1999).

The reporting of common physical complaints is associated with childhood illness behavior through processes of social learning. These include modeling, whereby the parents of somatizing children express somatizing behaviors in their own help-seeking (Benjamin and Eminson, 1992; Walker *et al.*, 1991), and the selective reinforcement of somatic complaints as opposed to communication about emotional states (Wilkinson, 1988). Certain forms of illness may also be reinforced on a societal level. In the context of the modern biomedical system based on the Cartesian dualism that separates mind and body (Kirmayer, 1988), patients may preferentially express distress with a physical symptom rather than with an overt psychological problem. This dualism also leads to the tendency for clinicians to tell patients who have no identifiable organic disease that there is "nothing wrong." This sort of superficial reassurance flatly contradicts patients' experience of distress and may be perceived as outright dismissal. Somatic distress remains a legitimate way to call attention to one's suffering, to have a symptom which is not simply "all in one's head" and which, therefore, does not impute lack of strength, will, or bad attitude. The irony is that precisely because hypochondriacal symptoms are not adequately grounded in a medical condition, they certify the patients' emotional distress and psychiatric condition.

Parsons (1951) described the classical model of the sick role as an essentially moral concept. The sick person has a right to be excused from usual social duties without blame, while in return he or she is expected to try to get well by seeking out medical help and following doctor's orders. This model works best in the case of identifiable medical conditions for which effective treatments are available. When a hypochondriacal patient presents with a physical complaint, the classic paradigm breaks down. In the absence of a known physical syndrome and the refusal to accept appropriate reassurances, the relationship between the hypochondriacal patient and the family physician often becomes conflictual and unsatisfactory (Barsky and Klerman, 1983) (see also Chapters 11 and 12).

An interesting question for future research concerns whether intensive efforts to investigate symptoms, while they lend authority to subsequent reassurances, might also convey the parallel contradictory message that one must be ill to warrant such elaborate diagnostic intervention. After all, some disease might still remain hidden, just beyond the reach of existing technology. There is evidence that the "pathologizing" attributions and "catastrophizing" cognitions of patients with functional gastrointestinal symptoms diminish over time with appropriate care by their physicians (Van Dulmen *et al.*, 1995). Decrease in "catastrophizing" cognitions was associated with continuity of care but not with intensity of investigations or frequency of visits. This points to the importance of the quality of the doctor–patient interaction as an important determinant of the outcome of illness worry in primary care.

## Treatment Approaches to Hypochondriasis in Primary Care

There is increasing evidence that hypochondriasis in primary care is a treatable problem with a good outcome for many patients (Barsky, 1996; Kellner, 1983; Robbins and Kirmayer, 1996). Although transient hypochondriacal worry may resolve spontaneously or with only routine investigation and reassurance by clinicians, there is much that the primary care provider can do to facilitate recovery (Kellner, 1992; Warwick, 1992). Careful management may reduce the risk of producing chronicity through too much investigation, ambiguous communication, and inconsistent support for anxious patients.

Some of the intensity and repetitiveness with which hypochondriacal patients express their concerns has to do with the perception that others do not believe they are ill or do not take their suffering seriously. Accordingly, there is a basic need to acknowledge suffering. Empathic listening and validation of the patient's anxiety as a legitimate problem in its own right can serve to engage the patient and establish a working relationship (Galatzer-Levy, 1980). The clinician can then explore the context of symptoms and anxiety, which will open up specific avenues for intervention.

---

### Case 1 (continued)

Ms. A. was asked to return 3 days after her initial visit to see the clinic nurse, and she had an appointment with the physician the following week. When her bruise disappeared she said she could cancel her appointment with the physician but was asked to keep the appointment. The physician expressed concern about her level of stress and the demands of caring for her mother alone. She was very appreciative of these empathic comments and although several times made motions to leave, she continued to talk at length of the obligation she felt to care for her mother.

Her mother was an elderly diabetic with severely limited vision and mobility due to retinopathy, glaucoma, and neuropathy affecting her extremities. She had lived with the patient for the past 4 years and had had a stroke 6 months earlier with residual paresis of her right side. She was able to ambulate and dress herself only with assistance. When not at work, the patient's life was devoted to caring for her mother.

When the patient was 3 years old, her father had had a stroke and was placed in a nursing home. She felt that he was poorly cared for and resented her mother for not caring for him herself. As a result, she made a firm commitment to care for her mother until her death.

On the day of her chest pain 6 months earlier, the patient's brother—who has chronic paranoid schizophrenia—was visiting for supper. After the meal, as the patient was leading their mother to the living room, her brother became acutely agitated, yelling at her and accusing her of trying to kill their mother. Unable to calm him down, she left the house for a walk, at which time she experienced the chest pain.

She responded well to empathetic comments during the session. Although she was relieved that the bruising had disappeared, she restated concern that her left arm still did not feel right and that she might have a cardiac condition. She agreed to wait and see the results of the cardiac stress test and a light exercise program.

---

As this case illustrates, empathic listening and careful exploration will identify many significant reasons for hypochondriacal patients' distress. At the same time, difficult life circumstances do not resolve simply because they have been uncovered. Indeed, it may be best to focus on enlarging patients' coping repertoire beyond help-seeking and illness preoccupation before challenging family or social arrangements that are central to a patient's identity or self-esteem.

Clinicians are heavily invested in the authority and completeness of biomedical explanation. Accordingly, they may overestimate the value of such information for patients and ignore other sources of health information—and anxiety—in the media as well as in the experience of the patient's family or friends. Reassurance must be consonant with prevailing social and cultural interpretations of symptoms. Clinicians who offer medical information that does not fit with the understandings of patients or their families may find that their information is ineffective.

Although many primary care patients with hypochondriasis have never received clear or systematic explanation and reassurance for their symptoms and concerns, in some cases continuous efforts to reassure have become part of the problem. In these situations, refusing to engage in reassurance may be helpful. In the 1920s the Japanese psychiatrist Shoma Morita developed a systematic treatment for hypochondriasis and related conditions. One component of Morita therapy, termed *fumon* therapy, consisted of ignoring patients' hypochondriacal complaints (Kitanishi, 1990). This pattern of systematic nonreinforcement (extinction), however, took place in the context of a milieu treatment conducted in Morita's own home, with his wife and daughter providing physical care for the patients. Thus, the strategic intervention of ignoring symptomatic behavior was coupled with a strong message of acceptance and support that gratified dependency needs. Simply ignoring symptoms without some evidence of an enduring commitment from the clinician is unlikely to have much beneficial effect.

Most hypochondriacal patients acknowledge that they are anxious and will accept interventions that address the anxiety provided their physical problems are also taken seriously. In some cases, the sources of anxiety are so profound and persistent that discussion, reassurance, and reattribution are not sufficient to diminish hypochondriacal symptoms. In such cases, more systematic and intensive cognitive-behavioral treatment may be needed (see also Chapter 14).

In Case 2, Mr. B. presented with more entrenched illness worries that were part of a lifelong pattern of health anxiety, medically unexplained symptoms, and help-seeking.

---

### Case 2 (continued)

Mr. B. was eventually referred for psychiatric assessment at a teaching hospital. He gave the history of the conviction of having HIV despite negative testing, continued experiencing physical symptoms, which he believed were manifestations of HIV infection, and exhibited ongoing help-seeking behavior. The psychiatric interview revealed a lifelong pattern of concern about his health, especially at times of stress. His earliest memory of this was of developing severe abdominal pain at the age of 7, after attending a funeral. He was hospitalized and had an exploratory laparotomy, during which a normal appendix was removed. His family was informed that his physical symptoms were "psychosomatic." He denied other serious physical problems or surgical interventions until 3 years prior to his presentation at the clinic. At that time, his father died soon after having been diagnosed with a gastric cancer. He recalled feeling very guilty at not having had a better relationship with his father and regretted not having taken the time to make amends before his death. He reported low mood, insomnia, and anorexia with a weight loss of 2.5 kilograms. He described occasional alcohol consumption. He denied family history of psychiatric treatment but suspected that his father had had an untreated depression.

He was diagnosed with major depression and hypochondriasis and was recommended a trial of an antidepressant. The family physician began sertraline 25 mg, which provoked numerous side effects (headache, nausea, and insomnia), but over several weeks these side effects abated and the dose was increased to 50 mg daily. Attempts to link the patient's preoccupation with illness to the significant losses in his life met with superficial agreement but no real interest in exploring these issues and no meaningful change in disease conviction.

The treatment plan has been to limit Mr. B.'s health care to one physician at the clinic, and to give him regular appointments in anticipation of his needs. New symptoms are assessed with a focused interview and physical exam, and investigations are done sparingly. This strategy has been successful in reducing his erratic use of emergency services but has not reduced his conviction of having HIV, or presenting new symptoms that he claims are related to HIV.

---

The primary care physician adopted the strategies established for the management of somatization disorder (Smith *et al.*, 1995). This reduced excessive health care utilization but did not diminish the cognitive symptoms of hypochondriasis. The delusional quality of Mr. B's concerns suggests that antipsychotic medication might be of help (Munro, 1988). It is also possible that a more systematic approach employing cognitive-behavioral interventions that target hypochondriacal beliefs and maladaptive coping strategies would result in a better outcome (Barsky *et al.*, 1988b; Clark *et al.*, 1998; Warwick *et al.*, 1996). This could be carried out by a family physician or nurse practitioner with appropriate training. Alternatively, health psychologists working in collaboration with family physicians can provide effective treatment for patients with persistent hypochondriasis.

Given the relatively small number of patients with severe hypochondriasis, specialized psychological treatments could be provided, ideally in a medical setting that does not unduly stigmatize or threaten the patient. Close collaboration between primary care providers and mental health experts is essential to find workable solutions for these most challenging situations.

## Conclusion

The primary care setting is unique in that clinicians see many milder, transient forms of illness worry. The WHO Collaborative Study on Psychological Problems in General Health Care concluded that the ICD-10 definition of hypochondriasis is too restrictive for use in primary care. It appears that the obstinacy, contrariness, or rejection of clinicians' opinion is not central to the most common forms of hypochondriasis in primary care, which tend to be more closely related to health anxiety. Moreover, it is unclear how often or how well doctors actually try to reassure their patients in primary care. A casual statement that "nothing is wrong" may provide little reassurance for a patient who is feeling manifestly unwell and who has many cues to worry about his or her health.

A dimensional approach to hypochondriasis in terms of illness worry, disease conviction, and functional somatic distress allows the clinician to identify specific cognitive and behavioral targets for intervention. Interaction with clinicians likely plays an important role in the outcome of hypochondriasis and, as with other somatoform disorders, continuity of care is particularly important to allay anxiety and avoid iatrogenic illness (see also Chapter 12).

Clinicians in primary care have the opportunity to intervene early and so may prevent chronicity. They are also well positioned to integrate medical and psychological care over the long term for patients who need more intensive treatment. The practitioner who is willing and able to take the time can do much to improve the condition of patients with hypochondriacal worry. Further research is needed to identify determinants of course and outcome, predictors of good response to treatment, and specific cost-effective treatment modalities suited to the primary care setting.

## Acknowledgments

We thank Dr. Melissa Hallman for the case examples and Suzanne Taillefer and Lucy Boothroyd for assistance with data analysis. This work was supported by grants from the Fonds de la recherche en santè du Quèbec.

### Notes

1. The Hypochondriasis Index omitted items related to having many symptoms as this conflates the notion of somatization disorder with hypochondriasis. Ratings of seriousness of illness referred to a generic rating for the most severe physical illness each patient reported (psychiatric disorders were not rated). This is very imprecise both because there is a wide range of severity associated with any given diagnosis and because multiple conditions may have an additive or multiplicative effect on patients' overall state of health. However, these methodological limitations do not affect the basic result that the level of hypochondriacal symptoms is not closely linked to concurrent medical illness.

2. The design of the study excluded patients who were called back by their physicians for a follow-up or regularly scheduled appointment. The sample, therefore, substantially underestimates the proportion of visits for health maintenance or monitoring of chronic illness.

3. Only normalizing and somatic attribution scales are used in the analysis because the study used the forced-choice version of the SIQ so that scores on any two scales completely determine the score on the third (Robbins and Kirmayer, 1991a).

### References

Adler G. 1981. The physician and the hypochondriacal patient. *New England Journal of Medicine* 304: 1394–1396.

American Psychiatric Association. 1994. *Diagnostic and Statistical Manual of Mental Disorders, Fourth Edition (DSM-IV)*. Washington, DC: American Psychiatric Press.

Barsky A.J. 1996. Hypochondriasis: medical management and psychiatric treatment. *Psychosomatics* 37: 48–56.

Barsky A.J., Klerman G.L. 1983. Overview: hypochondriasis, bodily complaints, and somatic styles. *American Journal of Psychiatry* 140: 273–283.

Barsky A.J., Wyshak G. 1990. Hypochondriasis and somatosensory amplification. *British Journal of Psychiatry* 157: 404–409.

Barsky A.J, Goodson J.D., Lane R.S., Cleary, P.D. 1988a. The amplification of somatic symptoms. *Psychosomatic Medicine* 50: 510–519.

Barsky A.J., Geringer E., Wool C.A. 1988b. A cognitive-educational treatment for hypochondriasis. *General Hospital Psychiatry* 10: 322–327.

Barsky A.J., Wyshak G., Klerman G.L., Latham K.S. 1990a. The prevalence of hypochondriasis in medical outpatients. *Social Psychiatry and Psychiatric Epidemiology* 25: 89–94.

Barsky A.J., Wyshak G., Klerman G.L. 1990b. Transient hypochondriasis. *Archives of General Psychiatry* 47: 746–753.

Barsky A.J., Wyshak G., Klerman G.L. 1990c. The Somatosensory Amplification Scale and its relationship to hypochondriasis. *Journal of Psychiatric Research* 24: 323–334.

Barsky A.J., Wyshak G., Klerman G.L. 1992. Psychiatric comorbidity in *DSM-III-R* hypochondriasis. *Archives of General Psychiatry* 49: 101–108.

Barsky A.J., Cleary P.D., Sarnie M.K., Klerman G.L. 1993a. The course of transient hypochondriasis. *American Journal of Psychiatry* 150: 484–488.

Barsky A.J., Coeytaux R.R., Sarnie M.K., Cleary P.D. 1993b. Hypochondriacal patients' beliefs about good health. *American Journal of Psychiatry* 150: 1085–1089.

Barsky A.J., Fama J.M., Bailey E.D., Ahern D.K. 1998. A prospective 4- to 5-year study of *DSM-III-R* hypochondriasis. *Archives of General Psychiatry* 55: 737–744.

Beaber R.J., Rodney W.M. 1984. Underdiagnosis of hypochondriasis in family practice. *Psychosomatics* 25: 39–45.

Benjamin S., Eminson D.M. 1992. Abnormal illness behaviour: childhood experiences and long-term consequences. *International Review of Psychiatry* 4: 55–70.

Clark D.M., Salkovskis P.M., Hackman A., Wells A., Fennell M., Ludgate J., Ahmad S., Richards H.C., Gelder M. 1998. Two psychological treatments for hypochondriasis: a randomised controlled trial. *British Journal of Psychiatry* 173: 218–225.

Costa P.T., McCrae R.R. 1985. Hypochondriasis, neuroticism, and aging: when are somatic complaints unfounded? *American Psychologist* 40: 19–28.

Escobar J.L., Rubio-Stipec M., Canino G., Karno M. 1989. Somatic Symptom Index (SSI): a new and abridged somatization construct. *Journal of Nervous and Mental Disease* 177: 140–146.

Escobar J.I., Gara J., Waitzkin H., Cohen Silver R., Holman A., Compton W. 1998. *DSM-IV* hypochondriasis in primary care. *General Hospital Psychiatry* 20: 155–159.

Fenigstein A., Scheier M.F., Buss A.H. 1975. Public and private self-consciousness: assessment and theory. *Journal of Consulting and Clinical Psychology* 43: 522–527.

Galatzer-Levy R.M. 1980. Beginning the treatment of hypochondriasis. *Archives of General Psychiatry* 37: 960.

García-Campayo J., Lobo A., Pérez-Echeverría M.J., Campos R. 1998. Three forms of somatization presenting in primary care settings in Spain. *Journal of Nervous and Mental Disease* 186: 554–560.

Gerdes T.T., Noyes R., Kathol R.G., Phillips B.M., Fisher M.M., Morcuende M.A., Yagla S.J. 1996. Physician recognition of hypochondriacal patients. *General Hospital Psychiatry* 18: 106–112.

Gureje O., Üstün T.B., Simon G.E. 1997. The syndrome of hypochondriasis: a cross-national study in primary care. *Psychological Medicine* 27: 1001–1010.

Hyler S.E., Redier R.O., Spitzer R.L., Williams J.B.W. 1983. *Personality Diagnostic Questionnaire* (PDQ). New York: New York State Psychiatric Institute.

Kellner R. 1983. Prognosis of treated hypochondriasis: a clinical study. *Acta Psychiatrica Scandinavica* 67: 69–79.

Kellner R. 1985. Functional somatic symptoms and hypochondriasis. *Archives of General Psychiatry* 42: 821–833.

Kellner R. 1986. *Somatization and Hypochondriasis*. New York: Praeger.

Kellner R. 1992. The case for reassurance. *International Review of Psychiatry* 4: 71–80.

Kellner R., Abbott P., Pathak D., Winslow W.W., Umland B.E. 1983. Hypochondriacal beliefs and attitudes in family practice and psychiatric patients. *International Journal of Psychiatry in Medicine* 13: 127–139.

Kellner R., Hernandez J., Pathak D. 1992. Hypochondriacal fears and beliefs, anxiety and somatization. *British Journal of Psychiatry* 160: 525–532.

Kirmayer L.J. 1988. Mind and body as metaphors: hidden values in biomedicine. In *Biomedicine Examined* (eds. Lock M., Gordon G.), Dordrecht: Kluwer.

Kirmayer L.J. 1999. Rhetorics of the body: medically unexplained symptoms in sociocultural perspective. In *Somatoform Disorders—A Worldwide Perspective* (eds. Ono Y., Janca A., Asai M., Sartorius N.), Tokyo: Springer-Verlag.

Kirmayer L.J., Robbins J.M. 1991. Three forms of somatization in primary care: prevalence, co-occurrence and sociodemographic characteristics. *Journal of Nervous and Mental Disease* 179: 647–655.

Kirmayer L.J., Taillefer S. 1997. Somatoform disorders. In *Adult Psychopathology, Third Edition* (eds. Turner S., Hersen M.), New York: John Wiley.

Kirmayer L.J., Robbins J.M., Dworkind M., Yaffe M. 1993. Somatization and the recognition of depression and anxiety in primary care. *American Journal of Psychiatry* 150: 734–741.

Kirmayer L.J., Robbins J.M., Paris J. 1994. Somatoform disorders: personality and the social matrix of somatic distress. *Journal of Abnormal Psychology* 103: 125–136.

Kitanishi K. 1990. Morita therapy from a transcultural psychiatric view. *Journal of Morita Therapy* 1: 190–194.

Lipman R.S., Covi L., Shapiro A.K. 1979. The Hopkins Symptom Checklist (HSCL): factors derived from the HSCL-90. *Journal of Affective Disorders* 1: 9–24.

MacLeod A.K., Haynes C., Sensky T. 1998. Attributions about common bodily sensations: their associations with hypochondriasis and anxiety. *Psychological Medicine* 28: 225–228.

Miller L.C., Murphy R., Buss A.H. 1981. Consciousness of body: public and private. *Journal of Personality and Social Psychology* 41: 397–406.

Munro A. 1988. Monosymptomatic hypochondriacal psychosis. *British Journal of Psychiatry* 153 (Suppl. 2): 37–40.

Noyes R., Kathol R.G., Fisher M.M., Philips B.M., Suelzer M.T., Holt C.S. 1993. The validity of *DSM-III-R* hypochondriasis. *Archives of General Psychiatry* 50: 961–970.

Noyes R., Kathol R.G., Fisher M.M., Phillips B.M., Suelzer M.T., Woodman C.L. 1994a. Psychiatric comorbidity among patients with hypochondriasis. *General Hospital Psychiatry* 16: 78–87.

Noyes R., Kathol R.G., Fisher M.M., Phillips B.M., Suelzer M.T., Woodman C.L. 1994b. One-year follow-up of medical outpatients with hypochondriasis. *Psychosomatics* 35: 533–545.

Noyes R., Holt C.S., Happel R.L., Kathol R.G., Tahla S.J. 1997. A family study of hypochondriasis. *Journal of Nervous and Mental Disease* 185: 223–232.

Parsons T. 1951. *The Social System.* Glencoe, IL: The Free Press.

Pennebaker J.W., Watson D. 1991. The psychology of somatic symptoms. In *Current Concepts of Somatization: Research and Clinical Perspectives* (eds. Kirmayer L.J., Robbins J.M.), Washington, DC: American Psychiatric Press.

Pilowsky I. 1967. Dimensions of hypochondriasis. *British Journal of Psychiatry* 113: 89–93.

Pilowsky I. 1997. *Abnormal Illness Behaviour.* Chichester: John Wiley.

Pilowsky I., Spence N.D. 1983. *Manual for the Illness Behaviour Questionnaire* (IBQ). Adelaide, Australia: University of Adelaide.

Robbins J.M., Kirmayer L.J. 1991a. Attributions of common somatic symptoms. *Psychological Medicine* 21: 1029–1045.

Robbins J.M., Kirmayer L.J. 1991b. Cognitive and social factors in somatization. In *Current Concepts of Somatization: Research and Clinical Perspectives* (eds. Kirmayer L.J., Robbins J.M.), Washington, DC: American Psychiatric Press.

Robbins J.M., Kirmayer L.J. 1996. Transient and persistent hypochondriacal worry in primary care. *Psychological Medicine* 26: 575–589.

Robins L., Helzer J.E., Croughan J. 1981. National Institute of Mental Health Diagnostic Interview Schedule: its history, characteristics, and validity. *Archives of General Psychiatry* 38: 381–389.

Robins L.N., Wing J., Wittchen H-U., Helzer J.E., Babor T.F., Burke J., Farmer A., Jablensky A., Pickens R., Regier D.A., Sartorius N., Towle L.H. 1989. The Composite International Diagnostic Interview: an epidemiologic instrument suitable for use in conjunction with different diagnostic systems and in different cultures. *Archives of General Psychiatry* 45: 1069–1077.

Rosenberg S.J., Hayes J.R., Peterson R.A. 1987. Revising the Seriousness of Illness Rating Scale: modernization and re-standardization. *International Journal of Psychiatry in Medicine* 17: 85–92.

Sensky T., MacLeod A.K., Rigby M.F. 1996. Causal attributions about somatic sensations among frequent general practice attenders. *Psychological Medicine* 26: 641–646.

Smith G.R., Rost K., Kashner M. 1995. A trial of the effect of a standardized psychiatric consultation on health outcomes and costs in somatizing patients. *Archives of General Psychiatry* 52: 238–243.

Strain J.J. 1986. The diagnosis, ontogenesis, and management of hypochondriasis. In *Emotional Disorders in Physically Ill Patients* (eds. Roessler R., Decker N.), New York: Human Sciences Press.

Van Dulmen A.M., Fennis J.F.M., Mokkink H.G.A., Vandervelden H.G.M., Bleijenberg G. 1995. Doctor-dependent changes in complaint-related cognitions and anxiety during medical consultations in functional abdominal complaints. *Psychological Medicine* 25: 1011–1018.

Walker L.S., Garber J., Greene J.W. 1991. Somatization symptoms in pediatric abdominal pain patients: relation to chronicity of abdominal pain and parent somatization. *Journal of Abnormal Child Psychology* 19: 379–394.

Warwick H. 1992. Provision of appropriate and effective reassurance. *International Review of Psychiatry* 4: 76–80.

Warwick H., Clark D.M., Cobb A.M., Salkovskis P.M. 1996. A controlled trial of cognitive-behavioural treatment of hypochondriasis. *British Journal of Psychiatry* 169: 189–195.

Watson D., Pennebaker J.W. 1989. Health complaints, stress, and distress: exploring the central role of negative affectivity. *Psychological Review* 96: 234–254.

Wilkinson S.R. 1988. *The Child's World of Illness: The Development of Health and Illness Behaviour*. Cambridge: Cambridge University Press.

World Health Organization. 1992. *The ICD-10 Classification of Mental and Behavioural Disorders: Clinical Descriptions and Diagnostic Guidelines*. Geneva: World Health Organization.

# II

# Theoretical and Etiologic Aspects

# 8

# Psychodynamic Perspectives on Hypochondriasis

## DON R. LIPSITT

> To evolve appropriate therapeutic tools, it is necessary to go beyond these limitations [of the phenomenological viewpoint] and enter another area of psychiatry: psychodynamics.
>
> Schäfer, 1982, p. 240

At a time when therapeutic paradigms focus largely on prompt, expeditious, limited, and (it its hoped) inexpensive intervention, attention to *psychodynamics* in this compendium of contemporary approaches to hypochondriasis may seem of only passing interest. Indeed, in many psychiatric training programs, educational observers have noted a dramatic shift of emphasis away from the study of psychodynamics toward the biological and neuroscientific (Jacobs *et al.*, 1997).

But if good treatment is based not only on the "what" and "how" of disease, but also on the "why," then it behooves practitioners to be aware of those factors that drive the hypochondriacal process and which can usefully inform any treatment approach. And, likewise, if the patient–physician relationship continues to be the bedrock of clinical practice, then comprehension of the psychodynamics of that relationship can lubricate the therapeutic interaction with hypochondriacal patients (Lipsitt, 1986; see also Chapter 12).

In this chapter, I will review the psychodynamic postulates that help elucidate well-described behaviors, traits, and symptoms of the hypochondriacal individual and attempt to correlate conventional clinical observation and therapeutic endeavors with theoretical constructs. For example, we may ask what light psychodynamic theory can shed on the hypochondriacal patient's fear of death, his often unshakable clinging to symptoms, his intense self-absorption with the body, his help-seeking/help-rejecting illness behavior, his refractoriness to treatment and reassurance, his capacity to evoke a negative reaction in physicians, and so on (Lipsitt, 1973).

## Definition of Psychodynamics

According to the *American Psychiatric Glossary*, "The science of psychodynamics assumes that one's behavior is determined by past experience, genetic endowment, and current reality" (Edgerton and Campbell, 1994, p. 171).

Although not specifically stated, it is generally assumed that intrapsychic conflict, mental mechanisms or defenses, and the unconscious are also important aspects of a psychodynamic approach. Behavior is believed to be motivated by drives with overt or covert goals or objectives, determined by the interplay of conscious and unconscious forces, capable of assessing reality, and occasionally resulting in regression of the individual's behavior and expression of emotion. In the psychodynamic approach, symptoms are generally thought to have symbolic meaning, with symptom "choice" determined by the interplay of all these factors, even when the mechanisms may not be apparent. Psychodynamic therapy attempts to alleviate symptoms through (*1*) elucidation of motives and defenses and (*2*) awareness of how the patient–therapist relationship, through transference and countertransference, can make conscious certain aspects of the individual's relationships with early significant figures that might be otherwise unconscious and conflictual.

## Early Beginnings of Psychodynamics

Certainly philosophers, psychologists, theologians, and others before Sigmund Freud's time had alluded to the unconscious and had offered creative explanations of behavior, but one cannot really speak of psychodynamic theory prior to Freud's discovery of the relationship of the unconscious to mental mechanisms and the topographical model of the mind.

The force and impact of Freud's ideas about emotional and behavioral vicissitudes dominated twentieth century thinking about human psychology. So compelling were his insightful formulations that they were applied to virtually every aspect of human endeavor. In this fervent climate of psychoanalytic exploration, one would naturally expect that Freud and his followers would have something pithy to say about a prevalent and ill-defined "condition" with a history spanning two thousand years. But, in fact, Freud wrote comparatively little of hypochondriasis. Even his own hypochondriacal proclivities did not entice him to explore it more fully in either his voluminous professional outpouring or in his personal autobiography (Schur, 1972). In one of his letters to Wilhelm Fliess (April 19, 1894), Freud wrote, "It is painful for a medical man, who spends all the hours of the day struggling to gain an understanding of the neuroses, not to know whether he is himself suffering from a reasonable or a hypochondriacal depression" (Bonaparte *et al.*, 1954, p. 82). His subsequent references to hypochondriasis appeared mostly in his investigations of narcissism, paranoia, and, briefly, "actual neurosis," that condition which he defined as similar to neurasthenia and anxiety neurosis, and which drew libido (sexual energy) away from external objects and attached it—to the point of "damming up"—to its own organs and self (Nunberg and Federn, 1962, p. 110).

Freud's first reference (in print) to hypochondriasis appeared in his earliest letter (November 24, 1887) to Fliess inquiring about the diagnosis and treatment of a patient whom Freud regarded as problematic. (Did Freud's curiosity begin with the so-called difficult or problem patient?) He confessed to Fliess of "the difficult task of differentiating between incipient organic and incipient neurasthenic affections," but added, "I have always held fast to one distinguishing characteristic. In neurasthenia a hypochondriacal element, an anxiety psychosis, is never absent, whether admitted or denied, and betrays itself by a profusion of new sensations, i.e., paresthesias" (Bonaparte *et al.*, 1954, p. 51).

In 1909, when members of the Vienna Psychoanalytic Society were considering printing a pamphlet to educate the public about psychoanalysis, Freud cautioned that they should not be too optimistic in their promotion as "the position of hypochondriasis is still suspended in darkness" (Nunberg and Federn, 1967, p. 76). At one point, he said that hypochondriasis was the somatic equivalent of paranoia (Nunberg and Federn, 1962, p. 110). But in 1911, the minutes of the Society record Freud's definition of hypochondriasis as "the state of being in love with one's own illness" (Nunberg and Federn, 1974, p. 243). Freud clearly indicated his intention to "draw away from the problem of neuroses . . . [and to] . . . come closer to ego psychology" (Nunberg and Federn, 1975, p. 192), and once having written his essay "On Narcissism" (S. Freud, 1914), he seems to have done just that.

Although his remarks about hypochondriasis anticipated fuller expansion in later writings, as he hypothesized about the relationship of hypochondriasis to neurasthenia and anxiety (the other actual neuroses), Freud wrote, "Let us . . . stop at this point. It is not within the scope of a purely psychological inquiry to penetrate so far behind the frontiers of physiological research" (Freud, 1914, p. 84). He explored the role of hypochondriasis quite extensively in the analysis of Schreber's memoirs (Freud, 1911) and an obsessional neurosis (the Wolf Man) (S.Freud, 1918[1914]), but there was in fact hardly another reference to hypochondriasis after his essay on narcissism in 1914.

This approach-avoidance behavior on Freud's part toward the complex subject of hypochondriasis mirrors the very kind of ambivalence we see in physicians confronting hypochondriacal patients in medical practice. And the see-sawing back and forth between psyche and soma (psychological:physiological) that punctuates the history of medicine to this day, characterized Freud's allusions to the topic. This dualism extends to the *DSM-IV* classification (American Psychiatric Association, 1994), which has made every effort to avoid psychodynamic elements in defining hypochondriasis.

When Freud's vacillation resolved in favor of his pursuit of a psychological theory of behavior, he showed preferential interest in applying the explanatory power of his ideas to hysteria; at the time, he felt that hypochondriasis was devoid of psychological meaning, less treatable, and therefore of less psychoanalytic interest. At the time Freud began working with Breuer on the epochal studies of hysteria (Breuer and Freud, 1893–95), hypochondriasis was regarded as largely an organic condition, although earlier medical literature had made reference to fears, "nervousness," and melancholia. Such characterizations, however, were little more than descriptive, phenomenological reports of a baffling affliction that only began to "make sense" when addressed with psychodynamic insights.

Despite Freud's curtailed interest in the condition, he contributed a number of valuable formulations toward an understanding of the dynamics of hypochondriasis. For example, the concept of "somatic compliance," in which there is "conversion of the excitation into a somatic innervation" (Breuer and Freud, 1893–95, pp. 122, 166; also S. Freud, 1905[1901], p. 40), laid the foundation for understanding all of the later-defined somatizing disorders. And later, in *The Ego and the Id,* although he did not mention hypochondriasis, Freud postulated that "the ego . . . is first and foremost a body-ego" (S. Freud, 1923, p. 27), an important tenet in explaining why regression evoked physical (somatic) responses. He defined the ego as "ultimately derived from bodily sensations, chiefly from those springing from the surface of the body" (S. Freud, 1923, p. 26).

Although Freud did seem to leave it to others to unravel the enigma of hypochondriasis, he did dwell on it to some extent in his analysis of the case of Schreber—an analysis, not of the person, but of the published memoirs of a man of high social standing who had suffered from severe psychiatric disorder for which he was hospitalized a total of 13 of 27 years following his initial hospitalization. His saga began with the onset of hypochondriacal delusions following his election to high political office in 1884 (Meissner, 1976). Schreber refers in his memoirs to his brief first illness only as hypochondriasis (Niederland, 1974, p. xiv). Ultimately, as disclosed in Freud's study, Schreber's severe hypochondriacal symptoms evolved into a florid psychosis. From his analysis of this case, Freud derived much of his theory of narcissism and described its relationship to both paranoid psychosis and hypochondriasis. According to Freud (1914, p. 83), hypochondriasis involves the narcissistic investment in bodily organs of libido, which is withdrawn from external objects and "dammed up" in the organs of the body, with a tension and "unpleasure"—but also sometimes with a paradoxical pleasure or "masturbatory equivalent" (Macalpine and Hunter, 1953)—that commanded the individual's full attention; the result was an "organ neurosis" or "actual neurosis."

It is this self-absorption in the body that so characterizes the hypochondriacal person, who is sometimes so consumed with his own body that he is unable to disengage long enough from it to comply with history-taking—or almost any other function, for that matter (Ladee, 1966). The paradoxical experience of simultaneous pleasure and pain has been noted by others (Edgcumbe and Burgner, 1973; Fenichel, 1945; Jacobson, 1953; Ritvo, 1981; Stekel, 1949) and has often been the basis of frustration in those physicians who attempt to "relieve" these patients of their "suffering." This formulation of simultaneity of pleasure and displeasure helps, in part, to understand the hypochondriacal patient's great reluctance (conscious or unconscious) to relinquish symptoms.

Freud was quite convinced from his clinical cases that hypochondriasis originated from some kind of sexual trauma early in life or as a result of those who masturbated excessively or practiced *coitus interruptus*. In a letter to Wilhelm Fliess on January 24, 1895, in which he discusses paranoia, Freud wrote that "the hypochondriac will struggle for a long time before he has found the key to his feeling that he is seriously ill. He will not admit to himself that it arises from his sexual life; but it gives him the greatest satisfaction to believe that his sufferings are not endogenous . . . but exogenous. So he is being poisoned" (Bonaparte *et al.*, 1954, p. 112). He wrote further that "In every case the delusional idea is clung to with the same energy with which some other intolerable, distressing idea is fended off from the ego. Thus these people love their delusion as they love themselves. Herein lies the secret" (Bonaparte *et al.*, 1954, p. 113). Clearly, Freud was more intent on addressing the psychodynamics of the paranoid state than on those of hypochondriasis itself, and it is this path of investigation and formulation that he pursued in the cases of Schreber and the Wolf Man (Meissner, 1976; 1977). From Freud's clinical observations, he remarked that "a specific process seems to turn the narcissist into a hypochondriac." (Nunberg and Federn, 1975, p. 192). We note from these cases that his attention was to the more extreme forms of hypochondriasis. Others have pointed out that this method of investigation regarding hypochondriasis gave short shrift to the lesser hypochondriacal states (Aisenstein and Gibeault, 1991).

Other psychodynamic principles explicated by Freud and later psychoanalytic writers include the role of guilt; clinging to symptoms; resistance to treatment and the negative therapeutic reaction; the fear of annihilation and death; the role of aggression and hostility; sadomasochistic interaction and illness as a defense. Although considerable overlap exists among them, each will be reviewed separately with reference to various psychoanalytic/psychodynamic theories.

## The Role of Guilt

In psychoanalytic theory, the child goes through phases of development from total dependency upon parental figures to eventual separation and identity-formation. These transitions will proceed smoothly provided the child's needs are empathically acknowledged and met by a relatively constant person (object). To the extent that this does not occur, it is expected that the child will experience anxiety, inner turmoil, a sense of betrayal, and fears of abandonment. When the infant is still merged with the parent, it cannot discern whether threatening or pleasurable stimuli come from within or without. The experience of deprivation, inadequate mothering, or separation is said to foster aggressive and sadistic fantasies, a residue of ambivalence in the child toward the parent (Levy, 1932). Because these imply danger and the expectation of retribution toward the child by the nurturing parent, such thoughts are repressed and substituted with guilt. According to most psychoanalytic writers, guilt was generated by the superego—the conscience—administering unconscious self-criticism. Freud called this unconscious guilt imposed by the superego on the ego "reproaches of conscience" (S. Freud, 1923, p. 53).

One way of retaining threatening fantasies in the unconscious repressed state is to transform them into conscious bodily expression. Because this process "plays a decisive economic part" (S. Freud, 1923, p. 27) in maintaining this compromised mental state, it often "puts the most powerful obstacles in the way of recovery" (S. Freud, 1923, p. 27). Others have regarded hypochondriacal symptoms as "a justification for guilt feelings" arising from hostile attitudes toward the object (Fenichel, 1945, p. 262); "the hypochondriacally affected organ represents . . . the object which . . . was introjected from the external world onto one's own body" (Fenichel, 1945, p. 263). Asking patients to assess the psychological meaning of their symptoms represents a threat of having to face their unconscious guilty feelings. It is probably less painful to acknowledge physical pain than the psychic fear of a more dreaded punishment. It is as though hypochondriacal individuals say to themselves "The powers that be will not destroy us as long as we punish ourselves" (Wahl, 1964, p. 207). (This is similar to Nietzsche's aphorism: "That which does not kill me makes me stronger.") It is this characteristic of hypochondriasis—the persistent need to diminish guilty feelings—that confers both masochistic and obsessional traits on the clinical portrait of the hypochondriacal patient (Stekel, 1949).

## Clinging to Symptoms

The need to keep negative affect at bay helps clarify the almost desperate need of the hypochondriacal patient to cling to his symptoms, which is, for primary care physicians, one of the most salient and vexing characteristics of the condition. In part, the affects replaced by these symptoms are not recoverable because they are preverbal (Valenstein, 1962, p. 322). In infancy, a broad spectrum of affect (anger, guilt, remorse, sadness, despair, affection) is expressed through the only means available at that stage of development—motor activity. This expression has communicational meaning and is responded to adaptively or not by those in the child's environment. If inner needs are not satisfied, the result is painful affects such as anxiety, anger, sadness, or depression. Painful adaptation in the form of physical symptoms "generally suggests a major problem in object tie from the first year of life and thereafter" (Valenstein, 1973, p. 373).

Most psychoanalysts attribute the hypochondriacal person's propensity for pain to the earliest experiences of life, usually traumatic environmental events or "poor parenting" that led to inadequate differentiation of the self from the object (parent) itself (Aisenstein and Gibeault, 1991; Ritvo and Solnit, 1958; Spitz, 1965). Patients later cling to painful affects "because they represent the early self and self-object. Giving up such affects . . . would be equivalent to relinquishing a part of the self and/or self-object at the level which those affects represent" (Valenstein, 1973, p. 376). Many clinicians have confirmed Valenstein's impression that "asking the patient to change the sense of his early self and self-objects . . . is asking a 'bit' much of any patient" (Valenstein, 1973, p. 376).

Some have hypothesized the patient's resistance to giving up symptoms as an anxious attempt to avoid "the regressive pull towards fusion with an early depressive, maternal object" (Olinick, 1964, 1970). The threat of regressing, according to Anna Freud (1952a) and others, "implies a threat to the intactness of the ego" through "a loss of personal characteristics which are merged with the characteristics of the love object. The individual fears this regression in terms of dissolution of the personality, loss of sanity, and defends himself against it by a complete rejection of all objects (negativism)" (A. Freud, 1952a, p. 259). Anna Freud calls hypochondriasis the "reestablishment of [the] earliest stage of the mother–child relationship" (A. Freud, 1952b, p. 80).

From her observations of war orphans and hospitalized children, Anna Freud concluded that these children "identify with the lost mother, while the body represents the child (more exactly: the infant in the mother's care)" (A. Freud, 1952b, p. 80). "The child actually deprived of a mother's care adopts the mother's role in health matters, thus playing 'mother and child' with his own body" (A. Freud, 1952b, p. 79). In other words, in caring for and comforting itself, the child identifies with the absent or emotionally unavailable mother. Thus the symptom is cherished for its connection with this comfort. For some children, returning to that stage was comforting, but threatening to others, especially when it implied a sense of loss of self-control; the child's lavishing attention on his or her own body is similar to that seen in adult hypochondriacal states.

Milrod describes this self-comforting behavior as "a return to a need-satisfying relationship in which both object and subject are within the self, . . . in other words, a narcissistic regression involving object relationships and the drives" (Milrod, 1972, p. 509), providing "a means of internally continuing the gratifying oedipal relationship on a relatively desexualized basis" (Milrod, 1972, p. 525), the gratification being "one important factor making this syndrome so difficult to treat" (Milrod, 1972, p. 526). Because, according to Milrod, "it is a universal experience to feel a heightened self-esteem and to expect love and approval with deprivation and pain" (p. 526), the person attached to pain prefers the certainty of that condition to the uncertainty of the parenting figure. Such individuals may even seek out pain "in order to enjoy the gratifications of comforting oneself" (Milrod, 1972, p. 526). In a clinical sense, the retention of symptoms is an economical compromise for the patient: The symptom assures access to those most identified as professional comforters (physicians), while avoiding an awareness of negative feelings or the threat of total abandonment. Unfortunately, this is usually an imperfect solution as most physicians do not offer a continuing relationship with a patient who "has nothing wrong." Refractoriness to medical reassurance may be seen as further testimony to the hypochondriacal individual's need to remain deeply attached to pain to maintain self-control, defend against narcissistic regression, and to avoid the fear of bodily disintegration (Starcevic, 1991; see also Chapter 13).

Because the hypochondriacal person, according to Vaillant (1977, p. 180), "has transformed covert rage into complaints of pain . . . [as a way of] . . . belabor[ing] others with his own pain or discomfort, . . . [he] is incapable of being comforted" (Vaillant, 1977, p. 180). Modern therapists have learned to be restrained in their endeavors to hastily "remove" symptoms from hypochondriacal patients (Lipsitt, 1975).

This ambivalent state of both wishing for and fearing the regressed stage of the mother–child relationship may help to explain why such patients are often described as "help-seeking, help-rejecting," the result of extreme neediness for human attachment, with ensuing anxiety over the likelihood that closeness could be "dangerous," not to be trusted, unlikely to be empathic, accepting or reliably available. "Doctor-shopping" (Lipsitt, 1968, 1970) for an idealized comforter is often the pattern that emerges.

## Negative Therapeutic Reaction; Resistance to Treatment

Early in his psychoanalytic studies, Freud had become aware of the hypochondriacal patient's attachment to symptoms and refractoriness to treatment and reassurance. He wrote of his treatment of the Wolf Man (S. Freud, 1918[1914]) that the patient had a "habit of producing transitory 'negative reactions'; every time something had been conclusively cleared up, he attempted to contradict the effect for a short while by an aggravation of the symptom which had been cleared up" (p. 69).

During their psychoanalytic treatment, these patients, when praised for their progress in treatment, "showed signs of discontent and their condition invariably [became] worse" (S. Freud, 1923, p. 49). Freud describes his first response, typical of that of most physicians, as seeing the patient as defiant or trying to "one-up" the physician. But more reflection led him to what he called the "negative therapeutic reaction" (S. Freud, 1923, p. 49), in which "every partial solution that ought to result, and in other people does result, in an improvement or temporary suspension of symptoms produces in them for the time being an exacerbation of their illness; they get worse during the treatment instead of getting better."

Freud hypothesized that the reaction of the patient to the possibility of recovery seemed so dreaded that it must be something more than merely that the "need for illness has got the upper hand," or that it can be explained by "narcissistic inaccessibility" (S. Freud, 1923, p. 49), defiance of the physician, or gain from illness. Rather, he postulated that what presented the "most powerful of all obstacles to recovery" was "a 'moral' factor, a sense of guilt," which "found its satisfaction in the illness and refuses to give up the punishment of suffering" (S. Freud, 1923, p. 49). So persuaded was Freud by this formulation that he wrote with great conviction "we shall be right in regarding this disheartening explanation as final" (S. Freud, 1923, p. 49). Although no mention was made of such reactions to attempted treatment of hypochondriacal patients, Freud did state that "this factor has to be reckoned with in very many cases, perhaps in all severe cases of neurosis" (S. Freud, 1923, p. 50).

Many others have since observed the results of the negative therapeutic reaction, as in the attachment to pain described by Valenstein (1973, p. 365), or the tendency in psychoanalyzed patients to experience a form of self-loss with development of transitory hypochondriacal states when they improve to the point of being able to pursue new activities (Kohut, 1971). Where Freud emphasized guilt at the core of the negative therapeutic reaction, Horney (1936) emphasized anxiety, suggesting that the hypochondriacal person most feared his own hostile destructiveness of others; she believed that patients showing the negative therapeutic reaction had a masochistic character structure and resisted therapeutic interpretations in competition with the analyst. Riviere wrote that cure to such patients represented the overwhelming and all-consuming responsibility to now make reparations to "all those he loved and injured" (Riviere, 1936, p. 318) and "from his unconscious depressive standpoint . . . his uncured status quo in an unending analysis is clearly preferable to such a conception of cure" (Riviere, 1936, p. 318).

## Fear of Death

Although the *DSM-IV* does not specifically allude to death anxiety as a cardinal symptom of hypochondriasis, certainly the ultimate fate of "serious disease" is potentially termination of life. In psychoanalytic and psychodynamic terms, the fear of death is virtually always present if mental mechanisms of defense are removed. Stolorow (1979) points out that "death anxiety has been interpreted as an expression of a variety of unconscious infantile fears—of castration (Bromberg and Schilder, 1933; S. Freud, 1923), of separation or object loss (Bromberg and Schilder, 1936), of one's own overwhelming sexual excitement or masochistic, self-destructive impulses (Fenichel, 1945) and of abandonment, persecution or Talionic punishments by the superego (Bromberg and Schilder, 1936; S. Freud, 1923)" (Stolorow, 1979, p. 201).

If, during the prolonged dependent phase of development, there is significant empathic failure or a thwarting of need-fulfillment, this may be experienced as a sense of loss, of abandonment, of diminished self-worth, or anxiety and anger or rage. Out of this context develops a fear in the child that he will lose the love of the people on whom he depends for nurturance, comfort, and protection against life's many dangers. One of these dangers is, in fact, punishment from the very people on whom he depends. Being "bad" in any way—including just the intention or thought of being bad—invokes the threat of parental disapproval, withdrawal of love, punishment or rejection. In the older child, it is the function of the superego to monitor behavior and thought and therefore to take over the parental role of punisher.

Freud had many times alluded to the fear of death as one of the reactions of his hypochondriacal patients (Bonaparte *et al.*, 1954, p. 78). According to Freud, it was the Oedipus complex, the child's fear of punishment for his incestuous-libidinal wishes toward the parent, that gave rise to castration anxiety, "reproaches of conscience" (S. Freud, 1923, p. 53) and ultimately to fears of annihilation and death, the same unconscious wishes that have been presumably directed toward others by the child. "Fear of the superego is finally transformed into fear of death; this takes place when it is projected onto the powers of destiny" (Furer, 1972, p. 20).

The tendency of patients in analysis to react to progress with mild hypochondriacal concerns, stemming from the guilt of oedipal triumph, has been noted by others besides Sigmund Freud (Fenichel, 1945; Kohut, 1971; H. Rosenfeld, 1965; Stolorow, 1979). It is theorized that the development of hypochondriacal symptoms defends against the potential fragmentation and disintegration of the self (A. Freud, 1952a; Guntrip, 1968; Kohut, 1971). Kohut (1971) proposes (pp. 216–217) that hypochondriacal preoccupation may be observed in both the physical and mental spheres (e.g., concern about body parts or worry over loss of one's intellect, mental function, and so on) and both may serve as a signal of impending danger. Stolorow defines the hypochondriacal fear of death as "a dreaded infantile danger situation [which] is replaced, through displacements, projections and other mechanisms, with a presumably more tolerable threat to life and limb," such as mutilation, pain, loss, and so on (Stolorow, 1979, p. 202). Proponents of Kleinian theory speculated that the death threat arose from fantasied attacks by internalized persecutory objects; physical symptoms are the result of the "good" objects winning out over the "bad" (Klein, 1948; H. Rosenfeld, 1965).

According to Stolorow, "hypochondriasis sounds the alarm when the regressive self-disintegration has actually begun, and the preoccupation with bodily organs or mental functions already contains a concretizing effort at self-restitution" (Stolorow, 1979, p. 211). The purpose of a signal is to announce that danger lurks close to the surface and can threaten the integrity of the self, especially in those instances of severe narcissistic vulnerability (Kohut, 1971; Stolorow, 1979). When the alarm does not "work," panic may set in, with its accompanying hypochondriacal fears and fear of death (Starcevic, 1989).

The level of narcissistic regression and vulnerability relative to ego maturity and stability will determine whether hypochondriacal symptoms will be mild and fleeting (e.g., in the course of therapy) or progress to prepsychotic forms (e.g., as prepsychotic phenomena and somatic delusions, as in the Schreber and Wolf Man cases) (Meltzer, 1964; D. Rosenfeld, 1984), or to complete structural decompensation (e.g., self-enucleation, self-castration, or self-amputation) (Stolorow, 1977).

The hypochondriacal elaboration of physical symptoms, in a psychodynamic sense, represents a sacrifice of the part for the whole, a kind of offering to the gods for protection against destruction or annihilation of the entire body or self. In this regard, it is similar to the autotomy seen in some animal species that can, for purposes of survival, sever a threatened part of the body to a predator.

On the theoretical assumption that hypochondriacal symptoms represent "protection" against further decompensation, removal, or "cure" in such cases—without other available support—would threaten the individual with fragmentation and disintegration of the self. Clinically, one sees the frequent recrudescence of new or old symptoms in patients whose symptoms have "accidentally" or "unexpectedly" abated. It has also been noted by many clinicians that these patients seem more likely to be intolerant of medication or to develop side effects necessitating their discontinuation (Lipsitt, 1970; Stekel, 1949; Wahl, 1964).

## Hostility

As noted previously, destructive, hostile aggressive feelings toward others are withdrawn from them and turned against the self as a way of relieving or expiating repressed guilt. Such a mechanism is perhaps observed most saliently in the masochistic character, in depression, and in hypochondriasis. The process by which this occurs has been formulated in a variety of ways: the product of fantasied attacks by internalized persecutory objects (Klein, 1948; H. Rosenfeld, 1958); results of a confusional state arising from early childhood in which the child is frustrated at not being able to differentiate its self from the parent-object, resulting in projection of oral sadistic parts of the self onto external objects, then reintrojected into the body and body organs (Klein, 1948; H. Rosenfeld, 1958); the dread of retaliation for sadistic fantasies turned into death anxiety, which then attaches to organs as a lesser threat to the intactness of the self (Kohut, 1971; Stolorow, 1979); the self-punishment by the superego (conscience) against the ego for permitting the breakthrough of id impulses (A. Freud, 1973; S. Freud, 1923). Riviere (1936) and others (Klein, 1948) emphasized the hypochondriacal experience of both love and hate toward an internalized object. Attempts to measure hostility have shown varying results, although correlation of anger and hostility with somatic symptoms has been noted (Barsky *et al.*, 1988; Kellner *et al.*, 1985; Mabe *et al.*, 1996; Noyes *et al.*, 1997).

Depending on the intensity of aggressive impulses or fantasies, they are variably referred to as *anger, hate, rage,* or *hostility.* Psychoanalytic literature often refers to oral or anal sadism or envy, depending on the developmental phase from which they derive. Milrod describes how self-pitying, self-comforting patients "inhibit the direct expression of hostile impulses while remaining surprisingly unaware of their less obvious, indirect or 'unintended' hostile behavior" (Milrod, 1972, p. 516).

## Sadomasochistic Interactions

For the most part, aggression, in psychoanalytic literature, is considered primarily an instinctual drive that remains unconscious until it manifests itself in acts, feelings, thoughts, or emotion. To the extent that aggressive impulses are often inhibited and unconscious, hypochondriacal patients will present as very needy, dependent, and demanding, but also passive in their response to proffered treatments, procedures, examinations, and so on. In this respect, they often enter a "corrupt bargain" with physicians to embark on extensive exploratory journeys, only to be ultimately and "justifiably" angered at the result.

At this point, the anger is projected onto the disappointing powerful figure and out of the self, only to be soon once again turned against the self to assuage the ensuing guilty feelings. In this manner, the cycle is repeated over and over again, projecting sadistic impulses onto others, then turning them once again on the self and inviting masochistic "retaliation" (Broden and Myers, 1981; A. Freud, 1923;

S. Freud, 1919). It is this thinly veiled anger that is generally experienced by physicians in repeated (or even first) contacts with hypochondriacal patients. Physicians express their frustration and counteraggression by using pejorative labels in referring to these patients (e.g., "crocks," "gourds," "turkeys," and so on) or describing how "They get under my skin" (or, in Britain, as "heartsink" patients who cause the physician's heart to sink when he sees their names on the daily list) (Mathers *et al.*, 1995; Lipsitt, 1970; see also Chapter 12).

Although one might expect that inwardly directed rage would spare others the exposure to the patient's anger, this anger is nevertheless readily experienced through the patient's persistent symptoms. Vaillant (1977, p. 180) describes hypochondriasis as "a profoundly irritating means of containing hostility," explaining that "rather than reproach others who in the past have failed to care for him, the hypochondriac berates the doctor." (We will recall Freud's designation of hypochondriacal symptoms as "self-reproaches.") It is this transformation of covert rage into complaints that Vaillant believes renders the hypochondriacal patient incapable of being comforted. In observing an aversion to explanation of symptoms in hypochondriacal patients, Wahl (1964, p. 203) notes that they "appear to be angered by attempts of the physician to assuage their fright or concern." This hostility to the physician has been observed by others as well. Valenstein notes how the hypochondriacal patient has a "predilection to exact a singular quality of pain from human relationships" (Valenstein, 1973, p. 366), an observation that helps explain the hostility attributed to hypochondriacal patients and the vexation experienced by their physicians.

In an unusually detailed case report of the psychoanalysis of a hypochondriacal woman, the psychoanalyst relates how the patient "made me feel anxious," describing the struggles with the patient that carried the risk of precipitating a sadomasochistic relationship in which each participant (patient and analyst) would express "insistence on one's own position as the only valid one" (Gutwinski-Jeggle, 1997, p. 56). In the medical setting, physician and patient each often has his own agenda, resulting in interaction of two individuals as though speaking different languages to one another.

## Defenses in Hypochondriasis

In a general sense, a *defense* is a mechanism of the ego that serves to protect the individual (self) from the emotional distress or trauma invoked by loss (of love or the object of love), by fears of imminent (internal or external) danger, or by the experience of "unpleasure" (A. Freud, 1973). When "prohibited" wishes, ideas, or feelings that are associated with real or imagined punishment threaten to break through into consciousness, an unconscious effort is made to repress them and, in the process, to substitute some other more acceptable—even if still bothersome—expression of the original mental phenomena. The ultimate expression is sufficiently disguised as guilt, pain, embarrassment, shame, depression or anxiety to distract one's full conscious attention from the "real" danger, while at the same time serving as a signal that such danger may be nearby. To the extent that the defenses "work," the individual may remain stably symptomatic or adapted; when they fail, affect can overwhelm the ego, leading to decompensation and ultimately fragmentation and disorganization (often referred to in lay language as "nervous breakdown").

In the theoretical formulations discussed above, one sees what a variety of defenses accomplish the work of hypochondriasis (Aisenstein and Gibeault, 1991). *Displacement* allows the individual to "disown" certain feelings, thoughts, wishes, and fantasies by *projecting* them onto others or onto the self (bodily organs). Awareness of guilt, aggression, and sexuality is diminished through *repression*. The mechanism of *introjection* permits the individual to internalize ambivalently held people (parents) from earliest life who, as sources of guilt, criticism, and punishment, must then be converted to less threatening forces, as physical symptoms, or expelled as other projections. Through *regression*, the individual retreats from a more to a less mature level of adjustment, which is not conflict free, but still less taxing than efforts at mature adaptation. *Splitting* occurs when the individual attempts to adapt by separating experiences and perceptions; the hypochondriacal patient uses this mechanism in characterizing doctors as "good" or "bad" according to how the patient's self-perceived needs are met, a mechanism frequently observed in borderline patients (Groves, 1978; Kernberg, 1975). Hypochondriasis itself is regarded by some as an immature mechanism of defense (Vaillant, 1977); as such, it allows "the transformation of reproach towards others arising from bereavement, loneliness, or unacceptable aggressive impulses into first self-reproach and then complaints of pain, somatic illness, and neurasthenia" (Vaillant, 1977, p. 384). Many other mechanisms of defense may be invoked in describing hypochondriasis: for example, symbolization, denial, distortion, passive-aggressive behavior, acting out, substitution, isolation, and so on.

## Conclusion

In hypochondriasis, the (unconscious) guilt over sexual (libidinous) and hostile (aggressive) wishes, fantasies, and feelings must be disguised to avoid overwhelming the individual (self, ego) with fears of (retaliatory) punishment, bodily damage ("castration"), and death. Thus, the illness of hypochondriasis, through its physical symptoms, permits the expression of all aspects of this constellation in something less than its full impact, namely the fear and conviction of serious disease (resisting reassurance), preoccupation with bodily functions (withdrawal from external interests), the persistence (chronicity) of symptoms, the unpleasure as well as pleasure (comforting the self, antagonizing others, secondary gain of illness), and the dependency on others (frequent medical visits). This "compromise formation" is achieved, in psychodynamic terms, through the work of defense mechanisms. The end result is the presentation of a physical complaint, generally (but not always) without concomitant physical findings.

The interplay of various defenses in the process of symptom formation is very complex. Nonetheless, an awareness of their role in hypochondriasis alerts the clinician to the strong possibility that the presenting complaint is frequently not the problem, but only a communicational representation of what may historically have preceded and, in fact, determined the current constellation of symptomatic features. Defenses can be adaptive or pathological, and identifying them as mature (altruism, humor, suppression, anticipation, sublimation), neurotic (intellectualization, repression, displacement, reaction formation, dissociation), or immature (projection, schizoid fantasy, hypochondriasis, passive-aggressive behavior, acting out) Vaillant (1977) helps to identify "where the patient is" in terms of severity of illness and adequacy of adaptation, and thus plays a significant role in the choice of therapeutic intervention (Diamond, 1987).

If understanding precedes empathy and compassion, then awareness of explanatory models for hypochondriacal syndromes may improve therapeutic efficacy, as well as patient and physician/therapist satisfaction. Gabbard has characterized psychodynamic psychiatry as "an approach to diagnosis and treatment characterized by a *way of thinking* about both patient and clinician . . . [including] . . . unconscious meaning and the reexperiencing of past relationships in the present with the clinician" (Gabbard, 1992, p. 991). If this orientation can enhance the clinician's interaction with the hypochondriacal patient, the beginnings of a therapeutic encounter can already begin (Lipsitt, 1986). In the process, much suffering and waste can be averted, while retaining the "complexity and richness of human functioning in the quicksand of neurotransmitters and molecular genetics" (Gabbard, 1992, p. 997) that tends to dominate medical progress. A psychodynamic perspective helps to retain meaning.

It must be kept in mind that no single model is adequate to explicate the complex interconnections of mind and body and their interaction with the social matrix that eventuates in something that for over two-thousand years has been called "hypochondriasis." The temporal interval between Freud's conception of "somatic compliance" and the entry into a new millennium has seen remarkable advances in neuroscience: genomic decoding, positron emission tomography (PET), magnetic resonance imaging (MRI), psychoneuroendocrinology, psychopharmacologic discovery, and so on, all of which can further our understanding of a most perplexing illness. We are now able to penetrate "far behind the frontiers of physiological research" where Freud left off (1914, p. 84) and to incorporate an almost infinite number of scientific insights into our clinical reasoning.

Our task is to acknowledge the contributions from every field and to integrate them in a manner that has the greatest likelihood of benefiting the patient. One model need not preclude another even when their respective languages may differ (Lipsitt, 1971). Psychoanalytic data and theory must ultimately be combined with physiological data to illuminate the mechanisms by which disease evolves (Reiser, 1968). It is toward that objective that I have attempted, in this chapter, to synthesize the psychoanalytic/psychodynamic insights that may assist us in the full understanding of hypochondriasis. Much remains to be clarified.

### References

Aisenstein M., Gibeault A. 1991. The work of hypochondria. *International Journal of Psycho-Analysis* 72: 669–681.

American Psychiatric Association. 1994. *Diagnostic and Statistical Manual of Mental Disorders, Fourth Edition (DSM-IV)*. Washington, DC: American Psychiatric Association.

Barsky A.J., Goodson J.D., Lane R.S., Cleary P.D. 1988. The amplification of somatic symptoms. *Psychosomatic Medicine* 50: 510–519.

Bonaparte M., Freud A., Kris E. 1954. *The Origins of Psycho-analysis: Letters to Wilhelm Fliess, Drafts and Notes: 1887–1902 by Sigmund Freud*. New York: Basic Books.

Breuer J., Freud S. 1893–95. Studies on hysteria. In *The Complete Psychological Works of Sigmund Freud, Standard Edition, Vol. 2:* 253–307. London: Hogarth Press, 1957.

Broden A.R., Myers W.A. 1981. Hypochodriacal symptoms as derivatives of unconscious fantasies of being beaten or tortured. *Journal of the American Psychoanalytic Association* 29: 535–557.

Bromberg W., Schilder P. 1933. Death and dying. *Psychoanalytic Review* 20: 133–185.

Bromberg W., Schilder P. 1936. The attitude of psychoneurotics toward death. *Psychoanalytic Review* 23: 1–25.

Diamond D.B. 1987. Psychotherapeutic approaches to the treatment of panic attacks, hypochondriasis and agoraphobia. *British Journal of Medical Psychology* 60: 79–84.

Edgcumbe R., Burgner M. 1973. Some problems in the conceptualization of early object relations. I. The concepts of need satisfaction and need-satisfying relationships. *Psychoanalytic Study of the Child* 27: 283–333.

Edgerton J., Campbell R.J. (eds). 1994. *American Psychiatric Glossary, Seventh Edition*. Washington, DC: American Psychiatric Press.

Fenichel O. 1945. *The Psychoanalytic Theory of Neurosis.* New York: Norton.

Freud A. 1923. The relation of beating phantasies to a daydream. *International Journal of Psycho-Analysis* 4: 89–102.

Freud A. 1952a. Notes on a connection between the states of negativism and of emotional surrender (Hörigkeit). *The Writings of Anna Freud, Vol. 4:* 256–259. New York: International Universities Press, 1968.

Freud A. 1952b. The role of bodily illness in the mental life of children. *Psychoanalytic Study of the Child* 7: 69–81.

Freud A. 1973. *Ego and the Mechanisms of Defense, Revised Edition.* New York: International Universities Press.

Freud S. 1905 [1901]. Fragment of an analysis of a case of hysteria. In *Standard Edition, Vol 7:* 3–122. London: Hogarth Press. 1953.

Freud S. 1911. Psycho-analytic notes on an autobiographical account of a case of paranoia (dementia paranoides). In *Standard Edition, Vol. 12:* 3–86. London: Hogarth Press, 1958.

Freud S. 1914. On narcissism: an introduction. In *Standard Edition, Vol 14:* 69–102. London: Hogarth Press, 1957.

Freud S. 1918 [1914]. From the history of an infantile neurosis. In *Standard Edition, Vol. 17:* 7–122. London: Hogarth Press, 1955.

Freud S. 1919. A child is being beaten. In *Standard Edition, Vol. 17:* 179–204, 1955.

Freud S. 1923. The ego and the id. In *Standard Edition, Vol. 19:* 3–69. London: Hogarth Press, 1961.

Furer M. 1972. The history of the superego concept in psychoanalysis: a review of the literature. In *Moral Values and the Superego Concept in Psychoanalysis* (ed. Post S.C.), New York: International Universities Press.

Gabbard G.O. 1992. Psychodynamic psychiatry in the "decade of the brain." *American Journal of Psychiatry* 149: 991–998.

Groves J.E. 1978. Taking care of the hateful patient. *New England Journal of Medicine* 298: 883–887.

Guntrip H. 1968. *Schizoid Phenomena, Object-Relations, and the Self.* New York: International Universities Press.

Gutwinski-Jeggle J. 1997. Hypochondria versus the relation to the object. *International Journal of Psycho-Analysis* 78: 53–68.

Horney K. 1936. The problem of the negative therapeutic reaction. *Psychoanalytic Quarterly* 5: 29–44.

Jacobs S.C., Hoge M.A., Sledge W.H., Bunney B.S. 1997. Managed care, health care reform, and academic psychiatry. *Academic Psychiatry* 21: 72–85.

Jacobson E. 1953. The affects and their pleasure-unpleasure qualities in relation to the psychic discharge processes. In *Drives, Affects, Behavior, Vol. 1* (ed. Lowenstein R.M.), New York: International Universities Press.

Kellner R., Slocumb J., Wiggins R.G., Abbott P.J., Winslow W.W., Pathak D. 1985. Hostility, somatic symptoms, and hypochondriacal fears and beliefs. *Journal of Nervous and Mental Disease* 173: 554–560.

Kernberg O. 1975. *Borderline Conditions and Pathological Narcissism.* New York: Jason Aronson.

Klein M. 1948. *Contributions to Psychoanalysis.* London: Hogarth Press.

Kohut H. 1971. *The Analysis of the Self.* New York: International Universities Press.

Ladee G.A. 1966. *Hypochondriacal Syndromes.* Amsterdam: Elsevier.

Levy D.M. 1932. Body interest in children and hypochondriasis. *American Journal of Psychiatry* 89: 295–315.

Lipsitt D.R. 1968. The "rotating" patient. *Journal of Geriatric Psychiatry* 2: 51–61.

Lipsitt D.R. 1970. Medical and psychological characteristics of "crocks." *Psychiatry in Medicine* 1: 15–25.

Lipsitt D.R. 1971. The relevance of psychoactive agents to psychotherapy. *Psychiatric Quarterly* 45: 76–86.

Lipsitt D.R. 1973. Psychodynamic considerations of hypochondriasis. *Psychotherapy and Psychosomatics* 23: 132–141.

Lipsitt D.R. 1975. The use of self-restraint in the practice and teaching of psychotherapy. *Psychotherapy and Psychosomatics* 25: 201–206.

Lipsitt D.R. 1986. Therapeutic alliance in psychiatric consultation. In *Psychiatry, Vol. 2* (eds. Michels R., Cavenar J.O., Brodie H.K.H.), Philadelphia: Lippincott.

Mabe P.A., Riley W.T., Jones L.R., Hobson D.P. 1996. The medical context of hypochondriacal traits. *International Journal of Psychiatry in Medicine* 26: 443–459.

Macalpine I., Hunter R.A. 1953. The Schreber case: a contribution to schizophrenia, hypochondria, and psychosomatic symptom-formation. *Psychoanalytic Quarterly* 22: 328–371.

Mathers N., Jones N., Hannay D. 1995. Heartsink patients: a study of their general practitioners. *British Journal of General Practice* 45: 293–296.

Meissner W.W. 1976. Schreber and the paranoid process. *The Annual of Psychoanalysis* 4: 3–40.

Meissner W.W. 1977. The Wolf Man and the paranoid process. *The Annual of Psychoanalysis* 5: 23–74.

Meltzer D. 1964. The differentiation of somatic delusions from hypochondria. *International Journal of Psycho-Analysis* 45: 246–250.

Milrod D. 1972. Self-pitying, self-comforting, and the superego. *Psychoanalytic Study of the Child* 27: 505–528.

Niederland W.G. 1974. *The Schreber Case. Psychoanalytic Profile of a Paranoid Personality*. New York: Quadrangle/The New York Times Book Company.

Noyes R. Jr., Holt C.S., Happel R.L., Kathol R.G., Yagla S.J. 1997. A family study of hypochondriasis. *Journal of Nervous and Mental Disease* 185: 223–232.

Nunberg H., Federn E. 1962. *Minutes of the Vienna Psychoanalytic Society: Vol. 1 (1906–1908)*. New York: International Universities Press.

Nunberg H., Federn E. 1967. *Minutes of the Vienna Psychoanalytic Society, Vol. 2 (1908–1910)*. New York: International Universities Press.

Nunberg H., Federn E. 1974. *Minutes of the Vienna Psychoanalytic Society, Vol. 3 (1910–1911)*. New York: International Universities Press.

Nunberg H., Federn E. 1975. *Minutes of the Vienna Psychoanalytic Society, Vol. 4 (1912–1918)*. New York: International Universities Press.

Olinick S.L. 1964. The negative therapeutic reaction. *International Journal of Psychoanalysis* 45: 540–548.

Olinick S.L. 1970. Panel report: negative therapeutic reaction. *Journal of the American Psychoanalytic Association* 18: 665–672.

Reiser M. 1968. Psychoanalytic method in psychosomatic research. *International Journal of Psycho-Analysis* 49: 231–235.

Ritvo S. 1981. Anxiety, symptom formation, and ego autonomy. *Psychoanalytic Study of the Child* 36: 339–364

Ritvo S., Solnit A.J. 1958. Influences of early mother–child interaction on identification processes. *Psychoanalytic Study of the Child* 13: 64–85.

Riviere J. 1936. A contribution to the analysis of the negative therapeutic reaction. *International Journal of Psycho-Analysis* 17: 304–320.

Rosenfeld D. 1984. Hypochondrias, somatic delusions and body scheme in psychoanalytic practice. *International Journal of Psycho-Analysis* 65: 377–387.

Rosenfeld H. 1958. Some observations on the psychopathology of hypochondriacal states. *International Journal of Psycho-Analysis* 39: 121–124.

Rosenfeld H. 1965. *Psychotic States.* London: Hogarth Press.

Schäfer M.L. 1982. Phenomenology and hypochondria. In *Phenomenology and Psychiatry* (eds. de Koning A.J.J., Jenner F.A.), London: Academic Press.

Schur M. 1972. *Freud: Living and Dying.* New York: International Universities Press.

Spitz R.A. 1965. *The First Year of Life.* New York: International Universities Press.

Starcevic V. 1989. Pathological fear of death, panic attacks, and hypochondriasis. *American Journal of Psychoanalysis* 49: 347–361.

Starcevic V. 1991. Reassurance and treatment of hypochondriasis. *General Hospital Psychiatry* 13: 122–127.

Stekel W. 1949. *Compulsion and Doubt, Vols. 1 and 2.* New York: Liveright.

Stolorow R.D. 1977. Notes on the signal function of hypochondriacal anxiety. *International Journal of Psycho-Analysis* 58: 245–246.

Stolorow R.D. 1979. Defensive and arrested developmental aspects of death anxiety, hypochondriasis and depersonalization. *International Journal of Psycho-Analysis* 60: 201–213.

Vaillant G.E. 1977. *Adaptation to Life.* Boston: Little, Brown.

Valenstein A.F. 1962. The psycho-analytic situation: affects, emotional reliving and insight in the psycho-analytic process. *International Journal of Psycho-Analysis* 43: 315–324.

Valenstein A.F. 1973. On attachment to painful feelings and the negative therapeutic reaction. *Psychoanalytic Study of the Child* 28: 365–392.

Wahl C.W. 1964. Psychodynamics of the hypochondriacal patient. In *New Dimensions in Psychosomatic Medicine* (ed. Wahl C.W.), Boston: Little, Brown.

# 9

# Meaning, Misinterpretations, and Medicine: A Cognitive-Behavioral Approach to Understanding Health Anxiety and Hypochondriasis

PAUL M. SALKOVSKIS
HILARY M. C. WARWICK

On an Internet bulletin board, someone reported that "my psychiatrist has just told me that I am suffering from *DSM-IV*." As therapists and researchers working with the problems characterized by severe and persistent health anxiety, we also suffer from *DSM-IV* (American Psychiatric Association, 1994), not least because it defines health anxiety as the somatoform disorder "Hypochondriasis." This classification is theoretically misleading, as it diverts attention away from the importance of anxiety and therefore threat, and onto more superficial characteristics of the problem. Still more problematic is the understandable dislike of the term by sufferers, who regard it as a pejorative label often equated with "imaginary illness" and malingering.

The alternative perspective, adopted as an integral part of the cognitive-behavioral approach to understanding and treating such problems, is to conceptualize hypochondriasis as the most extreme manifestation of severe and persistent anxiety focused upon health threat. This perspective not only has a normalizing influence that is helpful in therapy and personally empowering for the sufferer, but also allows the approach to be applied across a wider range of problems, including more transient forms of health anxiety; such an example is health anxiety as a response to medical procedures like health screening (Salkovskis and Rimes, 1997).

It is nevertheless instructive to examine the *DSM IV* definition, which presumably defines a group of people who suffer from particularly severe and persistent health anxiety, from the point of view of cognitive-behavioral theory. The main problem is defined as a preoccupation with *either* (a) the fear of having, *or* (b) the belief that one already has, a serious physical illness. These are quite different clinical presentations, and the distinction has profound implications both for the way the problem is conceptualized and for the ease of engagement in psychological or psychiatric treatment.

The fear of having a serious physical illness is likely to present as an explicitly psychological problem. For example, such a patient may present by saying, "I want you to help me with my fear of cancer." By contrast, the belief that one already has a serious physical illness tends to be presented with an explicit or implicit rejection of the notion of a psychological problem. For example, "I don't need psychological help. My problem is that I have cancer." This distinction closely corresponds to the notions of "illness phobia" and "disease conviction" (Bianchi, 1971). It is notable that most patients with disease conviction usually also show elements of illness phobia, although the converse is much less likely to be true (see also Chapter 2).

According to the *DSM-IV* diagnostic criteria, the preoccupation with health is based on the person's misinterpretation of bodily sensations. That is, the diagnosis depends on the detection of the presence of a cognitive distortion. Although welcoming the inclusion of the core cognitive factor in the definition, we believe it to be unduly restrictive to confine the misinterpretation criterion to bodily sensations. Patients anxious about their health tend to misinterpret other types of bodily *variations* as well, such as asymmetries in shape, skin blemishes, changes in bowel function, and so on. In addition, they also tend to misinterpret a range of other health-related information, including things doctors tell them, health information in the mass media, and the results of health screening programs.

To fulfill the criteria the problem is required to persist "despite medical examination and reassurance." The hidden implication of this criterion is that, to be diagnosed as suffering from hypochondriasis, reassurance has not only to have been offered, but also to have failed. This is an odd conceptualization, not least because it means that diagnosis depends on a physician delivering a form of psychotherapy (reassurance is the most widely used psychotherapeutic intervention in medicine; see Warwick and Salkovskis, 1985), and on this intervention being unsuccessful. Reassurance can take a wide range of forms, from "There's nothing medically wrong with you, so please leave my office" to a careful and detailed account of why the person cannot be suffering from the disease he or she fears. This second example highlights one of the fundamental problems of reassurance, which is that it aims to reduce people's fears by convincing them that they do *not* have a particular disease.

Given that there is evidence that reassurance is itself open to misinterpretation, we have suggested that, in some vulnerable individuals, the problem may persist *because* of medical examination and reassurance rather than *despite* it (Salkovskis and Warwick, 1986). By contrast to a "reassurance"-based intervention, the cognitive-behavioral approach to understanding and treating health anxiety suggests that the most appropriate way of dealing with fears is to help the person reconceptualize his or her problem in a positive way. That means helping the person understand both the specific and general ways in which anxiety can account for what he or she experiences. The cognitive-behavioral treatment approach is therefore based on the well-established notion that the best way to change a misinterpretation is to provide an alternative, more convincing (and possibly, but not necessarily, more accurate) explanation. If this alternative account is *sufficiently* convincing, then it is likely to displace the negative explanation.

## The Importance of Appraisal and Misinterpretation in the Experience of Health Anxiety

The cognitive theory of emotional problems developed by Beck and colleagues (1985) proposes that the misinterpretation of ambiguous situations or stimuli as more threatening than they really are is central to the experience and persistence of anxiety disorders. The meaning a person attaches to a stimulus or situation is therefore crucial in generating anxiety. For example, a person who experiences palpitations and believes these to be the early signs of heart disease is likely to become anxious and preoccupied with these concerns. When a man's family doctor sends him to see a cardiologist (the doctor's idea being to reassure him that all is well with his heart), he misinterprets the referral as an indication that the doctor believes him to have heart disease, and wishes to confirm this suspicion. The person understandably becomes anxious about and preoccupied with his health prior to the cardiology appointment. Unfortunately, his heightened anxiety also makes him more likely to misinterpret any ambiguous information in communications from the cardiology clinic, further increasing the person's belief that he has heart disease. The cognitive-behavioral hypothesis of hypochondriasis thus proposes that the central mechanism in people suffering from persistent health anxiety and hypochondriasis is a relatively enduring tendency to misinterpret bodily symptoms, bodily variations, and other information regarded as relevant to health as evidence of serious physical illness (Salkovskis, 1988a, 1989, 1996a; Salkovskis and Warwick, 1986; Salkovskis and Clark, 1993; Warwick and Salkovskis, 1990).

   The cognitive theory specifies that the impact of any misinterpretation is a function of the degree of threat perceived, which is in turn a function of at least four factors. The most obvious of these is the perceived likelihood of illness, which interacts with the perceived awfulness of that illness (this factor cannot only include factors such as the pain and suffering of being ill, but the more general consequences such as loss of role, upset and disturbance to loved ones, and so on). The other modulating factors are the extent to which the person perceives himself or herself as likely to be able to prevent the illness from worsening and the extent to which he or she is able to affect its course—that is, having effective means of coping with the perceived threat and the possibility of external factors intervening to help. In health anxiety, this latter aspect often focuses on the likely effectiveness of medical help. In the worst case, some patients perceive "rescue factors" as having a negative value; for example, believing that treatment of a cancer would be worse than the cancer itself. Taken together, the interaction among these different aspects of appraisal can be represented as:

$$\text{Anxiety} = \frac{\text{Perceived likelihood of illness}}{\text{Perceived ability to cope with the illness}} \times \frac{\text{Perceived cost, awfulness and burden of the illness}}{\text{Perception of the extent to which external factors will help (rescue factors)}}$$

An important implication of this analysis is that it is possible to be highly anxious about health with relatively low perceived likelihood of illness, given a relatively high perception of the awfulness of being ill (for example, people who believe that having cancer would result in being crippled by pain, disabled, becoming physically repulsive, being rejected and abandoned by those they love, and generally being dehumanized). Furthermore, a pattern of this kind coupled with a highly perceived likelihood of illness is likely to result in very extreme levels of anxiety. All four factors need to be taken into account both in the formulation of health anxiety and in any treatment interventions. It is also important to note that the factors identified here as important to health anxiety are those involved not only in other anxiety disorders, but also in normal anxiety (Beck et al., 1985); this allows an element of normalization to be included in treatment strategies (see also Chapter 14).

## The Origins and Maintenance of Misinterpretations

The cognitive theory suggests that the *origins and development* of the tendency to misinterpret health-relevant information can be understood in terms of the way in which knowledge and past experiences of illness (in self or others) leads to the formation of assumptions about symptoms, disease, health behaviors, the medical profession, and so on. Such general health-related assumptions can arise from a wide variety of sources, including early health- and illness-related experience, later events such as unexpected or unpleasant illness in the person's social circle, and information in the mass media. Figure 9.1 shows how the cognitive-behavioral approach conceptualizes the development of health anxiety.

Many of the assumptions learned are likely to be universal or shared by many others of similar cultural backgrounds. Socialized beliefs concerning possible sources of misinterpretation make the understanding of health anxiety relatively easier. The logic of misinterpretations is such that there are particular misinterpretations which are relatively likely for some stimuli and not for others. Examples of these are illustrated in Table 9.1.

It is proposed that the type of assumptions likely to lead to more severe and persistent health anxiety are those that are relatively rigid and extreme. For example, most people will share the assumption that "persistent and intense physical discomfort of an unusual and unexplained type could be a sign of ill health." The person prone to health anxiety, by contrast, will tend to believe that "any unexplained change in my body is always going to be a sign of serious illness." This former assumption is likely to be helpful in that it is likely to lead to an acceptable level of consultation motivated by health concern; the latter is more likely

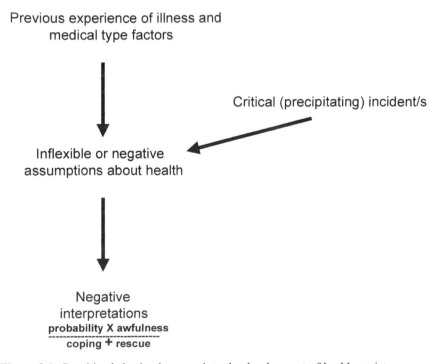

**Figure 9.1.** Cognitive-behavioral approach to the development of health anxiety.

**Table 9.1.** Meaning links bodily variations and misinterpretations

| Bodily variations | Misinterpretations |
| --- | --- |
| Heart racing, pounding, palpitations | "I'm having a heart attack; my heart will stop." |
| Lumps under skin | "I've got cancer." |
| Loss of sensation and tingling in arms and legs | "I've got multiple sclerosis." |
| Feeling dizzy, faint, weak legs | "I've got HIV, AIDS." |
| Feeling dizzy, heart pounding, chest tight and painful, palpitations | "I'm dying!" |
| Plus: | |
| Doctor sends you for further investigations | This means he or she believes, "I already have a serious illness." |

to lead to constant self-monitoring of bodily variations and both frequent medical consultation and extreme fear reactions motivated by overly negative interpretations of benign situations and stimuli. A further example of assumptions related to the way medical consultations are conducted is discussed elsewhere in this chapter.

Previous experience of physical ill-health in patients and their families and previous experience of unsatisfactory medical management may also be important in generating problematic assumptions about risks to health (see Bianchi, 1971). A striking example of the impact of media coverage of illness risk is provided by the increased occurrence of cases of "AIDS phobia" (Miller *et al.*, 1985) noted after the massive publicity campaign on this topic. More recently, media attention focused on the risk of "mad cow disease" has triggered persistent fears of and preoccupations with Creutzfeldt-Jakob disease in vulnerable individuals in the UK.

## General Health Assumptions Lead to Specific Misinterpretations

Examples of the type of potentially problematic assumptions that can lead to misinterpretations are "bodily changes are usually a sign of serious disease, because every symptom has to have an identifiable physical cause"; "if you don't go to the doctor as soon as you notice anything unusual, then it will be too late." Other beliefs relate to specific personal weaknesses and particular illnesses; for example, "There's heart trouble in the family," and "I've had weak lungs since I was a baby." Such beliefs may be a constant source of anxiety and/or may be activated in vulnerable individuals by critical incidents.

This type of assumption can also lead the patient to attend selectively to information that appears to confirm the idea of having an illness, and to selectively ignore or discount evidence indicating good health. A self-maintaining confirmatory bias can therefore occur once a critical incident has activated health-related assumptions and resulted in the misinterpretation of bodily variations or health information as indications of serious illness (Hitchcock and Mathews, 1992). Situations that constitute critical incidents and activate previously dormant assumptions include unfamiliar bodily sensations, hearing details of illness in a friend of a similar age, or new information about illness. Additional bodily sensations may then be noticed as a consequence of increased vigilance arising from anxiety. In patients who become particularly anxious about their health, such situations are associated with thoughts that represent personally catastrophic interpretations of the bodily sensations or signs. These misinterpretations drive and motivate a number of reactions that not only have the effect of maintaining the misinterpretations themselves but also of generating further stimuli that act as additional sources of misinterpretation.

Figure 9.2 shows the interaction between some of the factors involved in intensifying the perceived threat (and therefore anxiety), as well as the responses hypothesized to result in the persistence of such intense health anxiety. Elevations in the patient's perceived likelihood of being ill interacts and synergizes with the perceived awfulness of his or her feared illness, which in itself will often be inflated. At the same time, the health-anxious patient is likely to perceive himself or herself as unable to prevent the illness, and unable to affect its course (i.e., as having no effective means of coping with the perceived threat).

When patients become particularly anxious about their health, their preoccupation with such negative interpretations (experienced as personally catastrophic thoughts and images) will focus on bodily variations and other information that is appraised as relevant to their (ill) health. Catastrophic interpretations can in turn lead to one of two patterns of anxiety (or some combination). If the sensations or signs are *not* primarily those that increase as a direct result of the experience of anxiety (including, but not confined to, the consequences of autonomic arousal), or the patient does *not* regard the feared catastrophe as imminent (e.g., "These palpitations are the first sign of heart disease"), then the reaction will more likely be that typical of patients with a diagnosis of hypochondriasis. In contrast, if the symptoms that are misinterpreted are those which occur as part of anxiety-induced autonomic arousal *and* the interpretation is that the symptoms are evidence of *immediate* catastrophe (e.g., "These palpitations mean that I am having a heart attack right now"), a further immediate increase in symptoms will

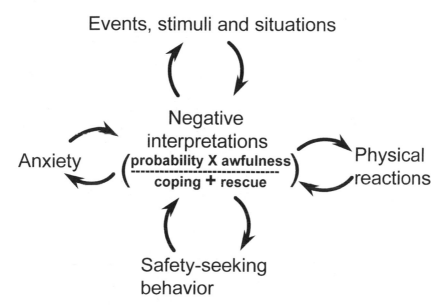

**Figure 9.2.** Factors involved in maintaining health anxiety.

result. If this process continues unchecked, it will spiral out of control, and a panic attack is the more likely response. There are reasons to consider that the two problems often overlap (see below); however, while the panic-type response is likely to be confined to sensations subject to rapid increase when anxious, both anxiety-related and anxiety-unrelated symptoms may play a part in the concerns of hypochondriasis patients.

## Specific Factors Involved in the Maintenance of Health Anxiety

Negative or even catastrophic interpretations of health-relevant information are commonplace. From time to time, the majority of people are liable to become briefly preoccupied with unexplained bodily variations. However, such episodes of health anxiety are usually transient. Symptoms fade, reassuring information from our doctor is absorbed with relief, and our anxiety about health declines and disappears. Clearly, the key to understanding and helping those in whom this health anxiety does not fade (or in whom it escalates to the point where it dominates the person's life) lies in understanding what it is that causes such anxiety to *persist*. The cognitive theory makes a simple prediction. The persistence of health anxiety is a result of processes that maintain the interpretations from which the anxiety arises. As each of these processes is motivated by threat beliefs, either as an automatic reaction or as strategically deployed responses to the perception of threat, vicious circles form. Some of the key processes that are hypothesized or known to operate to maintain negative appraisals are illustrated in Figure 9.2.

Although the relative contribution of each factor, and the specific details of those that are involved, vary from person to person, four main types of processes tend to be involved. These are: information-processing biases (particularly selective attention); physiological reactions (including, but not confined to, heightened experience of bodily sensations); safety-seeking behaviors (including avoidance, checking, and reassurance-seeking); and affective changes (particularly anxiety and depression).

## Biases in the Way That Threat Information Is Processed

Once a person begins actively to contemplate the possibility that he or she is suffering from a serious physical illness, the person's attention understandably turns to gathering evidence relevant to this possibility. Most people will have a tendency to err on the side of caution, as the consequences of a false negative decision (mistakenly believing that one is healthy when cancer is present, and therefore failing to take appropriate preventative action) are considerably more serious than the consequences of a false positive decision (deciding that one has cancer when this is not so). Patients with persistent health anxiety may be particularly aware of this difference and therefore consider inadequate anything less than *complete certainty* that they are healthy.

Attention is selectively focused on information that *could be* consistent with illness, whereas information inconsistent with illness beliefs tends to be disregarded as, at best, insufficient, and at worst, irrelevant. This phenomenon, often referred to as a *confirmatory bias*, is further bolstered by other assumptions prominent in health anxiety, such as "If I do not worry about my health, then I am likely to become ill." Selective attention is the most obvious manifestation of cognitive bias. Hypochondriacal patients notice (and attach special significance to) stimuli consistent with their health beliefs, and they either fail to notice or disregard inconsistent stimuli. Thus, patients concerned about their heart may notice palpitations that occur after they have gone to bed believing them a sign of cardiac weakness, but fail to notice that their heart responds appropriately (and imperceptibly) to their having to run to catch a bus.

Apart from resulting in increased preoccupation with bodily variations, selective attention can also operate to bias the impact of information provided by doctors in the course of medical consultation. For example, a patient was afraid that the symptoms he was experiencing were a sign of multiple sclerosis (MS). His doctor listed each symptom, indicating that it was not typical of someone with MS. At the end of the consultation, the physician summarized by saying that these symptoms would only be characteristic of MS "in extremely unusual cases." The patient focused on this statement, concluding that the symptoms he was experiencing could, in some cases, be symptomatic of MS, but of a type most doctors would fail to recognize. His disease conviction was therefore *increased* as a consequence of the way he weighted the information given in the consultation.

Once illness fears are activated, attention may be paid to previously unnoticed normal bodily changes (e.g., gastric distention after eating). The fact that they had not previously been noticed can lead the person to conclude that they are new phenomena, and therefore represent the effects of pathological processes. Focusing prompted by worries about health thus brings slight bodily variations to awareness at times when ideas about illness are already present, leading to a bias toward noticing information that is consistent with beliefs about being seriously ill.

## Interactions Between Misinterpretations and Bodily Sensations

Intense anxiety about the possible catastrophic meaning of health-related information and bodily variations will almost invariably result in physiological arousal as part of the normal reaction to stress. Those patients who then misinterpret an increase in symptoms as further evidence of illness will experience yet more anxiety and thus more symptoms, resulting in an upward spiral of symptoms, catastrophic misinterpretations, and anxiety.

Figure 9.3 shows a specific example of the type of cognitive-affective interaction that can generate panic. In this particular example, the negative interpretation also motivates a specific safety-seeking behavior that is likely to increase manifest symptoms. In other words, the belief "I will suffocate" leads to a safety-seeking behavior; patients try to prevent themselves from suffocating by struggling for breath. Unfortunately, the shortness of breath is a consequence of tightening of intercostal muscles, so as patients breathe more deeply, these muscles tighten yet more, generating chest pain and making it harder still to breathe. This safety-seeking behavior (struggling for breath), therefore, has two effects in this instance: It prevents patients from discovering that they will not suffocate, and actually increases breathlessness and sensations from their chest.

This type of pattern is characteristic of patients who experience panic attacks, but also occurs at a relatively lower level of intensity in patients who do not. When panic attacks are prominent, the sequence is almost invariably that if, and only if, bodily sensations are misinterpreted as a sign of a relatively imminent catastrophe, then the resulting anxiety will increase bodily sensations (Clark, 1988; Salkovskis, 1988a; Salkovskis and Clark, 1993). In a subset of patients,

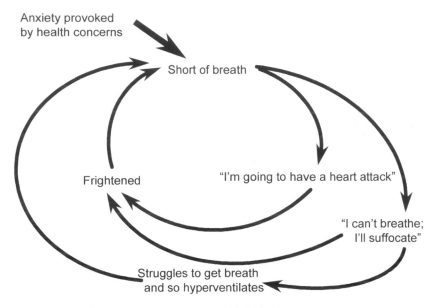

**Figure 9.3.** Example of a panic-type vicious circle/spiral.

this type of misinterpretation is almost immediately exacerbated by physiological processes, such as hyperventilation, as illustrated in Figure 9.3. The importance of processes such as hyperventilation has often been exaggerated (Salkovskis, 1988b). It is clear that seeking to teach patients controlled breathing as a way of combating hyperventilation is not an appropriate target for treatment. The problem is not hyperventilation (which occurs not only as part of panic in some patients, but commonly as a normal physiological response to excitement and anger) but rather the catastrophic meaning the patient attaches to his or her physiological responses. Note also that the vicious circles illustrated in Figure 9.3 would probably only constitute a subset (a "petal") of the processes illustrated in Figure 9.2.

Considerable specificity is often involved in psychophysiological reactions. For example, a patient who believed bowel disturbance indicated that he was developing Crohn's disease would experience abdominal symptoms as a reaction to stress, including the stress provoked by his health concerns. It also seems likely that some idiopathic pain problems might involve similar mechanisms (Salkovskis and Nouwen, in preparation).

There are further sets of effects that probably combine the interpretation/physiological response and interpretation/selective attention links. The meaning that people suffering from severe anxiety about health attach to bodily variations makes them attend more closely than usual to such variations. In doing so, they may develop a heightened ability to detect variations that most people simply would not notice. Patients suffering from severe health anxiety often say, "I'm certain that others are not plagued with a constant awareness of what their body is doing and the way it reacts." It is likely that this is true; individuals with health anxiety notice things that most other people simply would not. Unfortunately, this combination of somatically focused attention and greater awareness of physiological function related to their particular health concerns (Ehlers, 1997) has the understandable effect of further increasing their health concerns.

## Safety-Seeking Behaviors Motivated by Illness Beliefs

Recently, it has been suggested that the avoidance and escape behaviors characteristic of people suffering from anxiety problems can best be conceptualized from a cognitive perspective as "safety-seeking behaviors" (Salkovskis, 1991, 1996a, 1996b; Salkovskis *et al.*, 1996). It is an almost universal response to threat that one takes action intended to avert or reduce the likelihood and impact of perceived threat. Individuals who believe that they may be about to experience some catastrophe will seek to prevent it. The person afraid of having a heart attack refrains from exercising, the person who believes he or she is susceptible to cancer checks for early signs of disease and consults a doctor, perhaps insisting on examination or medical investigations. This type of behavior, by which the person seeks to avoid, check for, or totally exclude physical illnesses (e.g., avoiding physical exertion or contact with disease; reading medical textbooks; requesting frequent medical consultations; checking, manipulating, or inspecting the body), will maintain anxiety by increasing symptoms and preoccupation. Such behavior serves to focus the person yet more on the fears about which he or she worries, and this can thereby increase the degree of preoccupation experienced.

The safety-seeking behaviors used by patients may serve directly to increase the symptoms forming the focus of misinterpretation and, therefore, anxiety. For example, patients who believe that the discomfort they are experiencing indicates incipient disease may be motivated by these concerns to repeatedly prod areas of inflammation or pain, to take inappropriate medication, to focus excessive attention on particular bodily systems, and so on (Salkovskis and Bass, 1997; Warwick and Salkovskis, 1990). This behavior increases the discomfort that the patient has interpreted as a sign of illness and therefore fears. A patient with fears of MS believed that tingling in the fingertips was symptomatic of the diagnosis. He held out his hand, palm up and fingers bent, while focusing on his fingertips. When he did this he was alarmed to notice that he was experiencing tingling. He checked the sensitivity of his fingertips by repeatedly brushing his fingers over his clothes, and he found that the tingling got progressively more noticeable. The same patient believed that MS impaired his ability to become sexually aroused.

He would initiate lovemaking in order to check whether there was any sign of this happening to him. Not surprisingly, he found that sex was less stimulating than before, reinforcing his belief that he did indeed have MS.

Pain patients may adopt unusual ways of carrying out physical activity on the basis of the belief that "hurt equals harm." Unfortunately, some of the ways in which they seek to prevent further damage to themselves can have the effect of increasing muscle spasm and therefore pain. Paradoxically, this type of behavior often has the effect of making the person think thus: "It's this bad when I remember to be careful; it would be much worse if I did not."

Probably the most prominent and troublesome safety-seeking behavior in severe health anxiety is reassurance-seeking, which, as described above, is part of the definition of health anxiety. Several authors have proposed an important role for reassurance, although the possible mechanisms have seldom been discussed. Kenyon (1964) cites Wychoff, who argued that hypochondriasis is largely iatrogenic in the sense of being initiated or perpetuated by doctors, particularly by those ordering further physical investigations "just to make sure." This view is not supported by Pilowsky (1983) or Kellner (1982); the latter states that treatment strategies in hypochondriasis include "repeated physical examinations (with laboratory investigations when appropriate) and reassurance" (Kellner, 1982, p. 155).

The available data support the cognitive-behavioral view (Salkovskis and Warwick, 1986; Warwick and Salkovskis, 1985) that, although reassurance may be helpful in instances in which people have developed transient concerns about health, in people suffering from severe and persistent health anxiety it is likely to be useless at best and counterproductive at worst. Reassurance-seeking will undoubtedly have at least two further effects in many patients. First, it increases the likelihood of ambiguous or false positive results for medical investigations, which will be instituted by the doctor in an attempt to allay patients' fears. Second, it will result in the patients being given slightly different information by different physicians trying to reassure them, or different information by the same physician on different occasions. This usually undermines patients' confidence in their doctors' judgment. Direct contradictions of opinion between doctors have a particularly disastrous effect in this respect.

A substantial proportion of people suffering from health anxiety endorse high levels of belief in assumptions such as "If my doctor sends me for any further medical investigations, this means that he or she is doing so to confirm the suspicion that I am ill." This means that such patients are likely to interpret any investigation or referral to a specialist clinic as confirmation of their fears that their doctor believes them to be ill. If the effects of medical investigation can be so counterproductive, why do patients persist in seeking reassurance of this type?

We suggest that this is because of further assumptions typically held by patients suffering from health anxiety. For example, some patients believe that, because they have a history of anxiety, the doctor might withhold information about illness from them out of a misplaced sense of kindness. Note that this belief is often based on specific direct or indirect experience such as being involved in a decision to withhold information about a terminal diagnosis from an elderly relative. This is known to happen, particularly when it involves people considered by others to be psychologically vulnerable. It is therefore evident to the patients that they must assure themselves that this is not now happening to them, as they are usually aware that others regard them as psychologically vulnerable to potentially adverse health information.

Problematic assumptions may interact in counterproductive ways. Thus, many patients who believe that their doctor would only send them for investigation if there were good reason to believe that they were ill also believe that the only way to *really* rule out an illness is to have medical investigations. Understandably, such patients are reluctant to accept a clinical diagnosis of "wellness" that is not backed up by a specific test or investigation for the problem they fear.

Recently, we have noted that there may be some overlap between the reassurance-motivating beliefs of health-anxious patients and those of people suffering from obsessional problems. In obsessional problems, beliefs concerning the person's fears for being responsible for harm (including harm to themselves) appear to motivate checking and reassurance-seeking behavior (Salkovskis *et al.*, 2000). We believe that health-anxious patients have an inflated sense of responsibility for the way they interact with the physician during medical consultations. If this is so, then this might explain the way in which some patients, anxious about health, tend to irritate physicians by their overinclusive descriptions of the details of their symptoms, the circumstances in which they occur, and so on. Furthermore, such patients often express concern that their description of symptoms lacks sufficient detail for doctors to be able to make a diagnosis.

In a recent instance, one of us encountered a case in which it is clear why such beliefs developed. The patient described how, as a young man, he had believed himself to be "made of steel." He had no worries about his health and tended to ignore his safety in a wide range of health-relevant and health-irrelevant situations. One day, when he was 19, he experienced intense chest pains. Having been reassured by his family doctor that it was most likely caused by a pulled muscle, he ignored it for the remainder of the day. By evening, feeling considerably worse, he went to the emergency room, where the doctor diagnosed a collapsed lung and asked why the patient had not sought attention sooner. Explaining that he had seen his own doctor that morning, he was told that he must have failed to provide his doctor with the appropriate information. At that point, the patient developed the belief that at any time he could be afflicted by a dangerous medical condition, and that it was up to him to alert doctors to *all* relevant details of his condition, otherwise the appropriate diagnosis would not be made.

The most obvious effect of behavior is seen when the person believes that his or her safety-seeking behavior has the immediate and direct effect of preventing the feared catastrophe (as in the instance of individuals who believe they are in danger of having a heart attack if they do not succeed in reducing strain on their heart). In such instances, patients not only experience immediate relief because of the safety they believe they have achieved, but also inadvertently "protect" their belief in the potential for disaster associated with particular sensations. Each episode of anxiety, rather than being a disconfirmation, becomes another example of *nearly* being overtaken by a disaster: "I have almost died of a heart attack many times: I have to be more careful, or one of these times I won't be able to catch it in time." This in effect means that each episode of acute anxiety is perceived as a "near miss," which in itself increases the threat belief.

## Affective-Cognitive Interactions

The interaction between negative beliefs and disturbed mood, particularly anxiety and depression, is well established (Butler and Mathews, 1983; Teasdale, 1983). Affective disturbance increases negative thinking, which further increases affective disturbance, and so on. These processes probably also trigger ruminative worries about further implications of the feared consequences. For example, a woman feared that she had terminal cancer. When preoccupation with this belief became prominent, she would become both anxious and depressed. Her low mood would then bring on ruminations about how the family would cope (or not cope, in this instance) with her illness and subsequent death. She would imagine her husband and daughter struggling with the stress of losing her, and she would become preoccupied with the idea that their lives would be ruined by her death. Such rumination further increased her anxiety and depression, with subsequent escalation.

## Misinterpretations in Panic and Hypochondriasis

As described above, the cognitive theories of both panic disorder and hypochondriasis hypothesize that patients have an enduring tendency to misinterpret bodily sensations in a particularly threatening way, usually as a sign of illness. There is now compelling evidence for this hypothesis in patients suffering from repeated panic attacks relative to both nonclinical subjects and other anxious patients not suffering from panic (Clark *et al.*, 1997). However, hypochondriasis is also defined as preoccupation with illness belief that is based on misinterpretation of bodily sensations. In at least partial recognition of the potential for overlap, *DSM-III-R* (American Psychiatric Association, 1987) hypochondriasis was modified from the *DSM-III* (American Psychiatric Association, 1980) in order to exclude patients in whom the source of misinterpretations of illness exclusively arose from the symptoms of panic attacks. Thus, both conditions have in common the prominence of concerns about catastrophic internal events (illness) and the subjective basis of these concerns in misinterpretations of bodily sensations.

The cognitive hypothesis proposes a number of important ways that misinterpretations differentially affect patients with panic disorder and with hypochondriasis (Clark, 1988; Salkovskis, 1988a; Salkovskis and Clark, 1993; Warwick and Salkovskis, 1990). Salkovskis and Clark (1993) have described these in some detail, suggesting that the principal differences lie in (*1*) the type of symptoms misinterpreted, with panic patients more likely to misinterpret symptoms that can increase as a result of the experience of anxiety compared to hypochondriacal patients, whose focus of concern and misinterpretation covers a broader range of symptoms; (*2*) the time course represented by such misinterpretations, with panic patients being concerned about imminent catastrophes, and hypochondriacal patients tending to be concerned more about problems in the future; (*3*) linked to this, the type of consequent behaviors: Panic patients are more likely to engage in avoidant and escape behaviors, whereas hypochondriacal patients are more likely to use checking and reassurance-seeking behaviors.

In some patients, problems begin in the form of panic attacks, but their health concerns are not restricted to discrete panic episodes. Instead, these patients become preoccupied with broader health concerns, and they may begin to misinterpret nonautonomic symptoms. Such patients may experience both acute panic attacks and hypochondriacal preoccupations, although it could be argued that the hypochondriacal concerns are, in the first instance, secondary to panic (Noyes *et al.*, 1986). Probably less common, but equally interesting, are individuals in whom panic attacks develop as a secondary feature of general health/hypochondriacal preoccupations. This seems particularly likely when the person's fears begin to extend to autonomic sensations with a perceived possibility of more imminent catastrophes. Such people, as a result of having had a relatively long-standing belief concerning ill health, begin to believe that the illness they fear may claim them sooner rather than later.

It has been empirically established that panic patients have an *enduring* tendency to make catastrophic misinterpretations of bodily sensations so that these misinterpretations are not confined only to panic attacks (Clark *et al.*, 1997). This tendency to misinterpret was only found for physical sensations typical of panic; panic patients were not different from other anxious patients in the misinterpretation of other situations. The results remained unchanged once the effects of state anxiety at the time of testing were statistically removed, indicating that these findings could not be attributed to overall differences in anxiety. Some additional evidence shows that hypochondriacal patients differ from other anxious patients in terms of their *perception* and *misinterpretation* of normal bodily sensations (see also Chapter 10). One of the early studies to investigate the perception of bodily sensations was by Tyrer and colleagues (1980), who examined the awareness of pulse rate in cases of hypochondriasis, anxiety neurosis, and phobic anxiety. Subjective ratings of pulse rate were compared with ECG recordings taken during the viewing of films designed to induce varying levels of anxiety. There was a significantly higher correlation between subjective and measured pulse rates in cases of hypochondriasis *and* anxiety neurosis than in cases of phobic anxiety. Patients who originally expressed cardiac concerns had the highest awareness of pulse rate. Thus, the results obtained on this task did not differentiate between hypochondriasis patients and those suffering from anxiety neurosis, a category which incorporates current diagnoses of both panic disorder and generalized anxiety disorder.

In a more recent study (Salkovskis *et al.*, 1999), our group was able to demonstrate specificity in both misinterpretations and behavioral reactions along the lines predicted by cognitive-behavioral theory described above. As predicted, subjects with panic disorder were more likely to misinterpret symptoms that are increased by anxiety, while hypochondriasis subjects were likely to misinterpret a wider range of symptoms. Furthermore, patients suffering from panic attacks were more likely than other patients suffering from anxiety disorders to misinterpret anxiety-related sensations as a sign of immediate catastrophe.

By contrast, the misinterpretations made by hypochondriacal patients centered on catastrophes perceived as occurring at a time in the relatively distant future. It was notable that the substantial group of patients who suffer from both panic disorder and hypochondriasis show both types of misinterpretation, providing further evidence of the specificity of the time course in which the catastrophe is feared likely to occur. The time course of catastrophe was reflected in the type of corrective action chosen by these patients. Ratings of the likelihood of escape and checking behaviors were significantly higher in subjects with a diagnosis of hypochondriasis.

The specificity of misinterpretations predicted and found in severe and persistent health anxiety has important implications for treatment. A commonly used and particularly efficient strategy in the treatment of anxiety disorders such as panic disorder and social phobia involves helping patients to change their behavior in ways that lead to a clear disconfirmation of their threat beliefs (Clark, 1999; Salkovskis, 1991, 1996b; Salkovskis and Clark, 1995; Salkovskis *et al.*, 1999; Wells *et al.*, 1995).

It had previously been suggested that this type of treatment strategy would not be effective if the feared catastrophe were to be located in the more distant future, as disconfirmation would, in many instances, not be an option. It is usually possible to use a brisk run with the therapist to establish that a patient's chest pain is not the sign of an impending heart attack. Such a run would not be convincing for a patient who believes the occasional cardiac irregularity experienced is merely an early sign of a heart condition that will culminate in serious harm years later. Consequently, the cognitive therapist has to rely on providing the sufferers with a clear non-catastrophic alternative explanation of the patient's problem, and help to convince the patient that this alternative is true.

An example of a specific maintenance model worked out in the course of clinical assessment of a patient with fears of cancer is illustrated in Figure 9.4. Such a model would, for that patient, form the basis of the alternative account used in therapy.

If the alternative account is sufficiently convincing for the sufferer, it results in decreasing plausibility of the threatening explanation previously held by the patient (i.e., "I have the early signs of heart disease"). Clearly, alternative explanations based on more accurate understanding of the psychopathology of the problem concerned are more likely to be convincing to the sufferer, and they are particularly likely to survive the person's subsequent experience both in and out of therapy. We believe that the cognitive-behavioral approach is the best supported account of health anxiety, and it currently offers the most useful and ac-

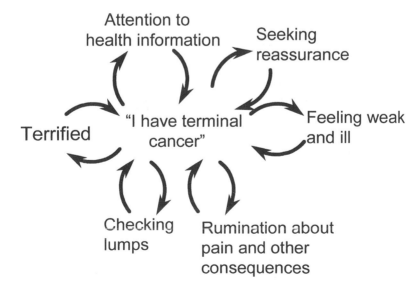

**Figure 9.4.** A specific maintenance model in a patient with hypochondriasis.

cessible way of helping people suffering from severe and persistent health anxiety to understand and deal with their problems.

## Conclusion

The cognitive-behavioral theory of hypochondriasis is firmly rooted in current cognitive approaches to emotional disorders in general (Beck, 1976). Moreover, it assumes that hypochondriasis represents the extreme (and handicapping) end of a continuum of normal health anxiety (Salkovskis, 1996a). This emphasis inevitably has a powerful normalizing influence reflected not only in the treatment (see Chapter 14) but also in the fact that the approach can readily be applied to understanding health anxiety in the context of somatic problems (Salkovskis, 1989, 1992) and the psychological reaction to health screening (Salkovskis and Rimes, 1997). A growing body of empirical evidence supports this view. We have argued here that the combination of further theoretical development and refinement will inevitably lead to more effective and efficient treatment.

## Acknowledgments

Paul Salkovskis is a Wellcome Trust Senior Research Fellow in Basic Biomedical Science.

## References

American Psychiatric Association. 1980. *Diagnostic and Statistical Manual of Mental Disorders, Third Edition (DSM-III)*. Washington, DC: American Psychiatric Association.

American Psychiatric Association. 1987. *Diagnostic and Statistical Manual of Mental Disorders, Third Edition Revised (DSM-III-R)*. Washington, DC: American Psychiatric Association.

American Psychiatric Association. 1994. *Diagnostic and Statistical Manual of Mental Disorders, Fourth Edition (DSM-IV)*. Washington, DC: American Psychiatric Association.

Beck A.T. 1976. *Cognitive Therapy and the Emotional Disorders*. New York: International Universities Press.

Beck A.T., Emery G., Greenberg R.L. 1985. *Anxiety Disorders and Phobias: A Cognitive Perspective*. New York: Basic Books.

Bianchi G.N. 1971. Origins of disease phobia. *Australian and New Zealand Journal of Psychiatry* 5: 241–257.

Butler G., Mathews A. 1983. Cognitive processes in anxiety. *Advances in Behaviour Research and Therapy* 5: 51–62.

Clark D.M. 1988. A cognitive model of panic. In *Panic: Psychological Perspectives* (eds. Rachman S.J., Maser J.), Hillsdale, NJ: Erlbaum.

Clark D.M. 1999. Anxiety disorders: why they persist and how to treat them. *Behaviour Research and Therapy* 37 (Suppl. 1): S5-S28.

Clark D.M., Salkovskis P.M., Ost L.G., Breitholtz E., Koehler K.A., Westling B.E., Jeavons A., Gelder M. 1997. Misinterpretation of body sensations in panic disorder. *Journal of Consulting and Clinical Psychology* 65: 203–213.

Ehlers A. 1997. *Perception of heartbeats and airway resistance in hypochondriasis.* Paper presented at the 3rd European Congress of Psychophysiology, Konstanz, Germany.

Hitchcock P.B., Mathews A. 1992. Interpretation of bodily symptoms in hypochondriasis. *Behaviour Research and Therapy* 30: 223–234.

Kellner R. 1982. Psychotherapeutic strategies in hypochondriasis. *American Journal of Psychotherapy* 34: 146–157.

Kenyon F.E. 1964. Hypochondriasis: a clinical study. *British Journal of Psychiatry* 110: 478-488.

Miller D., Green J., Farmer R., Carroll G. 1985. A "pseudo-AIDS" syndrome following from fear of AIDS. *British Journal of Psychiatry* 146: 550-551.

Noyes R., Jr., Reich J., Clancy J., O'Gorman T.W. 1986. Reduction in hypochondriasis with treatment of panic disorder. *British Journal of Psychiatry* 149: 631–635.

Pilowsky I. 1983. Hypochondriasis. In *Handbook of Psychiatry, Vol. 4* (eds. Russell G.E., Hersov L.), Cambridge: Cambridge University Press.

Salkovskis P.M. 1988a. Phenomenology, assessment and the cognitive model of panic. In *Panic: Psychological Perspectives* (eds. Rachman S.J., Maser J.), Hillsdale, NJ: Erlbaum.

Salkovskis P.M. 1988b. Hyperventilation and anxiety. *Current Opinion in Psychiatry* 1: 76–82.

Salkovskis P.M. 1989. Somatic problems. In *Cognitive Therapy for Psychiatric Problems: A Practical Guide* (eds. Hawton K., Salkovskis P.M., Kirk J., Clark D.M.), Oxford: Oxford University Press.

Salkovskis P.M. 1991. The importance of behaviour in the maintenance of anxiety and panic: a cognitive account. *Behavioural Psychotherapy* 19: 6–19.

Salkovskis P.M. 1992. Psychological treatment of noncardiac chest pain: the cognitive approach. *American Journal of Medicine* 92 (Suppl. 5a): 114S-121S.

Salkovskis P.M. 1996a. The cognitive approach to anxiety: threat beliefs, safety-seeking behaviour, and the special case of health anxiety and obsessions. In *Frontiers of Cognitive Therapy* (ed. Salkovskis P.M.), New York: Guilford Press.

Salkovskis P.M. 1996b. Resolving the cognition-behaviour debate. In *Trends in Cognitive-Behaviour Therapy* (ed. Salkovskis P.M.), Chichester: John Wiley.

Salkovskis P.M., Warwick H.M.C. 1986. Morbid preoccupations, health anxiety and reassurance: a cognitive-behavioural approach to hypochondriasis. *Behaviour Research and Therapy* 24: 597–602.

Salkovskis P.M., Clark D.M. 1993. Panic disorder and hypochondriasis. *Advances in Behaviour Research and Therapy* 15: 23–48.

Salkovskis P.M., Clark D.M. 1995. Linking theory, research and clinical practice in the cognitive-behavioural treatment of panic and hypochondriasis. In *25 Years of Scientific Progress in Behavioural and Cognitive Therapies* (ed. Kasvikis Y.), Athens: Ellinika Grammata.

Salkovskis P.M., Bass C. 1997. Hypochondriasis. In *The Science and Practice of Cognitive-Behaviour Therapy* (eds. Clark D.M., Fairburn C.G.), Oxford: Oxford University Press.

Salkovskis P.M., Rimes K.A. 1997. Predictive genetic testing: psychological factors. *Journal of Psychosomatic Research* 44: 477–487.

Salkovskis P.M., Clark D.M., Gelder M.G. 1996. Cognition-behaviour links in the persistence of panic. *Behaviour Research and Therapy* 34: 453–458.

Salkovskis P.M., Clark D.M., Hackmann A., Wells A., Gelder M.G. 1999. An experimental investigation of the role of safety-seeking behaviours in the maintenance of panic disorder with agoraphobia. *Behaviour Research and Therapy* 37: 559–574.

Salkovskis P.M., Wroe A.L., Gledhill A., Morrison N., Forrester E., Richards C., Reynolds M., Thorpe S. 2000. Responsibility attitudes and interpretations are characteristic of obsessive compulsive disorder. *Behaviour Research and Therapy* 38: 347–372.

Salkovskis P.M., Warwick H.M.C., Clark D.M. 1999. An evaluation of the specificity of reactions to bodily sensations in panic and hypochondriasis. (Manuscript submitted for publication.)

Teasdale J.D. 1983. Negative thinking in depression: cause, effect or reciprocal relationship? *Advances in Behaviour Research and Therapy* 5: 3–26.

Tyrer P., Lee I., Alexander J. 1980. Awareness of cardiac function in anxious, phobic and hypochondriacal patients. *Psychological Medicine* 10: 171–174.

Warwick H.M.C., Salkovskis P.M. 1985. Reassurance. *British Medical Journal* 290: 1028.

Warwick H.M.C., Salkovskis P.M. 1990. Hypochondriasis. *Behaviour Research and Therapy* 28: 105–117.

Wells A., Clark D.M., Salkovskis P.M., Ludgate J., Hackmann A., Gelder M.G. 1995. Social phobia: the role of in-situation safety behaviours in maintaining anxiety and negative beliefs. *Behavior Therapy* 26: 153–161.

# 10

# Somatosensory Amplification and Hypochondriasis

## ARTHUR J. BARSKY

The prominent disease fears, beliefs, and preoccupations of hypochondriacal patients are thought to stem from a misattribution of benign bodily symptoms and normal sensations to serious disease. The hypochondriacal patient misunderstands and misinterprets personal bodily experience as indicative of serious disease, when in fact there is no serious pathology present. This raises a fundamental question: What, exactly, is the sensory experience of hypochondriacal individuals? Does their perceptual experience differ from that of nonhypochondriacal patients; or alternatively, do they describe the same perceptual experience differently because they label and report bodily distress and sensation in more distressing and disturbing terms? In short, if a nonhypochondriacal man had the bodily sensations of a hypochondriacal person, how would he report that experience and to what degree would he develop the characteristic disease fears, beliefs, and bodily preoccupations?

## Background: The Concept of Amplification

Bodily sensation, of course, cannot be divorced from its cognitive appraisal, for the thoughts, beliefs, knowledge, and suspicions that one has about a sensation influence the sensation itself. Many observers, including Pennebaker (Pennebaker, 1982; Pennebaker and Brittingham, 1982; Pennebaker and Epstein, 1983; Pennebaker and Watson 1991), have pointed out this interaction and process of mutual reinforcement. Perception is not a process of passive registration but is actually an active process of stimulus selection, modulation, and assessment. This process is guided by cognitive factors such as explanatory beliefs concerning the perceptions and expectations about future perceptions. But while bodily perception and health-related cognition are inextricably intertwined, the fundamental question still remains: "How different is the hypochondriacal individual's perceptual experience and how different is his reporting style?" The following discussion focuses more on the perceptual and sensory component of hypochondriasis than on the cognitive processing and appraisal of sensation, but it is important to remember the two cannot be divorced from each other.

## Hypochondriacal Amplification

Hypochondriasis has been conceptualized as a disorder of bodily amplification, in which a wide range of somatic and visceral sensations are experienced as unusually intense, noxious, and disturbing. Thus, hypochondriacal individuals may be thought of as especially sensitive to, and intolerant of, bodily sensation in general. Such people may amplify normal physiological sensations (e.g., orthostatic dizziness or an ectopic cardiac beat), the somatic concomitants of intense affect, and the benign symptoms of trivial and self-limited infirmities (e.g., tinnitus, a twitching eyelid).

Hypochondriacal people, because their symptoms are so intense and uncomfortable, conclude that these sensations must be abnormal and pathological, rather than normalizing them by attributing them to a benign cause such as overwork, insufficient rest, inadequate exercise, or dietary indiscretion. A headache, for example, is attributed to a brain tumor rather than to "eyestrain," and a "cramp" is thought to indicate a heart attack rather than indigestion. Suspecting now that he is sick, the hypochondriacal person scrutinizes his body further for additional, confirmatory symptoms. He filters his somatic perceptions, selectively attending to those that confirm his hypothesis, while ignoring sensory input that does not confirm it (Leventhal, 1986; Pennebaker and Brittingham, 1982).

As a result, he now becomes aware of "new" symptoms that he had previously ignored or not consciously attended to, and these are incorrectly ascribed to the presumed disease. In addition, mounting anxiety itself generates autonomic symptoms, and these new symptoms are taken as additional evidence of an evolving disease process. Hence, initial, tentative suspicions about health gradually become organized into more firmly held beliefs about the presence of disease.

Empirical investigation of symptom amplification in hypochondriacal individuals has been relatively sparse, and it is difficult to draw any definitive conclusions from this literature. The results are sometimes contradictory; almost none of the studies employed clinically diagnosed hypochondriacal individuals but rather relied on volunteers such as college students; samples are often small and may be unrepresentative; psychiatric comorbidity is generally not measured; and variations in methodology make generalization across studies difficult. This literature includes a report that college students who are more hypochondriacal have a higher level of sensory arousal and greater sensitivity to paired flashes of light than do those who are less hypochondriacal (Hanback and Revelle, 1978). In more recent work, Gramling *et al.* (1996) subjected college students to a cold pressor test and found that the more hypochondriacal subjects terminated the task earlier and rated the pain as more unpleasant than did nonhypochondriacal subjects. They also exhibited objective differences in physiological reactivity in that the hypochondriacal subjects exhibited a greater increase in heart rate and decrease in hand temperature than did the controls.

Pauli *et al.* (1993), however, found that more and less hypochondriacal college students did not differ in their threshold for an experimental, thermally induced pain stimulus. Another study failed to find a relationship between hypochondriasis and a heightened awareness of internal bodily sensation—"private body consciousness" (Miller *et al.*, 1981). Normal subjects who are kinesthetic augmenters (overestimating the size of objects placed in their hands while blindfolded) score higher on hypochondriasis scales and have a lower tolerance for experimental pain (Petrie, 1978). In work with patients who had chronic, organic, nonmalignant pain, those with higher hypochondriasis scores rated their pain as more intense (Ziesat, 1978). Among a heterogeneous group of patients with pain complaints, those with disease conviction and disease phobia had lower thresholds and tolerance to experimental pain (Merskey and Evans, 1975), and psychiatric inpatients with disease phobias were also found to have lower thresholds for, and tolerance of, experimental pain (Bianchi, 1971, 1973).

Two studies suggest that hypochondriacal subjects are more sensitive to physiological sensations. In one, workers who reported respiratory symptoms disproportionate to their pulmonary function tests were found to be more hypochondriacal (Wright *et al.*, 1977). In the other study, conducted with psychiatric outpatients, those who were hypochondriacal estimated their pulse rate more accurately than did those who were phobic (Tyrer *et al.*, 1980).

## Amplification in the More General Phenomenon of Somatization

In its most limited and restricted sense, *amplification* could be a pathogenic mechanism of importance in only a single psychopathological condition, namely hypochondriasis. But the construct might also be helpful in understanding a variety of other clinical conditions in which patients complain of somatic symptoms that are medically unexplained or are disproportionate to demonstrable disease. Amplification could therefore play a role in the somatization seen in a number of

other psychiatric disorders (such as panic disorder), in the process of somatization more generally, and/or in the interindividual variability in somatic distress
seen among patients with serious medical morbidity.

Amplification may also have a role in many psychiatric conditions that are accompanied by functional somatic complaints, such as somatization disorder, somatoform pain disorder, depressive disorder, or panic disorder. Thus, it has been
found that the cortical-evoked potentials and changes in skin conductance produced by auditory stimuli are enhanced in somatization disorder patients (Gordon et al., 1986; Meares and Horvath, 1972). Similarly, idiopathic pain patients
with prominent anxiety and depression have lower thresholds for experimental
pain than do patients with chronic organic pain (Katon et al., 1981).

Amplification may influence the general process of somatization and a wider
range of medically unexplained complaints. A substantial body of literature
demonstrates a close relationship between psychological symptoms and psychological distress on the one hand and somatic symptoms and bodily distress on
the other. The tendency to experience and report a wide range of negative emotions, including anxiety, guilt, loneliness, and low self-esteem, has been termed
*negative affectivity* or *neuroticism*, and has been shown to be a reliable, valid,
and stable psychometric construct (Diener and Emmons, 1985; Watson and Clark,
1984; Watson and Tellegen, 1985).

Individuals who score high on self-report questionnaires of negative affectivity also report high levels of many somatic symptoms (Costa and McCrae, 1980,
1985; Pennebaker, 1982). This general association between emotional and bodily symptoms could reflect a true co-occurrence of psychiatric and medical morbidity in the same individuals. Another possible explanation (more relevant to the
present discussion) is that individuals high on negative affectivity may have a
tendency to recognize and report *both* psychological and somatic symptoms (i.e.,
to amplify all forms of distress).

Amplification may also influence another important clinical phenomenon,
namely the variability in symptom reporting among different individuals with the
same medical condition. Great differences exist in the intensity, number, and nature of somatic symptoms reported by different patients with the same medical
illness. For example, the presence of peptic ulcer disease, as documented endo-
scopically or radiographically, is only very weakly correlated with the presence
of symptoms (Bodemar and Walan, 1978; Peterson et al., 1977); arthritic joint
pain cannot be predicted on the basis of X-ray findings alone (Hussar and Guller,
1956) and is more closely associated with attitudes and beliefs about disease than
with severity of tissue pathology (Lichtenberg et al., 1986); dyspnea reported by
asthmatics corresponds poorly to measures of airway obstruction (Burdon et al.,
1982; Rubinfeld and Pain, 1976); and symptoms do not correlate with hemoglo-
bin levels in patients with mild to moderate anemia (Wood and Elwood, 1966).

Battlefield anesthesia furnishes a final, dramatic example of the variability in symptoms resulting from a given extent of tissue pathology. In a classic study of this phenomenon, Beecher (1956) compared battlefield casualties and civilian trauma victims and found that the former had substantially less pain and substantially lower narcotic requirements. Some of this interindividual variability could be due to differences in perceptual style or, more specifically, in the tendency to amplify, as well as in the specific setting.

Finally, amplification might prove conceptually useful in probing other psychiatric disorders in which distortions of body image and bodily perception occur. In the variants of monosymptomatic hypochondriasis—body dysmorphic disorder, olfactory reference syndrome, and delusions of parasitosis—there are obvious distortions in the perceptions of one's body. It might be productive to learn more about the extent to which these distortions in thinking and appraisal actually result from distortions of perception. In the case of body dysmorphic disorder, the patient's imagined defect or deformity is often based upon a minor or trivial and entirely normal, anatomical variation. One wonders about the degree to which this delusional belief stems from a distorted or amplified perception of this anatomical variation. Similarly in anorexia nervosa, there is a distorted perception of body size and shape, and it might be fruitful to investigate the degree to which the patient's beliefs are based upon an amplification of objectively verifiable, but much less extreme, bodily characteristics.

## Modulators of Amplification

Amplification theoretically has the properties of both a trait and a state. Some individuals are constitutionally more sensitive to bodily discomfort than others. Most of our work has examined these trait-like properties of amplification using the Somatosensory Amplification Scale (SSAS) (described below), which does appear to have a considerable degree of temporal stability. In this sense, it is a stable trait or enduring perceptual style. It could be learned in childhood in early formative experiences, or it could be constitutional, "hard wired" into the nervous system from birth. But one would also expect that the sensitivity to bodily sensation fluctuates within the same individual over time; like blood pressure, it must vary from time to time, while hovering in a relatively restricted range around the individual's characteristic baseline level.

What do we know about the precipitants, circumstances, events, and other proximate factors that modulate state amplification and make bodily sensations feel more intense and noxious and seem more alarming and ominous at some times and not at others? At least four factors influence the intensity of a given symptom at a given time: cognition, attention, context, and mood (Barsky, 1992).

## Cognition

Cognition is a potent modulator of symptoms. We experience and describe bodily sensations in terms of the information, beliefs, opinions, and ideas that we have about them. Etiological attributions are particularly important in this regard (Valins and Nisbett, 1971): A headache that an individual suspects is due to a brain tumor is much worse than one attributed to eye strain, and while the nociceptive sensation of a tight shoe and an osteosarcoma of the foot may be similar, the perceived experience is not. Symptoms are intensified when they are attributed to a serious disease rather than to more benign causes such as dietary indiscretion, lack of sleep, lack of exercise, or overwork. Thus, among patients with a comparable, acute viral illness, those who believe at the outset that their illness is more serious subsequently report more persistent and chronic symptoms (Cope et al., 1994; Dworkin et al., 1992; Vercoulen et al., 1996; Wilson et al., 1994).

## Attention

Attention to a symptom amplifies it, whereas distraction diminishes it. Thus, the more frequently postoperative patients are asked to rate their pain, the more intense they find it (Levine et al., 1982). In another example, subjects exercised on a treadmill while listening through headphones to either interesting bits of conversation or to their own labored breathing. Although they did not differ on physiological measures, group members hearing their own breathing reported significantly more fatigue, palpitations, and sweating (Pennebaker, 1982). Some symptoms, such as itching, coughing, and yawning, have been noted to have an "infectious" quality; once the symptoms are manifested by one member of a group, others soon experience them as well. The vector in these epidemics is attention: Someone's cough draws our attention to our own throats and we soon think we note a mild sensation of dryness or itchiness or scratchiness that was not there before (Barsky et al., 1988a; Pennebaker, 1982).

## Context

We also infer what we are perceiving from what we think we ought to be perceiving, and this depends largely on our circumstances and situation at the time (Barsky et al., 1988a). Situational context furnishes clues that are used to infer the meaning of and to decide on the significance of a bodily symptom, thereby influencing how intense and how noxious the symptom seems. If several family members have recently developed upper respiratory tract infections, then a benign sneeze will be noticed as the first evidence of having caught a cold rather than dismissed and ignored.

Circumstances and setting also influence perception by shaping our expectations of what we will be perceiving in the future. For example, waiting to meet someone who is late causes us to hear footsteps in the hallway outside that we would otherwise not have noticed. This is also illustrated by a multicenter study of aspirin treatment for unstable angina (Myers *et al.*, 1987). Patients enrolled at the centers whose informed consent forms explicitly mentioned possible gastrointestinal side effects had a significantly higher incidence of gastrointestinal symptoms, but not of confirmed gastrointestinal disease, than did the patients at the other sites (Myers *et al.*, 1987). The power of suggestion has also been shown to influence healthy subjects: Instructing them to attend to evidence of nasal "obstruction" as they breathe produces more symptoms than does instructing them to attend to the "free passage of air" (Pennebaker, 1982).

## *Mood*

Anxiety, depression, and other dysphoric mood states amplify bodily distress. Anxiety, for example, causes symptoms to be appraised as more ominous, dangerous, and alarming. Anxious people "catastrophize" bodily sensation, misattributing vague and ambiguous symptoms of unclear origin to serious diseases (Clark, 1986; Ottaviani and Beck, 1987). Anxiety also increases self-consciousness, and this apprehensive self-scrutiny amplifies preexisting symptoms and brings previously unnoticed sensations to conscious awareness. This is confirmed by experimental data showing that anxiety lowers the tolerance and threshold for a variety of unpleasant sensations and symptoms, including pain (Sternbach, 1978).

The situation with depression is analogous. Depressed individuals' negative and pessimistic cognition fosters the recall of illness-related memories, a negative view of their health and their future prognosis, and a heightened awareness of their unpleasant experiences. Depressed individuals believe they are defective and damaged. They imagine the worst, think about misfortune and death, and expect illness and suffering. Depression also directs one's attention inward, and this increased bodily preoccupation makes trivial and mild discomforts more disturbing.

## Development of a Self-Report Measure

In attempting to study the role of amplification in hypochondriasis, the first step our research group took was to operationalize the concept by developing a self-report questionnaire to assess it. Hypochondriacal patients in one sample were asked in unstructured interviews what symptoms and bodily sensations bothered them most. This generated a large item pool of complaints, which included normal bodily sensations, various minor and benign discomforts, and sensations not commonly thought to indicate serious disease (e.g., a bad taste in one's mouth, or yawning). A self-report questionnaire, using an ordinal response format, was then compiled. The questionnaire was administered to another sample of somatizing medical outpatients so that we could eliminate items that were redundant or failed to elicit the full range of responses. The result was the Somatosensory Amplification Scale (SSAS).

The SSAS asks the respondent the degree to which ten statements are "characteristic of you in general." Responses are rated on an ordinal scale from 1 ("not at all true") to 5 ("extremely true"). The items cover a range of uncomfortable bodily sensations and minor symptoms that generally do not connote serious disease. Two of the items ("hunger contractions" and "various things happening in my body") are similar to items in Miller's Body Consciousness Questionnaire (Miller et al., 1981).

We then administered this instrument to a random sample of primary care patients to study its psychometric properties. This provided preliminary evidence of the scale's test–retest reliability and internal consistency. The SSAS scores were not significantly related to sociodemographic characteristics or with aggregate medical morbidity.

## Self-Reported Amplification in Hypochondriasis

Once the psychometric properties of this instrument were established, we employed it in studying rigorously diagnosed hypochondriacal patients. A sample of patients meeting *DSM-III-R* (American Psychiatric Association, 1987) diagnostic criteria for hypochondriasis was obtained by screening consecutive attenders in the primary care clinics of the Massachusetts General Hospital. A comparison group was accrued, consisting of a random sample of all the remaining, nonhypochondriacal patients in the same setting. Patients completed the SSAS as part of an extensive research battery, and then completed it again 4 to 10 weeks later. The research battery also included measures of aggregate medical morbidity (using primary care physician ratings and a standardized audit of the patient's medical record); Axis I psychiatric disorder (using the Diagnostic Interview Schedule; Robins et al., 1981); Axis II disorder caseness (using a subscale of the Personality Diagnostic Questionnaire; Hyler et al., 1983); role impairment and disability (using the Functional Status Questionnaire; Jette et al., 1986); primary care physician ratings of the severity of the patient's hypochondriasis; and patient self-ratings of perceived overall health.

Hypochondriacal symptoms were measured with the Whiteley Index (Pilowsky, 1967, 1968, 1978) consisting of thirteen hypochondriacal attitudes, concerns, and beliefs. Responses are scored on an ordinal scale from 1 to 5. Principal-components analysis yields the following three factors: disease fear, disease conviction, and bodily preoccupation. Its test–retest reliability and discriminant and convergent validity have been established (Pilowsky, 1967, 1968, 1978). Hypochondriacal somatic complaints were assessed with the Somatic Symptom Index (SSI), comprised of twenty-six items drawn from the Minnesota Multiphasic Personality Inventory hypochondriasis subscale (Hathaway and McKinley, 1951) and the Hopkins Symptom Checklist somatization subscale (Derogatis, 1977; Derogatis *et al.*, 1974; Lipman *et al.*, 1977). Responses are scored on an ordinal scale from 1 to 5. This scale had a test–retest reliability of 0.86 (Pearson Product-Moment Correlation) and an intrascale consistency of 0.95 (Cronbach's alpha).

The SSAS was normally distributed in both samples, and was not significantly correlated with any sociodemographic characteristic. Test–retest reliability over a median interval of 74 days was 0.79 ($P = 0.0001$), and the internal consistency was 0.82 (Cronbach's alpha). The item-to-scale and item-to-item correlations and test–retest data are presented in Tables 10.1 and 10.2: item-to-scale correlations

**Table 10.1.** Psychometric characteristics of Somatosensory Amplification Scale in nonhypochondriacal comparison sample ($n = 75$)

| Item | Mean | Standard deviation | Item-to-scale correlation | | Test–retest reliability | |
|---|---|---|---|---|---|---|
| | | | r | P | r | P |
| 1. When someone else coughs, it makes me cough too | 1.16 | 0.47 | 0.37 | 0.001 | 0.30 | 0.080 |
| 2. I can't stand smoke, smog, or pollutants in the air | 2.44 | 1.29 | 0.55 | 0.0001 | 0.79 | 0.0001 |
| 3. I am often aware of various things happening within my body | 2.07 | 1.12 | 0.50 | 0.0001 | 0.50 | 0.0026 |
| 4. When I bruise myself, it stays noticeable for a long time | 2.11 | 1.27 | 0.62 | 0.0001 | 0.72 | 0.0001 |
| 5. Sudden loud noises really bother me | 1.33 | 0.79 | 0.31 | 0.007 | 0.65 | 0.0001 |
| 6. I can sometimes hear my pulse or my heartbeat throbbing in my ear | 2.23 | 1.32 | 0.64 | 0.0001 | 0.68 | 0.0001 |
| 7. I hate to be too hot or too cold | 1.73 | 0.98 | 0.56 | 0.0001 | 0.43 | 0.010 |
| 8. I am quick to sense the hunger contractions in my stomach | 2.91 | 1.24 | 0.66 | 0.0001 | 0.39 | 0.022 |
| 9. Even something minor, like an insect bite or a splinter, really bothers me | 2.30 | 1.08 | 0.39 | 0.0005 | 0.65 | 0.0001 |
| 10. I have a low tolerance for pain | 1.57 | 1.00 | 0.57 | 0.0001 | 0.59 | 0.0002 |

**Table 10.2.** Intercorrelations among SSAS items*

| | All subjects (N = 116) | | | | | | | | | |
|---|---|---|---|---|---|---|---|---|---|---|
| | 1 | 2 | 3 | 4 | 5 | 6 | 7 | 8 | 9 | 10 |
| 1. When someone else coughs, it makes me cough too | 1.0 / 0.000 | | | | | | | | | |
| 2. I can't stand smoke, smog, or pollutants in the air | 0.29 / 0.0043 | 1.0 / 0.000 | | | | | | | | |
| 3. I am often aware of various things happening within my body | 0.30 / 0.0023 | 0.30 / 0.0026 | 1.0 / 0.00 | | | | | | | |
| 4. When I bruise myself, it stays noticeable for a long time | 0.14 / ns | 0.32 / 0.0014 | 0.36 / 0.0003 | 1.0 / 0.000 | | | | | | |
| 5. Sudden loud noises really bother me | 0.18 / ns | 0.39 / 0.0001 | 0.14 / ns | 0.26 / 4.009 | 1.0 / 0.000 | | | | | |
| 6. I can sometimes hear my pulse or my heartbeat throbbing in my ear | 0.29 / 0.0042 | 0.32 / 0.0011 | 0.33 / 0.0009 | 0.26 / 0.0085 | 0.19 / NS | 1.0 / 0.000 | | | | |
| 7. I hate to be too hot or too cold | 0.12 / ns | 0.34 / 0.0006 | 0.27 / 0.0074 | 0.38 / 0.0001 | 0.43 / 0.0001 | 0.38 / 0.0001 | 1.0 / 0.000 | | | |
| 8. I am quick to sense the hunger contractions in my stomach | 0.10 / ns | 0.29 / 0.0042 | 0.37 / 0.0002 | 0.24 / 0.0169 | 0.25 / 0.0118 | 0.38 / 0.0001 | 0.45 / 0.0001 | 1.0 / 0.000 | | |
| 9. Even something minor, like an insect bite or a splinter, really bothers me | 0.21 / 0.037 | 0.32 / 0.0013 | 0.36 / 0.0003 | 0.41 / 0.0001 | 0.51 / 0.0001 | 0.33 / 0.0009 | 0.51 / 0.0001 | 0.34 / 0.0006 | 1.0 / 0.000 | |
| 10. I have a low tolerance for pain | 0.03 / ns | 0.07 / ns | 0.26 / 0.0102 | 0.32 / 0.0015 | 0.48 / 0.0001 | 0.12 / ns | 0.32 / 0.0013 | 0.25 / 0.0125 | 0.60 / 0.0001 | 1.0 / 0.000 |

*Pearson correlation coefficients.

varied from 0.66 to 0.31, and all were highly significant; item-to-item correlations varied from 0.60 to 0.03, but most were in the range of 0.35, and were highly significant.

The mean SSAS score was higher in patients meeting diagnostic criteria for *DSM-III-R* hypochondriasis than in the nonhypochondriacal comparison patients: 2.78 (*SD* = 0.67) versus 1.98 (*SD* = 0.58); *P* < 0.001. The relationship between amplification and hypochondriacal symptoms is explored in Table 10.3. In the comparison sample, (i.e., among patients who are not clinically hypochondriacal) amplification is highly correlated with hypochondriacal symptoms, particularly bodily preoccupation. Within the sample of *DSM-III-R* hypochondriacal patients, the correlations are somewhat weaker, and they fail to reach significance for disease conviction and somatic complaints. Among specific somatic symptoms, SSAS scores are most closely correlated with fatigue (*r* = 0.53; *P* = 0.0001) and weakness (*r* = 0.47; *P* = 0.0001). Chest pain and headaches are the weakest correlates.

Multiple stepwise regressions were performed (Table 10.4) using the Whiteley Index score as the dependent variable, and including as independent variables the SSAS score, sociodemographic descriptors, medical morbidity, total number of psychopathological symptoms (from structured diagnostic interview), personality disorder caseness, role impairment and functional status, patient-rated global health status, and ratings of the effectiveness of care by patient and doctor.

In the comparison (nonhypochondriacal) sample, amplification is the single most powerful correlate of the Whiteley Index score ($R^2$ = 0.318). A seven-step regression, including physician ratings of hypochondriasis, disability, and perceived global health status, attains a total $R^2$ of 0.633. In the hypochondriacal sample, the SSAS score again enters the equation first, accounting for 18.5% of

**Table 10.3.** Correlations of Somatosensory Amplification Scale (SSAS) and hypochondriacal symptoms (Whiteley Index)

|  | Comparison sample (*n* = 75) | | Hypochondriacal sample (*n* = 41) | |
| --- | --- | --- | --- | --- |
|  | *r* | *P* | *r* | *P* |
| Amplification and hypochondriasis (Whiteley Index) | 0.60 | 0.0001 | 0.43 | 0.005 |
| Amplification and disease conviction | 0.43 | 0.0001 | 0.15 | *ns* |
| Amplification and disease fear | 0.51 | 0.0001 | 0.35 | 0.023 |
| Amplification and bodily preoccupation | 0.54 | 0.0001 | 0.58 | 0.0001 |
| Amplification and somatization (Somatic Symptom Inventory) | 0.44 | 0.0001 | 0.20 | *ns* |

**Table 10.4.** Multiple stepwise regression, correlates of hypochondriacal symptoms*

| Step | Variable | Partial $R^2$ | Model $R^2$ |
|------|----------|---------------|-------------|
| **Comparison sample (n = 75)** | | | |
| 1 | Amplification (SSAS) | 0.318 | 0.318 |
| 2 | Physician-rated hypochondriasis | 0.142 | 0.459 |
| 3 | Diability | 0.072 | 0.532 |
| 4 | Patient-rated global health status (inverse) | 0.030 | 0.561 |
| 5 | Race | 0.039 | 0.600 |
| 6 | Physician-rated effectiveness of care (inverse) | 0.019 | 0.620 |
| 7 | Total psychopathological symptoms (DIS) $F_{7,61} = 15.02; P = 0.0001$ | 0.013 | 0.633 |
| **Hypochondriacal sample (n = 4)** | | | |
| 1 | Amplification (SSAS) | 0.185 | 0.185 |
| 2 | Age | 0.102 | 0.288 |
| 3 | Patient-rated global health status (inverse) | 0.076 | 0.364 |
| 4 | Physician-rated hypochondriasis | 0.060 | 0.423 |
| 5 | Sex $F_{5,35} = 8.48; P = 0.0001$ | 0.091 | 0.515 |

*Whiteley Index Score.

the variance. A five step equation, including age, sex (women being more hypochondriacal), patient-rated health status, and physician-rated hypochondriasis, explains 51.5% of the variance.

Thus, in both univariate and multivariate analyses, amplification is significantly associated with three different measures of hypochondriasis—a self-report symptom inventory, the *DSM-III-R* diagnosis, and primary physician ratings of hypochondriasis. Among the hypochondriacal symptoms, bodily preoccupation appears most closely associated with amplification. These associations are consistently more robust in the comparison than in the hypochondriacal sample. This is likely due to the much more restricted Whiteley Index scores in the hypochondriacal group, which weakens the power of the correlations found between the severity of hypochondriasis and the other measures.

Because amplification was associated with anxiety and depressive disorders as well as with hypochondriasis, this represents a possible confound in the association between hypochondriasis and amplification. An analysis of covariance (ANCOVA) was therefore performed, controlling for psychiatric comorbidity. The relationship between amplification and *DSM-III-R* hypochondriasis remained highly significant. The SSAS mean, adjusted for the total number of Axis I diagnoses, is 2.67 in the hypochondriacal sample and 2.04 in the comparison sample ($P = 0.008$). When adjusted for the presence of anxiety and depressive disorders, the SSAS mean is 2.54 in the hypochondriacal sample and 1.98 in the comparison group ($P = 0.001$). Medical morbidity is another possible confounder of the relationship between amplification and hypochondriasis, because medical illness might sensitize one to somatic sensation and foster bodily scrutiny. The SSAS, however, was unrelated to aggregate medical morbidity, whether measured with physician ratings or with a medical record audit.

The characteristics of the SSAS itself were interesting; in the comparison group the SSAS was significantly associated with anxiety and depressive disorders, but not with antisocial personality or alcohol or substance abuse. The same pattern of associations is seen in the hypochondriacal sample, but it does not reach statistical significance. This suggests some degree of discriminant validity of the SSAS, as it is the psychiatric disorders that are not typically characterized by prominent somatic symptoms, such as antisocial personality and alcohol or substance abuse, that remain unassociated with amplification (see also Chapter 3).

The association of the SSAS with hypochondriasis appears to be more specific and more powerful than with other psychiatric disorders; it persists after controlling statistically for other concurrent psychiatric comorbidity. Our findings are therefore consistent with the hypothesis that hypochondriasis involves a heightened sensitivity to benign bodily dysfunction and normal physiology. Although the SSAS and Whiteley Index appear to be closely related in this population, and to measure overlapping characteristics, they are not intended to tap the same theoretical construct. The Whiteley Index inquires into attitudes, concerns, beliefs, and fears about health and disease, while the SSAS asks about physical sensations, primarily sensations which are often benign, minor, and not generally regarded as symptomatic of serious medical disease.

A major limitation of this study is that amplification was measured with a self-report questionnaire. We are therefore dealing only with what patients say they perceive and not with an objective, independent measure of what they perceive. In addition, the cross-sectional nature of the study does not permit any conclusions about the direction of causality between hypochondriasis and somatosensory amplification; it is as likely that hypochondriasis causes amplification as it is that preexisting amplification causes patients to notice their somatic symptoms more and become more hypochondriacal.

## Longitudinal Studies

As our research continued, we were able to follow several hypochondriacal cohorts over time and could therefore examine the temporal stability and predictive power of the SSAS.

## Study 1

The initial work revealed considerable stability in SSAS scores over prolonged time periods. We studied medical outpatients who were referred for 24-hour ambulatory electrocardiographic monitoring to evaluate a chief complaint of palpitations (Barsky et al., 1995a). These patients were compared with nonpatient volunteers who had no cardiac complaints and no known history of cardiac disease. Both groups were studied with a battery of questionnaires including the SSAS and then underwent the same battery approximately 7 months later. In the nonpatient comparison group, the mean SSAS score was 2.03 at inception and 2.09 when tested 7 months later. In the palpitation patients the mean SSAS score at inception was 2.23, and at follow-up it was 2.26 (Barsky et al., 1995a). This suggests that amplification may be a fairly stable and enduring characteristic in nonhypochondriacal patients and in nonpatients.

Multiple stepwise regression was used to determine which clinical measures at inception predicted subsequent outcomes at follow-up. In the group with palpitations, SSAS scores at inception were associated with several outcomes at follow-up, but although these associations were statistically significant, they explained only a small proportion of the variance. At inception, SSAS scores, along with the number of psychopathological symptoms on structured diagnostic interview, did predict the continued presence of palpitations at 7-month follow-up; SSAS scores predicted impaired functioning in basic activities of daily living at follow-up; and amplification and psychiatric symptoms predicted utilization of the emergency department during the follow-up interval (Barsky et al., 1995a). But, as noted, while statistically significant, these associations were relatively weak.

## Study 2

We also conducted a 3-month follow-up of another series of medical outpatients complaining of palpitations (Barsky et al., 1996). In this sample, the interaction of amplification and life stress at inception was a significant predictor of palpitation severity 3 months later; in particular, a stepwise regression equation containing the interaction of the SSAS with minor, daily life stress (assessed with the Daily Hassles Scale) and the interaction of amplification with major, stressful life events predicted 21.4% of the variance in palpitation severity 3 months later. The number of emergency room visits was also predicted by the interaction of amplification and daily life stresses. These findings are compatible with the hypothesis that palpitations are more persistent in individuals who are both highly sensitive to bodily sensations *and* who experience a greater number of minor daily stressors and irritants. The existence of either predictor alone (i.e., ei-

ther an amplifying somatic style or a stressful daily life) is not sufficient to per-
petuate this functional somatic symptom; it is their combination that is salient.
Their interaction explains a significant proportion of the variance in palpitations
above and beyond the effect of each variable alone. The findings regarding medical utilization are compatible with those on symptom chronicity. The interaction
of amplification and daily stresses at inception also predicted the number of unscheduled emergency room and walk-in visits over the subsequent 3 months.

These results suggest at least two factors may be involved in precipitating and
perpetuating medically unexplained complaints: (*1*) a predisposing, trait-like amplifying somatic style in which a wide range of bodily sensations tends to be experienced as unusually noxious, and (*2*) precipitating current stressors, in
particular, minor irritants and hassles that recur in daily life. To the degree that
the SSAS is stable over months and even years, amplification could be viewed
as predisposing an individual to respond to life stress with a somatizing response.
People who amplify are continually barraged by uncomfortable bodily sensations
and might thereby be primed to become acutely symptomatic under stressful
circumstances.

## Study 3

We have also examined the temporal stability of amplification in hypochondriacal populations. In a longitudinal study of transient hypochondriasis, we found
that SSAS scores of transiently hypochondriacal medical outpatients remained
significantly higher than those of a nonhypochondriacal comparison group
(Barsky *et al.*, 1990). The hypochondriacal patients scored in the top 5% of patients on a hypochondriasis screening questionnaire, but 3 weeks later their hypochondriasis scores had fallen by 25% and they no longer met diagnostic criteria
for *DSM-III-R* hypochondriasis on a structured, diagnostic interview. When studied at this second point in time, the transiently hypochondriacal patients had SSAS
scores that were still significantly higher than those of the nonhypochondriacal
comparison group. These differences in amplification remained significant, even
after controlling for the greater aggregate medical morbidity found in the transiently hypochondriacal group, using an ANCOVA method (Barsky *et al.*, 1990).
These findings suggest the possibility that amplification might predispose one to
become hypochondriacal when threatened with a medical illness, although the
cross-sectional design of the study did not permit a test of this hypothesis.

## Study 4

When we compared the transiently hypochondriacal patients to nonhypochondriacal controls 22 months later (Barsky *et al.*, 1993a), they were still found to

have significantly higher SSAS scores. The multivariate analysis indicated that baseline amplification scores were a significant predictor of hypochondriacal symptoms at follow-up. This suggested that a preexisting, self-reported sensitivity to bodily sensation is associated with the subsequent persistence of hypochondriacal symptoms, even after the possible confounding effects of medical morbidity, psychiatric morbidity, and initial severity of hypochondriasis are taken into account (Barsky et al., 1993a).

*Study 5*

Finally, we also obtained SSAS scores on a hypochondriacal cohort over a 5-year interval (Barsky et al., 1998). In a group of 38 patients meeting *DSM-III-R* criteria for hypochondriasis, the mean amplification score was 3.01 ($\pm0.73$) at baseline and 2.99 ($\pm0.69$) 5 years later, thus demonstrating a considerable degree of temporal stability over a long period of time. Thirty-four percent of these patients no longer met *DSM* diagnostic criteria for hypochondriasis at 4-year follow-up. The SSAS scores of these patients (termed "remitters") were significantly lower at follow-up than were the SSAS scores of the patients whose hypochondriasis had not remitted. Thus, the clinical improvement in their condition was paralleled by a decline in amplification. Remitters and nonremitters did not differ in their amplification scores at inception, however. Amplification alone therefore did not predict subsequent course or remission status at follow-up. However, a three-way interaction, composed of amplification, normative health beliefs, and somatization (all measured at inception), was significantly associated with remission of hypochondriasis 4 years later.

## Objective Measures of Amplification

All the work presented so far is subject to the qualification that amplification has been measured with a self-report questionnaire, and there is no objective measure of the patient's perceptual acuity. That is, hypochondriacal patients report they are extremely sensitive perceivers of somatic and visceral stimuli. But are they? Are they in fact more sensitive interoceptors with unusually acute visceral discrimination?

We explored this question by examining whether hypochondriacal patients were actually more accurately aware of cardiac activity than nonhypochondriacal patients (Barsky et al., 1995b). The accurate awareness of resting heartbeat was determined with a laboratory heartbeat detection test (HBD), which requires subjects to judge the temporal relationship between an external stimulus (an audio tone) and any sensations they have of their heart beating. Subjects were connected to an electrocardiogram and seated in a dim, sound-attenuated room. They were then presented with a series of brief auditory stimuli, each of which was separated from the preceding electrocardiographic R-wave by one of six intervals (0, 100, 200, 300, 400, and 500 milliseconds). On each trial they were instructed to sample all the different R-wave-to-tone intervals, and then select the train of audio tones believed to be simultaneous with heartbeat sensations. A button was then pressed to register the choice and end the trial. Thirty such heartbeat detection (HBD) trials were completed, yielding a distribution of the number of times each interval was chosen. Subjects also completed the SSAS, a measure of state anxiety (the Spielberger State Anxiety Inventory; Spielberger *et al.*, 1970), a somatization scale, and a measure of the tendency to normalize ambiguous bodily sensations or alternatively to attribute them to disease.

The results appear in Table 10.5. Five and one-half percent of the hypochondriacal group were able to accurately detect the instant of cardiac contraction, as compared to 14.0% of the nonhypochondriacal comparison group, a difference not statistically significant ($P = 0.12$). In contrast to their objective performance, however, hypochondriacal patients had higher SSAS scores, rating themselves as significantly more sensitive to normal physiological sensations and minor bodily symptoms.

Thus, their self-ratings of perceptual sensitivity were not corroborated by this objective test of visceral interoception. The hypochondriacal sample contained more women, was significantly higher on state anxiety, and differed in ideal body weight. Because these characteristics have been shown in some studies to affect HBD performance, we compared the two groups again after controlling statistically for these differences, using logistic regression. The results did not change.

We then examined the relationship between hypochondriasis and cardiac perception further by examining the associations between hypochondriacal symptoms and HBD performance separately within each patient group. The HBD performance was not correlated significantly with amplification or somatization within either the hypochondriacal or the comparison group; HBD performance was *inversely* correlated with the severity of hypochondriacal symptoms in the hypochondriacal sample ($r = -0.32$; $P = 0.025$), but these measures were not significantly associated in the comparison sample ($r = 0.10$; $P = ns$). When the accurate and inaccurate cardioceptors within each sample were compared, they did not differ significantly in hypochondriacal concerns, somatization, bodily amplification, or childhood trauma.

Thus, *DSM-III-R* hypochondriacal patients were not found to be more accurately aware of their resting heartbeat than nonhypochondriacal patients from the same general medical setting. Nor was there evidence for a quantitative relationship between the accuracy of heartbeat awareness and the severity of hypochondriacal symptoms within each group. Indeed, among hypochondriacal

**Table 10.5.** The relationship between symptoms and perception in two groups
of hypochondriacal and nonhypochondriacal patients participating in a
Heartbeat Detection (HBD) Test

| Heartbeat Awareness | Hypochon- driacal Patients (n = 60) | | Nonhypochon- driacal Patients (n = 60) | | Statistical Test Applied | df | p |
|---|---|---|---|---|---|---|---|
|  | n | % | n | % |  |  |  |
| Overall accuracy HBD test | 3 | 5.5 | 7 | 14.0 | Fischer's Exact Test | NA | 0.12 |

| | Hypochon- driacal Patients (n = 60) Test Response Time (msec) | | Nonhypochon- driacal Patients (n = 60) Test Response Time (msec) | | Student's t-test | df | p |
|---|---|---|---|---|---|---|---|
|  | Mean | SD | Mean | SD |  |  |  |
| HBD test Mean inter- quartile range* | 266.9 | (54.4) | 276.9 | (62.6) | t = 0.87 | 103 | 0.38 |
| Somatization test (SSI) | 2.97 | (0.59) | 1.55 | (0.38) | t = 15.43 | 117 | 0.0000 |
| Amplification test (SSAS)† | 3.05 | (0.79) | 2.11 | (0.60) | t = 7.29 | 116 | 0.0000 |
| Test item: Can hear heart pounding in ears | 2.59 | (1.45) | 1.68 | (0.91) | t = 4.02 | 96 | 0.0000 |
| State anxiety test (STAI) | 2.22 | (0.54) | 1.70 | (0.35) | t = 6.10 | 98 | 0.0001 |
| Health norms test (HNST) | 14.8 | (5.07) | 17.8 | (3.99) | t = 3.68 | 118 | 0.0004 |

*Complete data obtained on 55 hypochondriacal patients and 50 comparison patients.
†Complete data obtained on 59 hypochondriacal patients and 59 comparison patients.

patients, there was a significant *inverse* correlation between hypochondriacal attitudes and concerns and HBD performance. Hypochondriacal patients are therefore not more accurate perceivers of cardiac activity; if anything, they may be
less sensitive discriminators.

In theory, the somatic complaints of hypochondriacal patients might result from
benign dysfunction, mild infirmities, and normal physiology, which are reported

because the hypochondriacal patient is more sensitive to them and better able to perceive them than is the nonhypochondriacal patient. This would imply that hypochondriacal individuals are able to make finer visceral discriminations and to detect more subtle cardiac irregularities than other individuals. Our findings suggest that this is not the case and imply instead that hypochondriacal cardiac symptoms may be better understood as resulting from a bias toward expressing bodily distress in general, a global proclivity to describe one's sensations as more uncomfortable. To use a signal detection paradigm, hypochondriacal complaints may result more from background noise, which the patient cannot distinguish from signal, than from unusually sensitive detection of weak signals.

These findings run somewhat counter to the literature, which suggests a positive association between hypochondriacal characteristics and sensitivity to pain, to paired flashes of light, and to kinesthetic stimuli (Gramling *et al.*, 1996; Hanback and Revelle, 1978; Petrie, 1978). These investigations, however, were not conducted on patients with diagnosed primary hypochondriasis. The work of Wright *et al.* (1977) and of Tyrer *et al.* (1980) is most similar to the present study. The latter reported that hypochondriacal patients estimated their pulse rates more accurately than did phobic patients. Pulse estimation, however, differs from the cardioceptive task we employed and is subject to knowledge and guessing.

## Studies of Amplification in Other Populations

The concept of amplification has led us in two additional research directions. In one, we probed the relationship between self-reported amplification (measured with the SSAS) and cardiac awareness in nonhypochondriacal populations. In the other, we studied the amplification of symptoms that had a demonstrable medical basis to see whether the construct might shed some light on the wide interindividual variability in symptoms seen among different individuals with the same severity and extent of tissue pathology.

### *Cardiac Awareness*

Studies of ambulatory medical patients with palpitations, and a nonpatient convenience sample, confirmed our earlier finding that SSAS scores were *not* significantly associated with awareness of resting heartbeat. Patients completed the same resting heartbeat detection task described earlier. Heartbeat awareness was unrelated to SSAS scores (i.e., subjects who reported they were unusually sensitive to bodily sensations were no more accurately aware of the instant of ventricular systole than subjects who were not self-reported amplifiers) (Barsky *et al.*, 1993b). Interestingly, however, a statistically significant correlation existed between their response to the single SSAS item "I can sometimes hear my pulse or my heartbeat throbbing in my ear" and accurate heartbeat awareness.

Subjects also underwent continuous, round-the-clock ambulatory electrocardiographic (ECG) monitoring and kept symptom diaries in which they recorded the precise onset of all palpitations experienced. These records enabled us to establish whether or not diary reports of palpitations coincided temporally with changes in cardiac activity. The findings with respect to the accuracy of palpitations noticed during ambulatory monitoring differed from those on heartbeat awareness: SSAS scores showed significant *inverse* correlation with accuracy of symptom reports. That is, the palpitations reported by amplifiers were significantly *less* likely to be accompanied by changes in cardiac rate or rhythm than the palpitations reported by subjects who scored low on the SSAS.

Thus, it appears that the subjective sense that one is exceptionally sensitive to a wide range of nonpathological bodily discomforts is not associated with a more accurate awareness of heartbeat, and is negatively associated with the accuracy of cardiac symptom reporting. Amplifiers were hypothesized to be more accurate interoceptors who are more sensitive to normal physiology and benign dysfunction. But it appears that amplifiers are, if anything, less accurately aware of cardiac activity. This suggests that, in signal detection terms, rather than being extremely sensitive detectors who are able to discern and discriminate individual, weak, or ambiguous bodily sensations, amplifiers and hypochondriacal patients are actually less able to distinguish these signals from background noise—that is, they are flooded with a multitude of uncomfortable stimuli that nonamplifiers and nonhypochondriacal individuals are able to disregard or "gate out."

The fact that different results were obtained with the HBD task and the diary recordings of palpitations is not as surprising as it might at first appear. Performance on laboratory tests of visceral interoception generally differs from performance measured *in vivo*, during everyday life (Pennebaker, 1995; Pennebaker and Watson, 1988; Pennebaker et al., 1985; Tyrer et al., 1980; Whitehead et al., 1977). (An analogous picture emerges in pain research, where the sensitivity to experimental and pathological pain differ [Jamner and Schwartz, 1986; Sternbach, 1974].)

First, the detection of *resting* heartbeat is a different psychophysical task from the detection of irregularities in and departures from that baseline. In other words, people may be better able to perceive changes in a physiological system than to perceive the steady state itself (Pennebaker, 1982, 1995). Second, we know that bodily perception is affected by the context in which it occurs (Pennebaker, 1982), and the circumstances and setting of the experimental laboratory differ markedly from those of the natural environment. In daily life, external stimuli compete for attention, and it is more difficult to focus one's attention internally, different situational feedback occurs, and different cues and external information are available to interpret one's sensory experience. This point has been made by Pennebaker (1995) and Pennebaker and Watson (1988) in studying the awareness of blood pressure and blood sugar. Finally, bodily perception is profoundly influenced by the beliefs, ideas, and expectations we have about what we perceive. The implications of an arrhythmic sensation, with its alarming and ominous threat to health, are very different from the meaning and significance we attach to sensing one's normal, resting heartbeat.

### The Amplification of Organic Disease

We have also been interested in the role of somatosensory amplification in influencing the intensity of somatic symptoms caused by demonstrable medical disease. Clinicians have long been aware of the wide range in symptom severity experienced by patients with comparable disease processes (i.e., with the same extent of organ or tissue pathology).

One might hypothesize that amplifiers, when medically ill, would experience more severe symptoms than nonamplifiers with the same disease process. We have examined this in a study of ambulatory medical patients with upper respiratory tract infections (URIs) (Barsky et al., 1988b). Consecutive patients seeking treatment for URIs completed self-report questionnaires measuring amplification (the SSAS), URI symptoms, functional impairment, and psychological distress. The URI severity was assessed with a standardized physical examination. Using multiple stepwise regression analysis, amplification emerged as a significant correlate of the severity of URI symptoms ($R^2 = 0.11$). Amplification was more powerful in this respect than was the patient's physical examination score. Also, SSAS scores were significantly correlated with disability, even after controlling for medical morbidity. A regression equation including somatic symptoms, global discomfort, and amplification explained 42% of the variance in disability (Barsky et al., 1988b). These findings suggest that a general tendency to amplify bodily sensation may contribute to the interindividual variability in symptoms and disability seen among patients with the same, self-limited medical illness.

## Conclusion

Clinical observation of hypochondriacal patients and the nature of their complaints suggests that they misinterpret the significance of minor bodily sensations and misattribute them to serious disease. A self-report questionnaire was developed to assess this tendency to amplify benign bodily sensation. Studies using this instrument reveal it to be highly correlated with several different measures of hypochondriasis, even after taking into account the possible confounding effects of psychiatric comorbidity, medical disease, and sociodemographic characteristics. Prospective, longitudinal studies indicate that amplification is temporally stable in both hypochondriacal and nonhypochondriacal populations, and that it generally tracks with the severity of hypochondriasis over time. Transiently hypochondriacal patients have persistently higher amplification scores than do nonhypochondriacal patients, and long-term follow-up has indicated that remitted hypochondriacal patients have lower amplification scores than do patients whose hypochondriasis has not remitted.

There remains, however, the important question of the nature of hypochondriacal patients' bodily perceptions. We therefore undertook to study their accurate awareness of resting heartbeat. This work revealed that hypochondriasis is unrelated to heartbeat detection. In addition, in a sample of medical outpatients amplification was actually *inversely* related to the likelihood that palpitations noted during daily life were accompanied by any change in cardiac rate or rhythm. Though far more study of bodily interoception in hypochondriasis is needed, these findings at least suggest that hypochondriacal patients are not actually better detectors or more accurate discriminators of cardiac stimuli. Rather than focusing on a single, subtle visceral sensation and amplifying it, hypochondriacal patients may better be thought of as flooded with a wide range of "background noise" that they are unable to damp down, ignore, or "gate out."

Finally, it is clear that amplification has both trait and state properties, and further study of the latter may be helpful in understanding a wide range of clinical conditions characterized by bodily symptoms that are disproportionate to demonstrable disease.

## References

American Psychiatric Association. 1987. *Diagnostic and Statistical Manual of Mental Disorders, Third Edition, Revised* (*DSM-III-R*). Washington, DC: American Psychiatric Association.

Barsky A.J. 1992. Amplification, somatization and the somatoform disorders. *Psychosomatics* 33: 28–34.

Barsky A.J., Geringer E., Wool C.A. 1988a. A cognitive-educational treatment for hypochondriasis. *General Hospital Psychiatry* 10: 322–327.

Barsky A.J., Goodson J.D., Lane R.S., Cleary P.D. 1988b. The amplification of somatic symptoms. *Psychosomatic Medicine* 50: 510–519.

Barsky A.J., Wyshak G., Klerman G.L. 1990. Transient hypochondriasis. *Archives of General Psychiatry* 47: 746–752.

Barsky A.J., Cleary P.D., Sarnie M.K., Klerman G.L. 1993a. The course of transient hypochondriasis. *American Journal of Psychiatry* 150: 484–488.

Barsky A.J., Cleary P.D., Brener J., Ruskin J.N. 1993b. The perception of cardiac activity in medical outpatients. *Cardiology* 83: 304–315.

Barsky A.J., Cleary P.D., Coeytaux R.R., Ruskin J.N. 1995a. The clinical course of palpitations in medical outpatients. *Archives of Internal Medicine* 155: 1782–1788.

Barsky A.J, Brener J., Coeytaux R.R., Cleary P.D. 1995b. Accurate awareness of heartbeat in hypochondriacal and non-hypochondriacal patients. *Journal of Psychosomatic Research* 39: 489–497.

Barsky A.J., Ahern D.K., Bailey E.D., Delamater B.A. 1996. Predictors of persistent palpitations and continued medical utilization. *Journal of Family Practice* 42: 465–472.

Barsky A.J., Fama J.M., Bailey E.D., Ahern D.K. 1998. A prospective 4- to 5-year study of *DSM-III-R* hypochondriasis. *Archives of General Psychiatry* 55: 737–744.

Beecher H.K. 1956. Relationship of significance of wound to pain experienced. *Journal of the American Medical Association* 161: 1609 1613.

Bianchi G.N. 1971. Origins of disease phobia. *Australian and New Zealand Journal of Psychiatry* 5: 241–257.

Bianchi G.N. 1973. Patterns of hypochondriasis: a principal components analysis. *British Journal of Psychiatry* 122: 541–548.

Bodemar G., Walan A. 1978. Maintenance treatment of recurrent peptic ulcer by cimetidine. *Lancet* I: 403–407.

Burdon J.G.W., Juniper E.F., Killian K.J., Hargreave F.E., Campbell E.J.M. 1982. The perception of breathlessness in asthma. *American Review of Respiratory Disease* 126: 825–828.

Clark D.M. 1986. A cognitive approach to panic. *Behaviour Research and Therapy* 24: 461–470.

Cope H., David A., Pelosi A., Mann A. 1994. Predictors of chronic "postviral" fatigue. *Lancet* 344: 864–868.

Costa P.T., Jr., McCrae R.R. 1980. Somatic complaints in males as a function of age and neuroticism: a longitudinal analysis. *Journal of Behavioral Medicine* 3: 245–257.

Costa P.T., Jr., McCrae R.R. 1985. Hypochondriasis, neuroticism, and aging. When are somatic complaints unfounded? *American Psychologist* 40: 19–28.

Derogatis L.R. 1977. *SCL-90. Administration, Scoring and Procedures Manual. Clinical Psychometric Research.* Baltimore, MD: John Hopkins University School of Medicine.

Derogatis L.R., Lipman R.S., Rickels K., Uhlenhuth E.H., Covi L. 1974. The Hopkins Symptom Checklist (HSCL): A self-report symptom inventory. *Behavioral Science* 19: 1–15.

Diener E., Emmons R.A. 1985. The independence of positive and negative affect. *Journal of Personality and Social Psychology* 47: 1105–1117.

Dworkin R.H., Hartstein G., Rosner H.L., Walther R.R., Sweeney E.W., Brand L. 1992. A high-risk method for studying psychosocial antecedents of chronic pain: the prospective investigation of herpes zoster. *Journal of Abnormal Psychology* 101: 200–205.

Gordon E., Kraiuhin C., Meares R., Howson A. 1986. Auditory-evoked response potentials in somatization disorder. *Journal of Psychiatric Research* 20: 237–248.

Gramling S.E., Clawson E.P., McDonald M.K. 1996. Perceptual and cognitive abnormality model of hypochondriasis: amplification and physiological reactivity in women. *Psychosomatic Medicine* 58: 423–431.

Hanback J.W., Revelle W. 1978. Arousal and perceptual sensitivity in hypochondriacs. *Journal of Abnormal Psychology* 87: 523–530.

Hathaway S.R., McKinley J.C. 1951. *Minnesota Multiphasic Personality Inventory*. New York: The Psychological Corporation.

Hussar A.E., Guller E.J. 1956. Correlation of pain and the roentgenographic findings of spondylosis of the cervical and lumbar spine. *American Journal of Medical Science* 232: 518–527.

Hyler S.E., Redier R.O., Spitzer R.L., Williams J.B.W. 1983. *Personality Diagnostic Questionnaire (PDQ)*. New York: New York State Psychiatric Institute.

Jamner L.D., Schwartz G.E. 1986. Self-deception predicts self-report and endurance of pain. *Psychosomatic Medicine* 48: 211–223.

Jette A.M., Davies A.R., Cleary P.D., Calkins D.R., Rubenstein L.U., Fink A., Kosecoff J., Young R.T., Brook R.H., Delbanco T.L. 1986. The Functional Status Questionnaire: reliability and validity when used in primary care. *Journal of General Internal Medicine* 1: 143–149.

Katon W., Williamson P., Ries R. 1981. A prospective study of 60 consecutive psychiatric consultations in a family medicine clinic. *Journal of Family Practice* 13: 47–55.

Leventhal H. 1986. Symptom reporting: a focus on process. In *Illness Behavior; A Multidisciplinary Model* (eds. McHugh S., Vallis T.M.), New York: Plenum Press.

Levine J.D., Gordon N.C., Smith R., Fields H.L. 1982. Post-operative pain: effect of extent of injury and attention. *Brain Research* 234: 500–504.

Lichtenberg P.A., Swensen C.H., Skehan M.W. 1986. Further investigations of the role of personality lifestyle and arthritic severity in predicting pain. *Journal of Psychosomatic Research* 30: 327–337.

Lipman R.S., Covi L., Shapiro A.K. 1977. The Hopkins Symptom Checklist (HSCL): factors derived from the HSCL-90. *Psychopharmacology Bulletin* 13: 43–45.

Meares R., Horvath T. 1972. "Acute" and "chronic" hysteria. *British Journal of Psychiatry* 121: 653–657.

Merskey H., Evans P.R. 1975. Variations in pain complaint threshold in psychiatric and neurological patients with pain. *Pain* 1: 73–79.

Miller L.C., Murphy R., Buss A.H. 1981. Consciousness of body: private and public. *Journal of Personality and Social Psychology* 41: 397–406.

Myers M.G., Cairns J.A., Singer J. 1987. The consent form as a possible cause of side effects. *Clinical Pharmacology and Therapeutics* 42: 250–253.

Ottaviani R., Beck A.T. 1987. Cognitive aspects of panic disorders. *Journal of Anxiety Disorders* 1: 15–28.

Pauli P., Schwenzer M., Brody S., Rau H., Birbaumer N. 1993. Hypochondriacal attitudes, pain sensitivity, and attentional bias. *Journal of Psychosomatic Research* 37: 745–752.

Pennebaker J.W. 1982. *The Psychology of Physical Symptoms*. New York: Springer-Verlag.

Pennebaker J.W. 1995. Beyond laboratory-based cardiac perception: ecological interoception. In *From the Heart to the Brain: The Psychophysiology of Circulation-Brain Interaction* (eds. Vaitl D., Schandry R.), Frankfurt, Germany: Peter Lang Publishers.

Pennebaker J.W., Brittingham G.L. 1982. Environmental and sensory cues affecting the perception of physical symptoms. In *Advances in Environmental Psychology* (eds. Baum A., Singer J.E.), Hillsdale, NJ: Erlbaum.

Pennebaker J.W., Epstein D. 1983. Implicit psychophysiology: effects of common beliefs and idiosyncratic physiological responses on symptom reporting. *Journal of Personality* 51: 468–496.

Pennebaker J.W., Watson D. 1988. Blood pressure estimation and beliefs among normotensives and hypertensives. *Health Psychology* 7: 309–328.

Pennebaker J.W., Watson D. 1991. The psychology of somatic symptoms. In *Current Concepts of Somatization: Research and Clinical Perspectives* (eds. Kirmayer L.J., Robbins J.M.), Washington, DC: American Psychiatric Association Press.

Pennebaker J.W., Gonder-Frederick L., Cox D.J., Hoover C.W. 1985. The perception of general vs. specific visceral activity and the regulation of health-related behavior. In *Advances in Behavioral Medicine* (eds. Katkin E.S., Manuck S.B.), Greenwich, CT: JAI Press.

Peterson W.L., Sturdevant R.A.L., Frankl H.D., Richardson C.T., Isenberg J.I., Elashoff J.D., Sones J.Q., Gross R.A., McCallum R.W., Fordtran J.S. 1977. Healing of duodenal ulcer with an antacid regimen. *New England Journal of Medicine* 297: 341–345.

Petrie A. 1978. *Individuality in Pain and Suffering, Second Edition*. Chicago: University of Chicago Press.

Pilowsky I. 1967. Dimensions of hypochondriasis. *British Journal of Psychiatry* 113: 89–93.

Pilowsky I. 1968. The response to treatment in hypochondriacal disorders. *Australian and New Zealand Journal of Psychiatry* 2: 88–94.

Pilowsky I. 1978. A general classification of abnormal illness behaviours. *British Journal of Medical Psychology* 51: 131–137.

Robins L., Helzer J.E., Croughan J. 1981. National Institute of Mental Health Diagnostic Interview Schedule: its history, characteristics, and validity. *Archives of General Psychiatry* 38: 381–389.

Rubinfeld A.R., Pain M.C.F. 1976. Perception of asthma. *Lancet* I: 882–884.

Spielberger C.D., Borsuch R.L., Lushene R.E. 1970. *State-Trait Anxiety Inventory*. Palo Alto, CA: Consulting Psychologists Press.

Sternbach R.A. 1974. *Pain Patients: Traits and Treatments*. New York: Academic Press.

Sternbach R.A. 1978. Psychological dimensions and perceptual analyses, including pathologies of pain. In *Handbook of Perception* (eds. Carterett E.D., Friedman M.D.), New York: Academic Press.

Tyrer P., Lee I., Alexander J. 1980. Awareness of cardiac function in anxious, phobic and hypochondriacal patients. *Psychological Medicine* 10: 171–174.

Valins S., Nisbett R.E. 1971. Attribution processes in the development and treatment of emotional disorder. In *Attribution: Perceiving the Causes of Behavior* (eds. Jones E.E., Karouse D.K., Kelley H.H.), Morristown, NJ: General Learning.

Vercoulen J.H.M.M., Swanink C.M.A., Fennis J.F.M., Galama J.M.D., van der Meer J.W.M., Bleijenberg G. 1996. Prognosis in chronic fatigue syndrome: a prospective study on the natural course. *Journal of Neurology, Neurosurgery and Psychiatry* 60: 489–494.

Watson D., Clark L.A. 1984. Negative affectivity: the disposition to experience aversive emotional states. *Psychological Bulletin* 96: 465–490.

Watson D., Tellegen A. 1985. Toward a consensual structure of mood. *Psychological Bulletin* 98: 219–235.

Whitehead W.E., Drescher V.M., Heiman P., Blackwell B. 1977. Relation of heart rate control to heartbeat perception. *Biofeedback Self-Regulation* 2: 371–392.

Wilson A., Hickie I., Lloyd A., Hadzi-Pavlovic D., Boughton C., Dwyer J., Wakefield D. 1994. Longitudinal study of outcome of chronic fatigue syndrome. *British Medical Journal* 308: 756–759.

Wood M.M., Elwood P.C. 1966. Symptoms of iron deficiency anaemia. A community survey. *British Journal of Preventive and Social Medicine* 20: 117–121.

Wright D.D., Kane R.L., Olsen D.M., Smith T.J. 1977. The effects of selected psychosocial factors on the self-reporting of pulmonary symptoms. *Journal of Chronic Disease* 30: 195–206.

Ziesat H.A., Jr. 1978. Correlates of the tourniquet ischemia pain ratio. *Perceptual and Motor Skills* 47: 147–150.

# 11

# Hypochondriasis, Abnormal Illness Behavior, and Social Context

## ISSY PILOWSKY

Until the psychiatric profession emerged as an independent medical discipline, and, even more recently, found a role in general hospitals, it was not possible for hypochondriasis to be comprehensively considered from a "psychiatric" viewpoint. Before then, when psychiatrists (or "alienists" as they were known) practiced almost exclusively in "asylums," the only occasions on which they encountered hypochondriacal phenomena were when they were part of a psychotic illness such as schizophrenia or affective disorder. The patients with nonpsychotic hypochondriasis were seen, in the main, by physicians who were not necessarily inclined to write about or research the subject, with occasional notable exceptions.

The social milieu in which medical practice was conducted changed to a considerable degree during the first half of the twentieth century, with the establishment of private and state health insurance programs and prepaid health insurance programs. As a result, the doctor–patient relationship was exposed to many social forces and institutions that wanted to know, because they were paying the doctor's bill, what they were paying for and whether the same outcomes could be achieved at lower cost. One may speculate whether the Cochrane movement ("evidence-based medicine"), whose purpose is to establish the comparative value of various treatments, is, in part, a response to the questions being asked by governmental and private insurers.

In this new climate of concern over burgeoning health care costs, the hypochondriacal patient could come to be regarded as a virtual enemy of the state. Unfortunately, the fear of hypochondriasis and its confusion with malingering could sometimes result in "malingerophobia" and consequent errors of judgment about a patient's need for help, leading to an upsurge in litigation against doctors. The media have frequently reported cases of individuals being sent home and later dying of a myocardial infarction.

It is no wonder, then, that a negative attitude toward hypochondriacal patients has prevailed. This has been well illustrated by Singh *et al.* (1981), particularly the remarkable lack of constraint shown by medical writers in revealing hostile and, indeed, unethical attitudes toward hypochondriacal patients. For example, Hutchison (1934) stated that a "hypochondriac" could be viewed as akin to a stamp collector, collecting symptoms rather than stamps and happy doing so. Thus, why not leave him as he is, observed Hutchison; and in any event, why kill the goose that lays the golden egg? This is only one of a number of cases of doctors who were ready to publish views blatantly disrespectful of patients. Their preparedness to do this and the readiness of editors of medical journals to publish such outpourings suggest a medical and a social climate conducive to open condemnation of such patients. Still, why did hypochondriacal patients' behavior elicit so much hostility?

## Attitudes Toward Hypochondriacal Patients

We may also ask how it comes about that a doctor's altruistic drives may sometimes become so distorted as to suggest hostility rather than concern toward the patient. This question has been explored previously in the sociobiological and social psychological literature (Pilowsky, 1977). What emerged was that in practically all species studied, and certainly in humankind, the altruistic impulse is exquisitely ambivalent and sensitive to factors in the environment for the nature of its final expression. A universal concern is the fear of the "cheater" who works out ways of evoking altruism, thus gaining an evolutionary advantage for his genes to the disadvantage of the "altruist." Thus, sociobiologists see an advantage for species survival to be derived from the ambivalence of altruism.

Against this background, the tendency to perceive the patient with inexplicable physical symptoms as a possible malingerer may be seen as virtually a "normal" or invariable reaction. Nonetheless, it is part of doctors' professional and fiduciary responsibility to patients to be aware of such negative responses and to be in control of them.

## Social Construction of Hypochondriasis

Although *hypochondriasis* is an ancient term with a history of at least two thousand years, it was not until the early nineteenth century that its meaning began to approach the one it has today. Reasons for the shift in the conceptualization of hypochondriasis can be found in the changes both in the medical and psychiatric professions, and in social factors (see also Chapter 1). The latter pertain to the changing roles of physicians in the society, new aspects of the relationship between physicians and patients, and changing conceptualizations of and attitudes toward the "sick role." These will be discussed below.

The "status" of hypochondriasis and related conditions, such as hysteria (proclaimed by Dover in 1733 [q.v., 1733] to be the same as hypochondriasis, except that it occurred in women, whereas hypochondriasis was found in men), became a subject of many debates, reflecting, among other things, the social concerns and structure of medical services delivery systems of the time. This is illustrated by comments on hysteria made by Elliot Slater, an eminent psychiatrist at the London National Hospital for Nervous Diseases.

Slater's genetic and clinical studies led him to the conclusion that "hysteria" did not exist (Slater, 1961, 1965). When psychiatrists in St. Louis, Missouri, advanced the view that hysteria or Briquet's syndrome, as they preferred to name it, did indeed exist as a distinct clinical entity, Slater argued thus:

> Quite recently we have seen the revival of an old French diagnosis, Briquet's syndrome, which is now called *St. Louis hysteria*, because of the work done on it by the psychiatrists at St. Louis, Missouri. The symptoms are of any imaginable kind. They have nothing characteristic about them and they can affect any bodily system. Their one characteristic is that the single patient has many symptoms. However, as the number of symptoms found depends on the doctor's enthusiasm in eliciting them, the making of the diagnosis will depend on his commitment. Unless he is convinced that the syndrome exists he will never see it, just as ghosts are only seen by those who believe in them. (Slater, 1982, p. 38).

Slater went further, noting that the vast majority of these patients are women:

> The great majority of doctors who had to deal with these women were, of course, male. Men have little instinctive aptitude for empathy for women; and they are in any case liable to write off specifically feminine ways of thinking, feeling and acting as "hysterical." Faced by symptoms they do not understand, in women who do not engage their sympathy, the male doctors find an easy way out in relegating them to a category, to a diagnosis, "hysteria," which follows these hapless patients from one centre to another and becomes a self-fulfilling prophecy. I greatly fear that St. Louis hysteria is a product of machismo, of male chauvinism, of which one can find many other examples in medicine. (Slater, 1982, p. 39).

Although Slater does not seem aware of it, his engagement in this debate is illustrative of the way in which illnesses are socially constructed.

In addition to hysteria and hypochondriasis, there are many well-known examples of conditions that have initially been refused social recognition as illnesses and then accepted, or vice versa. For example, in ancient Rome, epilepsy was known as the "sacred disease" and sufferers were regarded as being struck down by the gods, who then communicated special messages through them to the mortals. Of course, this attitude toward epilepsy has subsequently changed. A more recent example is that of alcoholism: Many years passed before the societal establishment accepted alcoholism as an illness, also because of its devastating social consequences. As a result, the patient who accepts a diagnosis of alcoholism and agrees to be treated for it becomes entitled to a "sick role" and its attendant privileges (see below).

## The Doctor–Patient Relationship in the Diagnosis of Hypochondriasis

The focus on the role of the doctor in the diagnosis of hypochondriasis refers not only to the professional role but also to the societal role and thus establishes a bridge between the individual's psychopathology and society's attitudes toward illness. The concept that makes the physician's social role quite clear is that of the "sick role," introduced by the sociologist Talcott Parsons in 1964 (Parsons, 1951). As with any role, it carries obligations and privileges.

The obligations to be fulfilled for granting of the sick role are these:

1. The role must be regarded as essentially undesirable;
2. the individual must recognize an obligation to cooperate with others in order to achieve "health" and thus eventually divest oneself of the sick role; and
3. the individual must utilize the services of those regarded by society as competent to diagnose and treat the illness.

The privileges associated with the sick role are these:

4. The person is not regarded as "responsible" for the state (that is, he or she cannot produce or terminate it by a conscious act of will and thus is not malingering);
5. the person is accepted as someone requiring care; and
6. the person is entitled to exemption from normal obligations, taking into account age and the nature of the impairment.

On the basis of this formulation I have suggested (Pilowsky, 1978) that an "illness" be defined as follows: "An organismic state which fulfills the requirements of a relevant reference group for admission to the sick role."

This definition produces the natural link between the intrapsychic life of the individual and the demands of society placed on anyone claiming the sick role. Consideration of the sick role formulation, especially the obligations (*2*) and (*3*) stated above, makes clear that the doctor plays a crucial part in the legitimization of illness in the process of granting the sick role. Doctors are reluctant to grant the sick role to hypochondriacal patients mainly because these patients are perceived as uncooperative and because they utilize medical services inappropriately. Both of these are often seen as a consequence of the difficulty of hypochondriacal individuals to accept reassurance from their doctors as to the innocuous nature of their complaints.

## Sick Role, Response to Reassurance, and Hypochondriasis

It can be argued from an historical perspective that as long as the hypochondriacal phenomena encountered were delusional in form and part of psychotic illnesses, it did not seem necessary to focus on the nature of reassurance, given that the abnormality of ideation was so self-evident. Therefore, emphasis on the lack of adequate response to medical reassurance appears to be a relatively recent development, and there is now little disagreement over the salience of this feature of hypochondriasis.

As a consequence, current definitions of hypochondriasis include a lack of response to adequate medical reassurance, although the criteria for considering the reassurance to be adequate have rarely been enunciated (see also Chapters 2 and 13).

The requirement of a lack of response to medical reassurance for the diagnosis of hypochondriasis seems to accompany the idea that patients gain some kind of pleasure from their symptoms and resist giving them up. This was implied by Kraepelin (1904) when he wrote that hypochondriacal patients probably tolerate their symptoms "with a sort of secret pride," that their illness "becomes a source of entertainment," and that "not infrequently, they sabotage the doctor's prescription and show some satisfaction in having succeeded" (Kraepelin, 1904, p. 327).

However, the response of hypochondriacal patients to reassurance may have deeper implications. Thus, Wahl (1963) stated that "these patients appear to be angered by attempts of the physician to assuage their fright or concern" (p. 10). If we regard hypochondriasis as an individual's psychological strategy for remaining unaware of intrapsychic conflicts or external threats that threaten psychological equilibrium, then we cannot be surprised to find that they resist suggestions that such conflicts may be present.

This feature makes referral to a psychiatrist very difficult unless the process is carefully and sensitively managed (Pilowsky, 1997, p. 97). The difficulty in

achieving referral to a psychiatrist has been investigated empirically by Clarke
*et al.* (1991). They found that general hospital patients who scored high on the
General Health Questionnaire (Goldberg and Williams, 1988) (i.e., those who
were highly likely to suffer from a nonpsychotic psychiatric disorder) were more
likely to be referred to a psychiatrist than a low scoring group. But within the
high scoring group, patients were less likely to be referred to a psychiatrist if
their scores on the Disease Conviction scale of the Illness Behaviour Questionnaire (Pilowsky and Spence, 1994) indicated a tendency to hypochondriasis.

The presence of a need within the hypochondriacal patient to view the problem as a somatic one, without a psychological cause, is not based on a misunderstanding or a personal whim. It is as much a symptom of psychological
disturbance as pyrexia is of infection, joint stiffness is of arthritis, and abdominal rigidity is of peritonitis. It is a surface manifestation of an attempt to prevent
or alleviate an internal pain. Thus, it is not surprising that the patient resists probing of the tender personal areas as much as the arthritic person resists movement
of the tender joint and the patient with peritonitis reflexively resists having the
abdomen palpated. It is little wonder that this resistance may be expressed with
anger, as Wahl (1963) had suggested, especially, one may add, if reassurance is
offered in a tactless manner.

Issues surrounding reassurance often introduce complications in the process
of diagnosing hypochondriasis, and there is general agreement between clinicians
that the diagnosis of hypochondriasis is not easy. The difficulty stems in part
from the fact that the diagnosis emerges from a development at some point in
the doctor–patient relationship. More precisely, the diagnosis of hypochondriasis
becomes possible if there is a fundamental disagreement between the doctor and
the patient (see also Chapter 12). Only when the physician feels confident enough
to offer the patient a definitive opinion as to the nature of the sick role can a diagnosis of hypochondriasis be entertained. If the patient holds a strong belief that
a disease is present which merits a different sick role and attendant privileges,
and this belief cannot be altered by what the doctor believes are the "objective
data" (Pilowsky, 1969), then there will be tension between doctor and patient.
Nevertheless, it is particularly important to establish patients' subjective feelings
and ideas about their state of health.

There is another point to be made about the issue of reassurance and the basis upon which it can be safely offered. This concerns historical and cultural influences on the doctor–patient relationship. Some clinicians may maintain that
the relationship has become altered, if not distorted, by the fact that many of these
patients are seen in a medicolegal context where the purpose is not management
of the condition but rather the provision of a report to the patient's legal advisers who will in any event give it to their client to read. Furthermore, in the
medicolegal context, neither the patient nor his legal advisers may wish to hear

that the physical discomforts are "nothing to worry about." We should also bear in mind that some courts might come to accept hypochondriasis as an illness that should be compensated if it has been precipitated by an industrial accident.

One may also argue that the reassurance issue has only arisen since doctors have felt able to take responsibility for offering a diagnosis and advice about a treatment program and patients have felt that they have a right to this information. Such a right also pertains to a patient's interest in knowing what the financial cost of the treatment program is—an interest also shown by medical insurers.

## Phenomenologically-Based Diagnostic Criteria for Hypochondriasis

The core features of hypochondriasis are described variously as a fear of disease, a preoccupation with ideas of disease, and a belief in the presence of physical disease (even where none exists). In the fourth edition of the *Diagnostic and Statistical Manual of Mental Disorders* (*DSM-IV*; American Psychiatric Association, 1994), hypochondriasis is defined as the "preoccupation with fears of having, or the idea that one has, a serious disease" (p. 465), which "persists despite appropriate medical evaluation and reassurance" (p. 465). The latter part of this definition (Criterion B) is an example of the only condition in which appropriate behavior on the part of the medical profession is required for the making of a diagnosis. Under these circumstances, I have suggested (Pilowsky, 1997) that matters might be improved by the use of diagnostic criteria for hypochondriasis that were consistently phenomenological, as follows:

A. An uncomfortable awareness of bodily sensations is present most (>50%) of the time.

B. Fears and concerns about health and disease are present most of the time.

C. An awareness of an inability to accept reassurance from doctors who have offered clear information, associated with the concern that doctors have not done everything possible to detect disease or are withholding information and/or treatment which could be helpful. There may also be a concern that one is being accused of malingering.

D. An awareness of an inability to accept the suggestion that non-physical— i.e., psychosocial—factors may be relevant to one's condition, and the experience of marked emotional discomfort when this possibility is raised.

It may also be helpful to express these experiences from the patient's viewpoint. Thus, a patient may say:

- "I notice things in my body such as pains or palpitations and I worry about my health all the time. I think I might have cancer or I'm going to have a heart attack or a stroke. Sometimes I think I'm silly, but I still go on worrying."
- "Even though my doctor has investigated everything very thoroughly, I can't accept what he says about there being nothing to worry about—at least not for long."
- "When a doctor says my symptoms may be due to an emotional problem and that we should talk about possible worries with my family or job, I get very upset and annoyed because I don't think I have any problems at all. Then I can find myself worrying about my health even more. In fact, I often wonder if I am being accused of malingering."

Clinical experience indicates that many patients can provide such a description of their experiences if given the opportunity to do so. Furthermore, they are rarely, if ever, offended by an initial question such as, "Do you suffer from hypochondriasis?" or "Have your symptoms made you hypochondriacal?" The invariable response is to ask for an explanation of the word *hypochondriasis*, which can then be given in terms of the aforementioned criteria. Interestingly, whether or not patients agree that they are themselves hypochondriacal, almost all seem to know someone—usually a relative—who is "a hypochondriac."

## Abnormal Illness Behavior

The concept of abnormal illness behavior was originally introduced (Pilowsky, 1969) in the hope of clarifying the relationship between conditions such as "hysteria" and "hypochondriasis" in the context of the psychiatric assessment of chronic pain. It was hoped that this would obviate the frequent use of these terms as pejorative labels. Because clinical experience suggests that abnormal illness behavior has been appropriated for similar uses, as were the aforementioned terms, it is crucial to define a condition such as hypochondriasis as precisely as possible. I have tried to achieve this within the framework of the concept of "abnormal illness behavior." Let us therefore consider the definition of *abnormal illness behavior*.

Abnormal illness behavior is defined as an inappropriate or maladaptive mode of experiencing, evaluating, or acting in relation to one's own state of health; this maladaptation persists, despite the fact that a doctor (or other recognized social agent) has offered accurate and reasonably lucid information concerning the person's health status and the appropriate course of management (if any), with provision of adequate opportunity for discussion, clarification, and negotiation based on a thorough examination of all parameters of functioning (physical, psychological, and social), taking into account the individual's age and educational and sociocultural background.

In 1984, at a meeting of the European Society for Psychosomatic Research in London, Heinz Wolff described this definition as a "dangerous idea." In so doing, he directed attention to a core issue, and indeed the reason why it is so crucial to define abnormal illness behavior. It seemed that he was articulating a concern held by many about a blatantly iatrocentric definition that seems to regard the doctor's opinion as a "gold standard" against which to judge the patient's ideas, because, after all, doctors could be mistaken.

I am well aware that many doctors will fall short of what is required by the definition, but it should be self-evident that the definition refers to an "ideal-type" doctor just as the definition as a whole is of an ideal-type syndrome (as indeed are all descriptions and definitions of illnesses). It is very rare, however, that a condition encountered in a patient is precisely the same as described in textbooks. Insofar as physicians are engaged in a pattern-recognition exercise, they are looking for the diagnosis that most closely approximates the classic description. Thus, the doctor essentially deals with probabilities while the patient seeks or expresses certainties. One of the key features of hypochondriasis is that one can never be sure that the hypochondriacal patient may not turn out to be right about his or her disease fears and beliefs. Therefore, the physician's appropriate behavior is not to adopt an attitude of absolute certainty, but rather to offer an opinion based on probabilities. The patient leans toward certainty with even less basis than does the doctor.

Few, if any, would wish to offer an argument for regarding doctors as infallible, and this is certainly not my intention. However, hypochondriasis is an unusual and perhaps unique condition in that the validity of the patient's ideas can only be tested against a "recognized" medical opinion since the patient's ideas are in themselves a medical opinion. Here it should be emphasized that we are not referring to the patient's symptoms, but rather to the manner in which they are focused on and interpreted. In other words, we base our diagnostic decision on the patient's ideas, attitudes, and opinions, not on the nature of the symptoms.

Patients in general are probably seeking and will accept reassurance, which would be judged adequate by peer review. There is no absolute or "gold" standard for the quality of the reassurance, but it would be at a level of suitability, which a particular doctor's peers would presumably consider adequate. Standards are usually set by a panel of a doctor's peers, especially if there are complaints about a doctor's behavior or competence.

I have classified hypochondriasis (Pilowsky, 1993) as a form of abnormal illness behavior, which has the following characteristics:

1. It is somatically focused;
2. it is illness-affirming;
3. its motivation is predominantly unconscious; and
4. it can be manifested either as a neurotic (somatoform) disorder or as a psychotic condition if hypochondriacal delusions are present.

It is more likely for secondary and psychotic abnormal illness behavior to be seen in psychiatric hospitals, whereas the primary care physicians and general hospital psychiatrists or consultation-liaison psychiatrists will more often see abnormal illness behavior in the form of causal misattribution, primary hypochondriasis, and other somatoform disorders. The differing claims concerning the nosological status of primary hypochondriasis between Kenyon (1964) and Pilowsky (1970) may well be explained by the fact that the work of the former had been done with patients referred to a psychiatric hospital, while the work of the latter had been done with patients seen in a general hospital.

## Cross-Cultural Aspects of Hypochondriasis

Is hypochondriasis confined mainly to modern, "Western" societies? This issue has received little attention, but it is plausible that the differences in the nature of the doctor–patient relationship and in the cultural expectations between modern and traditional societies play a role in the "forms" of hypochondriasis and hypochondriasis-like disorders that may be seen in various parts of the world.

For example, there is a striking difference between the role of the modern doctors and that of Zulu traditional healers in southern Africa. The latter do not offer a diagnosis and a treatment plan as do the former because, as can be seen from the description below, in the traditional healers' interview technique, the Zulu patients' opinion about their diagnosis and treatment is not sought. In fact, the patients have to respond to the prescribed treatment using the vocabulary of agreement, and they participate in the treatment ritual regardless of their complaints. Presumably, this allows them to retain their status within their tribal group should they wish to be supported by it. Therefore, an illness akin to "modern" hypochondriasis (particularly its aspect of diagnostic and treatment "disagreement" between the traditional healer and the patient) may be rarely if ever encountered among the Zulu patients in the tribal setting. Such a "disagreement" might be labeled as reflecting hypochondriasis if these patients were to seek help in a Western medical setting.

The Zulu traditional healers fulfill their function as intermediaries to the spirit world. Their task is to ascertain the way in which the sufferer has offended an ancestor and to report what sort of sacrifice should be made in expiation. The so-called witch-doctor takes a history by rapidly reciting a list of statements or propositions to all of which the sufferer and his relatives, if present, must respond with the words "I agree" or by clapping their hands. The "witch-doctor" presumably draws her conclusions from the way this phrase is uttered or the hands are clapped. After this, she enters into a trance and when she emerges she conveys her message from the world of the ancestors. Commonly, the sufferer may have to sacrifice a goat or some other domestic animal such as a fowl in order to appease the ancestors. The "witch-doctor" is usually a woman because both genders can speak frankly to a woman, while women cannot use certain words in the presence of a man. A homosexual male can also fill the role.

There may be certain similarities between the seeking of health care in traditional and modern societies, including a tendency toward excessive health care seeking. It remains to be elucidated whether the latter signifies mistrust in the healers of patients from traditional societies or whether patients are seeking to establish which healer is regarded the most appropriate by healers themselves, by the patient's family and, of course, by the sufferer. Thus, it is not unusual for sufferers in traditional societies to consult an herbalist and a Western-trained doctor at the same time, in much the same way as a "Western" patient may consult simultaneously an orthopedic surgeon, a chiropractor, a health food store, and a pharmacist.

In Qatar, a "culture-bound neurosis" (El-Islam, 1975) similar to hypochondriasis was described in women who do not fulfill their traditional, prescribed female roles (e.g., in those who do not marry or who "fail" to have children). The condition consists of numerous "unexplainable" somatic symptoms for which the women undergo many examinations, looking for a presumed organic etiology. Such women receive attention and care, and they are regarded as invalids who are therefore "excused" from a failure to fulfill their socially imposed "duties" and as too physically ill to marry or reproduce. It should be noted that in certain times and places these women might be diagnosed as having "hysteria."

Kirmayer (1996) has suggested that strict and rigid culturally imposed beliefs and rules contribute to a "blurring of the distinction between anxious preoccupations and delusions" (p. 152), which may explain the frequency with which cases of monosymptomatic, delusional, or quasi-delusional hypochondriasis are reported in some developing countries (Osman, 1991).

A recent cross-national study of hypochondriasis in primary care conducted in fifteen cities around the world (Gureje *et al.*, 1997) did not reveal large differences between the developed and developing nations in the occurrence of hypochondriasis, including medical help-seeking and refusal to accept medical reassurance. Although the authors of the study emphasized that the fifteen sites were selected to "represent broad diversity in culture and socioeconomic development" and that the participating clinics were regarded as "representative primary care centres in the various countries" (p. 1002), the fact is that the study was conducted in large cities of a few developing countries, and that it excluded significant segments of the rural population in which traditional medicine is more likely to be practiced, and traditional values, beliefs, and roles more strictly upheld. In addition, with this kind of study, it is difficult to know the nature of the reassurance and the precise context in which it was given.

## Conclusion

Hypochondriasis is a condition that can act as a litmus test of the standard of medicine being practiced in any community, in particular the nature and quality of the doctor–patient relationship. For example, if a particular doctor or group of doctors are diagnosing abnormal illness behavior, namely "hypochondriasis" or "hysteria," far more often than other doctors, we may find on careful examination of the circumstances that they do not understand the cultural background of their patients and are using the diagnosis in a dismissive way. Alternatively, the doctor may be working under excessive pressure (the difficult circumstances of seeing too many patients in too short a time).

It can be argued that hypochondriacal individuals are apt to influence the diagnostic and treatment agenda by insisting that their symptoms are due to somatic problems and by rejecting the suggestion that psychosocial factors may have a part to play. It does not take much imagination to suppose that some doctors will be more compliant than others with the patient's wishes.

Thus, it is well known that there are doctors (perhaps more often, although certainly not invariably) of an older generation who are reluctant to accept the legitimacy of psychiatry's contribution to medicine as a whole, and are themselves as influenced as the general population by the stigma attached to psychiatric illness. They may therefore empathize with the patient who does not wish to see a psychiatrist and act accordingly. Although it is reasonable not to expect every student to become a psychiatrist, one of the aims of clinical teaching is for students to know enough psychiatry to be able to detect the possible presence of emotional disorder and, at the very least, not to stand in the way of the patient being seen by a psychiatrist.

Of course, it is crucial that referral to a psychiatrist not be perceived by the patient as a rejection. This is readily avoided if the referring physician continues to see the patient while utilizing the advice of the psychiatric consultant in the treatment process. Above all, one should not abandon all interest in the somatic dimension of the patient's functioning, but should carry out periodic physical examinations as required.

## References

American Psychiatric Association. 1994. *Diagnostic and Statistical Manual of Mental Disorders, Fourth Edition* (*DSM-IV*). Washington, DC: American Psychiatric Association.

Clarke D.M., Minas I.H., McKenzie D.P. 1991. Illness behaviour as a determinant of referral to a psychiatric consultation/liaison service. *Australian and New Zealand Journal of Psychiatry* 25: 330–337.

Dover T. 1733. *The Ancient Physician's Legacy to His Country*. London: Printed for the relict of the late R. Bradley.

El-Islam M.F. 1975. Culture-bound neurosis in Qatari women. *Social Psychiatry* 10: 24–29.

Goldberg D.P., Williams P. 1988. *A User's Guide to the General Health Questionnaire*. Windsor, England: NFER-Nelson.

Gureje O., Üstün T.B., Simon G.E. 1997. The syndrome of hypochondriasis: a cross-national study in primary care. *Psychological Medicine* 27: 1001–1010.

Hutchison R. 1934. Hypochondriasis: individual, vicarious and communal. *British Medical Journal* I: 364–367.

Kenyon F.E. 1964. Hypochondriasis: a clinical study. *British Journal of Psychiatry* 110: 478–488.

Kirmayer L.J. 1996. Cultural comments on somatoform and dissociative disorders: I. In *Culture and Psychiatric Diagnosis: A DSM-IV Perspective* (eds. Mezzich J.E., Kleinman A., Fabrega H., Parron D.L.), Washington, DC: American Psychiatric Press.

Kraepelin E. 1904. *Klinische Psychiatrie*. Leipzig: Verlag von Johann Ambrosius Barth.

Osman A.A. 1991. Monosymptomatic hypochondriacal psychosis in developing countries. *British Journal of Psychiatry* 159: 428–431.

Parsons T. 1951. *The Social System*, Glencoe, II: The Free Press

Pilowsky I. 1969. Abnormal illness behaviour. *British Journal of Medical Psychology* 42: 347–351.

Pilowsky I. 1970. Primary and secondary hypochondriasis. *Acta Psychiatrica Scandinavica* 46: 273–285.

Pilowsky I. 1977. Altruism and the practice of medicine. *British Journal of Medical Psychology* 50: 305–311.

Pilowsky I. 1978. A general classification of abnormal illness behaviours. *British Journal of Medical Psychology* 51: 131–137.

Pilowsky I. 1993. Aspects of abnormal illness behaviour. *Psychotherapy and Psychosomatics* 60: 62–74.

Pilowsky I. 1997. *Abnormal Illness Behaviour*. Chichester: John Wiley.

Pilowsky I., Spence N.D. 1994. *Manual for the Abnormal Illness Behaviour Questionnaire* (*IBQ*), *Third Edition*. Adelaide: University of Adelaide, Department of Psychiatry.

Singh B., Nunn K., Martin J., Yates J. 1981. Abnormal treatment behaviour. *British Journal of Medical Psychology* 54: 67–73.

Slater E. 1961. The Thirty-fifth Maudsley Lecture: Hysteria 311. *Journal of Mental Science* 107: 359–381.

Slater E. 1965. Diagnosis of "hysteria." *British Medical Journal* I: 1394–1399.

Slater E. 1982. What is hysteria? In *Hysteria* (ed. Roy A.), Chichester: John Wiley.

Wahl C.W. 1963. Unconscious factors in the psychodynamics of the hypochondriacal patient. *Psychosomatics* 4: 9–14.

# III

# Treatment Considerations

# 12

# The Patient–Physician Relationship in the Treatment of Hypochondriasis

## DON R. LIPSITT

> The significance of the intimate personal relationship between physician and patient cannot be too strongly emphasized, for in an extraordinarily large number of cases both diagnosis and treatment are directly dependent on it, and the failure of the young physician to establish this relationship accounts for much of his ineffectiveness in the care of patients.
>
> Peabody, 1927, p. 878

> While the precise nature and extent of the influence which psychoanalysis and so-called psychodynamic psychiatry have had on modern medicine are debatable, it seems . . . that the most decisive effect has been that of making physicians explicitly aware of the possible significance of their relationship to patients.
>
> Szasz and Hollender, 1956, p. 585

Of the hundreds of thousands of patient–physician interactions occurring worldwide, probably a relatively small number would be characterized as "difficult." Nonetheless, this group would appear to be most taxing of the physician's tolerance, patience, understanding, and clinical skill. If, as the literature suggests, somatizing patients are especially high utilizers of medical services (Barsky *et al.*, 1996; Escobar *et al.*, 1987; Katon *et al.*, 1990; Lin *et al.*, 1991), then it can be expected that every practicing physician will experience the often vexing challenge of treating patients whose primary or secondary condition is hypochondriasis (Kaplan *et al.*, 1988).

Much can be learned about the patient–physician relationship in examining more closely how physicians and hypochondriacal patients relate to one another

(Peters *et al.*, 1998). And because the management of hypochondriacal patients is so rooted in the patient–doctor relationship, the better we understand the nuances of that relationship, the more effective we may expect our treatment to be.

In this chapter I will briefly review pertinent literature about patient–doctor relationships, describe more specifically the illness behavior of the hypochondriacal patient (phenomenologically and psychodynamically) and the physician's corollary response, and offer suggestions—based on clinical report, research, and theory—for working with hypochondriacal patients. Other parts of this volume address important definitional, diagnostic, and therapeutic aspects of the hypochondriacal patient; the approach taken here assumes that the patient–doctor/ therapist relationship is the matrix of all relevant interventions.

## Background

In the workaday world of most physicians, the "doctor–patient relationship" is taken for granted, an assumption of a working arrangement that embraces most interactions with patients. Throughout civilization, physician/healers have been imbued with great power and authority, and the sick have usually depended on them for solace, compassion, and (hopefully) cure (although the Hippocratic Oath makes no mention of cure). For most physicians, the "doctor–patient relationship" is considered sacrosanct, although for some it has become mere shibboleth for political, economic, and behavioral agendas. Nonetheless, it is, for the most part, acknowledged as the *sine qua non* of diligent, committed, appropriate doctoring (Bloom, 1963; Stoeckle, 1987), the very foundation of medical practice, and imbued with social status that sanctions rights and privileges accorded no other profession. It is this richly textured format that both physician and patient willingly enter, with its great potential for both beneficial and harmful outcomes.

In characterizing the modal doctor–patient relationship, we would say that each partner seeks some kind of connectedness—the patient to be understood, comforted, treated, and to be made well; the physician, through empathy and skill, to correct a perceived disruption in the patient's life and to be realistically appreciated and rewarded for his or her dedication and skill. The physician must be nurturant without expecting reciprocity, be intimate without violating the delicate boundary between patient and physician. The patient must be able to be temporarily dependent without compromising separateness. Together, patient and physician must be able to "read" each other, communicate effectively, and work cooperatively toward the intended goal. All in all, this is not an easy set of tasks, now made more challenging by changes in medical practice wherein others (e.g., insurers, managed-care companies, regulators, and so on) become part—for better or worse—of the doctor–patient relationship (Barsky and Borus, 1995). Communication, already complicated, can become even more entangled.

What does each participant bring to the relationship that will influence the twists and turns it will take? Both come from backgrounds often of widely diverse education, socioeconomic status, religion, race, culture, personal developmental history, beliefs, attitudes, wishes, expectations, disappointments, experience, and vulnerabilities (Vaillant, 1972). Despite this marked variability, physicians are trained, implicitly or explicitly, to show no discrimination in the application of their learned skills to those individuals who are in need. But the fullness of this relationship is seldom achieved in practice; indeed, deviations from its idealized form have been acknowledged in the negative responses of doctors to frustrating interactions with troublesome patients (Anstett, 1980; Drossman, 1978; George and Dundes, 1978; Grant, 1980; Groves, 1978; Hahn *et al.*, 1994, 1996; Jeffery, 1979; John *et al.*, 1987; Lipsitt, 1970; Longhurst, 1980; Martin, 1955; Mathers *et al.*, 1995; Stern, 1984).

A best-selling novel (Shem, 1978) portrays the sadistic ward behavior of house staff toward bothersome patients: The senior resident, indoctrinating his new intern into the "real world of ward medicine," says, "There is a finite number of House gomers, and since gomers don't die, they rotate through the House several times a year. . . . You get to know them by their particular shrieks." The resident caricatures the patient as having congestive heart failure, pneumonia, sepsis, dementia, an unobtainable blood pressure, and refusing to eat and wanting to die. He informs the intern that the first thing one does with such patients is to place them somewhere else. Accused by the intern of being heartless and treating the patient like a piece of luggage, the resident replies, "Oh? I'm crass, cruel and cynical, am I? I don't feel anything for the ill? Well, I do; I cry at movies. But a gomer in the House of God is something else. You'll find out for yourself tonight" (Shem, 1978, p. 77). While this interchange burlesques reality to some degree, it is not so far removed from the way attitudes toward patients are transmitted in postgraduate medical training.

## Medical Education

It is not only in recent times that physician–patient relationships have been found deficient, sometimes blamed on excessive paperwork, severe regulation, external control, and overwork (Bosc, 1979; Brandt and Kutner, 1957; Cousins, 1981; Gorlin and Zucker, 1983). More than 70 years ago, F.W. Peabody, a revered professor of medicine wrote that "young graduates have been taught a great deal about the mechanism of disease, but very little about the practice of medicine— or, to put it more bluntly, they are too 'scientific' and do not know how to take care of patients" (Peabody, 1927, p. 877). Peabody held that "The practice of medicine in its broadest sense includes the whole relationship of the physician with his patient" (p. 877) and singled out for discussion "patients who have 'nothing the matter with them,' " that "large group of patients who do not show objective organic pathologic conditions." (p. 878). Although not designated as such at the time Peabody wrote, it is likely that the patients he was referring to we would now recognize as somatizers, those patients whose physical complaints seldom are supported by objective findings. Regarding treatment of these patients, Peabody observed that "it is not the disease but the man or woman who needs to be treated" (p. 880).

Virtually every decade since Peabody's admonitions, medical literature has critically reflected disappointment in the capacity of medical education to adequately prepare graduating physicians for the interpersonal aspects of medical practice, especially for the care of those patients regarded as "difficult" (Becker and Geer, 1958; Engel, 1977; Fox, 1957; Gallagher, 1978; Henderson, 1935; Merton *et al.*, 1957; Moos and Yalom, 1966; Mumford, 1970; Reynolds and Brice, 1971; Rezler, 1974; Ries *et al.*, 1981; Schwenk and Romano, 1992; Schwenk *et al.*, 1989; Sharpe *et al.*, 1994; Starr, 1982; Strauss, 1978).

A physician's sensitivity to the nuances of his or her relationship with patients was such a rarity in earlier times that physicians attentive to relational matters were upheld as the titans of the medical profession. Medical schools, for their part, espouse the importance of doctor–patient relationships as the foundation of medical practice but crowd their curricula with so many other "essentials" of a superior medical education that little time remains for this important aspect of training.

An appreciation of the role of affect in medical education is especially neglected (Davis, 1968). Because the educational process for physicians is rooted historically in anatomy, histology, biology, and "scientific" medicine, there remains a strong bias toward the biomedical side of medicine. The affective or psychosocial dimension of medicine is characteristically shunned or even derided as "soft and fuzzy" (Fredericks and Mundy, 1976; Glauber, 1953; O'Malley, 1970; Zabarenko and Zabarenko, 1978).

Medical school admissions committees telegraphed a preference for "objective" orientation when they previously admitted mainly students who had majored in the biological and chemical sciences. Students learned from the start to revere objectivity over subjectivity, to search for certainty and "cure"; disappointment runs high when neither is forthcoming (Fox, 1957). The deleterious impact of "dualism," the fragmentation of medical study into focus on *either* psyche *or* soma, is a characteristic of medical training and practice that has been stubbornly resistant to change (Lipsitt, 1983). Where affect is missing, dehumanization is apt to occur. Medical students are said to pass through an educational process ("from 'pre-cynical' to 'cynical' years") that transforms them from sensitive, compassionate people on entry to medical school to cold and cynical graduate physicians (Becker and Geer, 1958; Eron, 1955; Ort *et al.*, 1964).

Sociologists have studied this interesting transformational process extensively (Becker and Geer, 1958; Bloom, 1979; Knight, 1973; Merton *et al.*, 1956, 1957; Shapiro and Lowenstein, 1979). Throughout medical training, there are abundant overt and covert messages that affect should be controlled (Daniels, 1960; Lipp, 1977; Mizrahi, 1986). The implied risk of responding negatively to highly affective situations has been demonstrated repeatedly. One study (Ort *et al.*, 1965) showed that students would be biased toward patients with chronic illness, with the expectation that such patients would be hostile, rebellious, or demanding and would jeopardize the (student) physician's control of the relationship. Such biases, left unattended, would carry over into later practice (Parets, 1967; Smith and Zimny, 1988).

Even more than chronic illness, mental illness generates negative affects in student and graduate physicians (Hooper *et al.*, 1982; Moos and Yalom, 1966; Tucker and Reinhardt, 1968). Nonpsychiatrist physicians readily acknowledge discomfort with psychiatric patients and avoid psychiatric wards; likewise, the difficulty many physicians have in tolerating a patient's tears has been observed commonly by consultation-liaison psychiatrists. It is not surprising that most physicians, trained in Western medicine, find greater comfort in their commerce with physical medicine, with "objective" findings that have applicable and demonstrable remedies.

In some sense, physicians are like patients in their preference for physical complaints; in both, the language of emotion is less well-learned, "alexithymic" (no words for feelings), so to speak. In the life experience of most people, one's childhood hurts and annoyances have usually been assuaged with physical remedies (a drink of water, a cookie, a turned on light, a bandage, a kiss, and so on), a possible early antecedent for what might be a later preference for physical explanation of perceived distress. Subsequent efforts to "translate" somatic expression into emotional language may encounter major obstacles. A physician untutored in the language of emotion will have great difficulty penetrating beyond his or her patient's concrete somatic symptom to unravel the more troublesome disturbance (Parets, 1967; Smith and Zimny, 1988).

## Early Studies

Inquiry into the earliest studies of doctor–patient relationships almost certainly leads to Freud's original studies of the psychoanalytic process, in which he discovered that the very relationship between patient and analyst could enhance or impede therapeutic outcome. From this awareness came elaboration of the dynamics of transference (Freud, 1912a), "a cathexis which is held ready in anticipation . . . directed to the figure of the doctor" (p. 100). This varied from one individual to another and derived from "the combined operation of [his] innate disposition and the influences brought to bear on him during his early years" (p. 99).

In outlining recommendations for psychoanalytic technique, Freud paid the utmost respect to *transference*, acknowledging that it could account for changes in patients irrespective of the content of sessions or their interpretations. Observing the importance of the impact of transference, Freud cautioned that the "doctor should hold himself in check, and take the patient's capacities rather than his own desires as guide" and that "as a doctor, one must above all be tolerant of the weakness of a patient" (Freud, 1912b, p. 119). It was the bond of transference, according to Freud, that permitted effective treatment to occur at all: "Not until an effective transference has been established in the patient, a proper rapport with him . . ." can treatment be said to begin (Freud, 1912c, p. 139), for "it remains the first aim of the treatment to attach [the patient] to it and to the person of the doctor" (p. 139). Before long, Freud also acknowledged the potential of the physician to unwittingly and negatively influence the treatment through the effect of the patient on the doctor's own unconscious processes, an accompaniment of treatment Freud termed *countertransference* (Freud, 1910).

Because every psychoanalytic treatment included scrutiny of the transference, psychoanalytic literature provides a rich lode of data regarding patient–physician interaction (see, for example, Gutwinski-Jeggle, 1997, and Valenstein, 1973). It is not the purpose or place to review this literature here, but only to allude to psychoanalytic observations that can illuminate techniques for working with hypochondriacal patients (see also Chapter 8).

Although Freud's insights about the role of transference in the therapeutic relationship were available early in the twentieth century, it was not until the 1950s and 1960s that marked interest emerged in their application to understanding the doctor–patient relationship (Bloom, 1963; Szasz and Hollender, 1956). While transference implied an essentially unconscious process, "therapeutic or working alliance" connoted a more conscious aspect of doctor–patient relationships, primarily in psychoanalysis but also more broadly applied to all treatment encounters (Brenner, 1979; Lipsitt, 1986).

References to the nature and importance of the doctor–patient relationship appeared episodically in the medical literature (Henderson, 1935; Lewin, 1946; Nunberg, 1938; Peabody, 1927; Simmel, 1938), but it was not formally codified before Talcott Parsons's social analysis in 1951. Parsons (1951a) saw the relationship between physician and patient as a social system revolving around the "sick role," embedded in which are the reciprocal obligations of both. In legitimate sickness, society confers immunity from normal social responsibility and blame on the patient. It is the inherent task of the sick person to strive to become well, to seek technically competent help and to permit temporary dependency on others in the process of recovering. It is the physician's complementary role to validate or legitimize the patient's right to the sick role, to exercise his or her skills as a physician in altruistically aiding the patient's recovery, and to help enlist the patient's family in marshalling support toward the same health-restoring goals. For Parsons, the sick role implied deviance but did not emphasize the extreme forms observed in some patients called "difficult." He did, however, acknowledge the significance of transference and the imperative for the physician/ psychotherapist to be cautious of recrimination, reciprocity, or judgment of the patient's deviant behavior (Parsons, 1951b).

Subsequent to Parsons's important contribution and in recognition of the varieties of relationships experienced in doctor–patient encounters, later theorists described various models of doctor–patient relationships, attending for the most part to the degree of control and authority exercised by the physician and the relative activity and passivity of the participating actors (Bennett, 1976; Bloom and Wilson, 1972; Gallagher, 1978; Siegler and Osmond, 1974; Szasz and Hollender, 1956; Thomasma, 1983), sometimes influenced by cultural or subcultural factors (Bloom, 1963; Kleinman, 1978; Mechanic, 1972). It was recognized that different circumstances in the patient's illness called for the use of different models of the relationship and that individual physicians, because of their own predilections and backgrounds might be more at ease with one model than with another. Although the importance of communication was not fully addressed in these early models, subsequent focus on this important variable has been robust for its relevance to treatment outcome as well as for compliance with medical recommendations (Bennett, 1976; Docherty and Fiester, 1985; Epstcin *et al.*, 1993; Hall *et al.*, 1981; Roter and Hall, 1992; Waitzkin and Stoeckle, 1972).

The "fit" of patient and doctor in arriving at mutually workable models was (and is) often haphazard or random; a physician's adaptability is always most tested by those patients who most deviate from the idealized sick role. In the case of hypochondriasis, the "diagnosis" is most often made in the pejorative breech (George and Dundes, 1978; Leiderman and Grisso, 1985; Lipsitt, 1970) than in careful application of true diagnostic criteria (i.e., *DSM-IV*, American Psychiatric Association, 1994).

The following section examines the unique aspects of the doctor–patient relationship that emerge with patients whose "true" diagnosis is hypochondriasis as well as with those who are simply called "hypochondriacs" out of frustration in the encounter. This exploration begins with assessing what each participant brings to the relationship.

## What the Doctor Brings

What motivates one to enter the medical profession is not always easy to ascertain, but sociological studies suggest that there is usually at least a wish to help sick people (Menninger, 1957; Rogoff, 1957); one survey posed the following question to entering medical students: "Do you think you would get more personal satisfaction from successfully solving a relatively simple medical problem for a patient who expresses great appreciation, or from successfully solving a very complicated problem for a patient who expresses no appreciation whatever?" (Rogoff, 1957, p. 128). In this study, most of the students showed a preference for an appreciative patient over the reward of the intellectual satisfaction of solving a challenging medical problem. If this response is generalizable and enduring, one might expect this to exert a profound impact on a physician's attitudes and emotional responses to one's patients.

Clearly, not all patients are liked. Likability depends upon many characteristics of both patients and their physicians (Groves, 1978; Hall *et al.*, 1993; Hooper *et al.*, 1982; Mally and Ogston, 1964; Martin, 1957; Papper, 1970; Stern, 1984; Walker *et al.*, 1997). One physician's least-liked patients may be those whose major problem is substance abuse, obesity, mental illness, malingering or chronic disease, or those who are seductive and openly hostile or psychotic. Even with these *overt* "objectionable" characteristics, these patients do not challenge the traditional doctor–patient relationship in the same way as the more *covertly* angry, character-disordered, factitious, or somatizing patients, especially those whose illness involves chronicity, pain, and hypochondriasis, with their known refractoriness to treatment. It is these conditions, where the nuances of the doctor–patient relationship "go underground," so to speak, that elicit the most acute affective responses in physicians. And, as described above, medical education poorly prepares physicians to understand or tolerate such tension, uncertainty and affectivity. It is not that physicians are unaccustomed to listening sympathetically to patients with the most inordinate hardship and pain, but that certain types of patients present their suffering in ways that alienate the best instincts of the physician.

Physicians have a wish to heal, to cure, to see results for their efforts and expect patients to be satisfied with and appreciative of the results (Konner, 1987). Because none of these outcomes is very likely in the treatment/management of hypochondriacal patients (at least early in its course), these patients provoke disappointment, frustration, and rejection out of feelings of ineptness, helplessness, and diminished self-esteem as a physician. Symptoms that cannot be substantiated with physical findings tend to be called "not real," and therefore convey disbelief in the patient's own perception of distress; the implication is that he or she is malingering. The notion that a physical symptom could be generated unconsciously is not part of a physician's customary repertoire.

For the most part, physicians seek connectedness to their patients through empathy and caring. But when these initial impulses are thwarted, there is a sense that physicians have been betrayed by the patient. This is especially so in those situations where a patient's very sad story, multiple problems, and desperate need initially mobilize the physician's natural indulgence of "rescue" fantasies. Inability to accomplish the objective of symptom alleviation can evoke guilt and anger in the physician who takes this failed outcome as a statement about his or her personal competence, dedication, and skill. Some physicians defend themselves against such emotional trauma by developing a doubting, distant, and hesitant approach to their patients, and may be described by patients as "cold" or "in a shell."

Physicians tend to be most comfortable in positions of authority, control, and activity. This has great appeal for patients who wish to be attended by someone who is decisive, strong, and directive. But patients who themselves have a pronounced need for control, autonomy, and dependency often clash with such physicians. The hypochondriacal patient confronts the physician with the dilemma of needing both activity and passivity, autonomy and dependence, at different times and thus is unpredictable. Unpredictability breeds chaos in the patient–physician relationship and is not easily tolerated by the physician; the urge to be rid of such patients is promptly summoned in the physician (Mizrahi, 1986).

In postgraduate education in internal medicine, the overburdened, harried, and tired resident portrays himself or herself as "doing battle." In this setting, one study described how interns saw patients: "The patient, the embodiment of a recalcitrant and impenetrable system, many characterized as the ultimate enemy. Apathy about, if not apathy toward, patients was expressed by most of the cohort completing internship" (Mizrahi, 1986, p. 33). The training experience, the process of "socialization" into the profession of medicine, has been characterized by many as one that leaves physicians poorly prepared for interaction with patients by fostering such distancing mechanisms as escaping into work (Coombs and Goldman, 1973), or emphasizing technique in preference to patient contact (Light, 1980).

Curiously, even though physicians know that illness heightens dependency upon others and that they expect patients to depend on them, dependency becomes burdensome when it exceeds a certain threshold (Gallagher, 1978). Even the most nurturant of physicians will refer to patients who exceed this threshold as "demanding" or "needy." The line between acceptable dependency and excessive demand may be thin and vulnerable to easy "violation." Any threat of crossing the boundary may elicit both appropriate and inappropriate distancing maneuvers on the part of the physician. The labeling of patients by pejorative terms like "crock" (Lipsitt, 1970) and "gomer" (George and Dundes, 1978) helps the physician deflect self-criticism for intolerance and simultaneously widens the distance between oneself and the patient.

For many physicians, the contradictions inherent in working with the hypochondriacal patient hamper establishment of a working alliance: The physician must speak with patients of physical distress while believing that their problem is psychological; they must accept a patient's reluctance to relinquish a symptom even while desperately requesting help; they must acknowledge that the reassurance most patients seek seems ineffective with the hypochondriacal patient; they must realize that some patients who come to doctors simply do not want to get well; and they must entertain the idea of a long-term relationship with patients they are inclined to be rid of. Few physicians come to practice with either the knowledge or intuition of how to treat hypochondriasis. Advising physicians of the importance of listening to these patients is anathema, for they already pride themselves on this basic function of the physician; it is said, however, that a physician's usual listening time lasts about 18 seconds before interrupting the patient's narrative.

## What the Patient Brings

The hypochondriacal patient initially brings to the relationship what every patient brings to a physician—a chief complaint. But it is often a well-worn complaint, one that has been presented to other physicians, emergency rooms, clinics, and hospitals in the past. Despite its chronicity, the complaint has a sense of urgency about it, whether from anxiety, frustration, or low expectation. These patients have been noted by a number of often illustrious physicians to amplify or "catastrophize" minor perturbations (Barsky, 1979; see also Chapter 10). From disappointment with prior medical experience, patients may carry a "chip on the shoulder" attitude, one that signals growing tension, doubt, and distrust in the relationship.

Although the presentation may be assertive and "needy," there is a sense of passive submission, an offering up of oneself for trials of treatment. This demeanor may forecast a struggle for control within the relationship, with the patient appearing alternately dependent, then energetically "independent."

It is often in this context that struggles ensue over compliance with recommendations or medication. Eventually, it appears that the patient is engaging in flawed attempts to make a meaningful connection with the physician, a relationship, nonetheless, of great importance to the patient but which eludes the patient as he or she alternates between requesting (seeking) help and avoiding (rejecting) it. The physician may give up after feeling helpless to relate to such patients (Adler, 1972; Goodwin et al., 1979; Myerson, 1979).

The patient manifests a persevering attachment to the symptoms (Valenstein, 1973). Even with the physician's earnest attempt to "go beyond the presenting complaint," there is a reluctance in the patient to drift very far from it. When the physician makes the observation of slight improvement over time, it is minimized or denied by the patient. Treatment with medications seems to yield little other than objectionable side effects and magnified complaints. The patient frequently compares the current physician's ministrations—favorably or unfavorably—to those of the many doctors who have been part of the patient's continuous odyssey in search of help, a search wherein the symptom is the currency of interaction. Repeated encounters with the physician often heighten a sense of frustration, amplify the complaint, and increase anxiety. These patients perceive themselves as gravely ill, while the physician sees them as relatively healthy or "worried well." The patient is experienced by the physician as self-defeating, irritating, unlikable, abrasive, obnoxious, and masochistic. Described by Horowitz and Marmar (1985), patients who relate with difficulty commonly have borderline or narcissistic personality organizations. These patients tend to have "high state mobility . . . and to present in polysymptomatic syndromes over time" (Horowitz and Marmar, 1985, p. 574).

Although experienced otherwise by physicians, these patients do not knowingly come to bedevil or annoy the doctor. They present themselves as entitled to care because of their extraordinary suffering, often portrayed as the result of fate, but not infrequently precipitated by the individual himself. In a typology of personality styles as they relate to medical management (Kahana and Bibring, 1964), the "long-suffering, self-sacrificing (masochistic) patient" most clearly describes the profile of the hypochondriacal patient. Their misfortunes are displayed exhibitionistically, sometimes evoking initial sympathy but more often a sense of guilty discomfort. Although seemingly searching desperately for acceptance and caring, the result is almost inevitably the opposite. Efforts to console, reassure, or praise seem perversely met with irritation, distrust, and greater suffering. It is this intense conviction of "sickness" and the accompanying inability to be reassured that mark the special features of the truly hypochondriacal patient, who, it has been said, brings to every medical encounter a deeply entrenched low self-esteem and profound sense of incompleteness (Adler, 1981).

## The Relationship

The encounter of the hypochondriacal patient with the somatically oriented physician eventually arrives at a cataclysmic juncture. As I have written elsewhere (Lipsitt, 1986):

> Failure to reach an understanding with the patient of the 'true' nature of the complaint sows the seeds of a dysfunctional relationship. It is then but a short step to the labeling of patients as 'difficult' or 'problematic.' The patient who persists in the wish to be listened to and understood may be perceived ultimately as 'demanding,'

'manipulative,' and 'complaining.' The enduring complaint of pain, the meaning of which eludes both patient and physician, failing of proper 'translation,' is described ultimately as 'not founded in physical disease,' therefore 'hypochondriacal,' and the patient's behavior, because of failure to improve, as 'help-rejecting.' " (p. 4).

Attempts to comprehend these dysfunctional relationships can be addressed both phenomenologically (Hellstrom *et al.*, 1998) and psychodynamically (Lipsitt, 1973; Wahl, 1963).

## Phenomenology

Of the many millions of people who awake each day with all varieties of aches and pains, only a small percentage will find their way to a doctor's office; it is only at that point that they become patients. For the most part, these will be individuals who tend to react sensitively to physical discomfort, who may be predisposed to worry about their health, or who have other reasons to be concerned that "all is not right," such as family history of specific illnesses, recent trauma, or atypical bodily distress. After a few minutes with their physician, a brief history, appropriate physical examination, and perhaps some basic laboratory tests or X-rays, the largest numbers of these individuals will feel comforted with symptomatic treatment, the physician's explanatory words, or the reassurance that their distress does not portend anything serious. But for a very small number, the traditional medical approach will be insufficient to calm the patient's anxieties. Despite medical reassurance, the patient with hypochondriasis will persist in the fear and belief that a serious disease accounts for the distress for months or even years, secretly assuming that it is only a matter of time before the physician will detect the true nature of the ailment. Here the process begins of what may in time be a most difficult experience for both patient and physician.

Patients very quickly get categorized, either consciously or intuitively, into "good" (compliant) and "bad" (difficult) (Lorber, 1975). It is well-known that both physician and patient prefer the "physical" mode of interaction, with patient presenting a clearly definable locus of distress, and the physician readily elaborating clinical "hunches" that can easily be confirmed (or ruled out) by physical examination and selected laboratory studies. Both participants in this process "speak the same language," as it were. If the physician proposes a formulation and diagnosis that approximates what the patient more or less expected, each is pleased. Expectations have been met, treatment is begun, and outcome gratifies doctor and patient in this medical encounter. They have established a concordant relationship, one in which the requisites of the "sick role" have been met, bringing satisfaction to both patient and physician. In contradistinction to those who do not fit so nicely into traditional patterns, this patient might be called "easy."

Those patients who do not conveniently conform to expectable illness behavior may find that the physician's ministrations and reassurances generate in them disbelief, disappointment, puzzlement, and increased concern. In subsequent visits, patients may report failure of medication treatment, intensified symptoms, and increased demandingness for help. At least for a time, the physician, pridefully intent on plying his or her skill, may try one and another therapeutic interventions, sometimes resulting in what has been anonymously called *furor therapeuticus.* Patient and physician feel as though they are working at cross-purposes. Communication is flawed, expectations are not met, intense frustration is expressed by word and gesture, and ultimately the patient feels not understood, while the physician feels his or her time has been improperly used or wasted.

What had begun as a well-intentioned encounter with such patients may readily deteriorate into a discordant relationship in which the physician begins to feel irritated, baffled, angry, impatient, and burdened. He or she is loath to confer the benefits of the "sick role" on these patients, out of a sense that "nothing is wrong." In this context, patients may feel reprimanded and accused of fraudulence. Patients begin to be seen by their previously well-meaning physicians as clinging, dependent, entitled, "not sick." In such cases, it is as though patient and physician have been speaking two different languages. Both parties feel misunderstood and even victimized. Both begin to experience each other as "bad," with the physician assuaging his or her anger and feelings of ineptitude with pejorative labels for the patient, the patient looking elsewhere for help, solace, understanding, and comfort ("doctor-shopping"). Terms applied to the patient include "crock," "turkey," "problem patient," and even "hypochondriac," the latter applied more as opprobrium than diagnostic term.

## Psychodynamics

The relationship of hypochondriacal patient and physician is best understood psychodynamically as a sadomasochistic interaction (Lipsitt, 1973). It is perhaps one of the most difficult interpersonal encounters to comprehend since it presumes that these patients, unlike most, do not wish to get well. Recognition of this anomaly has given rise to the expression "illness as a way of life" (Ford, 1983).

As described elsewhere in this book (see Chapter 8), hypochondriacal symptoms are held to be manifestations of unconscious guilt, serving as a defense against awareness of hostile aggressive impulses toward important people in one's life. These are people who have the power and ability to deny fulfillment of the child's basic needs. The resulting hostile feelings experienced from this deprivation are projected out onto others, feared for their destructive intent, then quickly turned against the self, with the "offering" of a physical "impairment" as expiation for guilt and a bid for love. Removal of the symptom exposes the individual to the raw experience of guilt, the destructive rage of the powerful figures, and the consuming fear of annihilation and death. It is this "tug-of-war" of patient and physician, the former desperately seeking to cling to symptoms and the physician just as desperately searching for a "cure," that gives the relationship its sadomasochistic cast.

The relationship is further confounded by the patient's apparent perverse ability to find "pleasure" in suffering. This behavior is not readily understood unless it is recognized that it is not the suffering *per se* that patients seek but rather the love, comfort, and potential for feeling worthy that suffering may assure (both "primary" and "secondary" gain of illness). Where guilt plays a prominent part, self-sacrifice in and of itself may assume a "pleasurable" role in reducing the pain of suffering; such is the depiction of martyrs.

Important traumatic experiences of childhood may be played out in the patient–physician relationship, especially when patients are most regressed in their help-seeking endeavors. Hypochondriacal patients display great sensitivity to deprivation as well as overgratification, as they may have experienced in early childhood. Feelings and expressions of anger or love have often been repressed and viewed as dangerous. Punitive parents (or physicians) are preferred to being neglected or ignored; punishment may be welcomed and, at times, even experienced with pleasure.

The masochistic traits of the patient almost invariably will elicit corresponding sadistic responses in the physician. Attempts to comfort or reassure the patient are disregarded or rejected by the patient; symptoms are intensified, leading almost invariably to the anticipated irritation in the physician, perhaps erupting in outright rejection. This response "justifies" the patient's belief that the physician (parent) is a "bad" person. Reciprocal aggression in the physician will increase the patient's tension, in turn leading to worsening of symptoms. Paradoxically, what the patient seeks and which is unfamiliar to the physician is praise for the capacity to bear suffering with great strength. It is only when the physician can be trusted to take notice of the patient's suffering and "understands" that any degree of recovering from the pain will be a difficult task, that the patient may "dare" to begin to form a working alliance, a process that may require an extended time. Reassurance can only take place in this trusting, enduring relationship (Starcevic, 1990, 1991; see also Chapter 13).

## Application of the Patient–Physician Relationship to Treatment of the Hypochondriacal Patient

Very few of a physician's patients will actually meet the full diagnostic (*DSM-IV*) criteria of hypochondriasis. But many of those who present with somatizing disorders are at risk of being mislabeled "hypochondriacs." Appreciation of the nuances of an appropriate patient–physician relationship with all these patients will facilitate accurate diagnosis, more effective management, potentially beneficial outcome, and enhanced gratification for the physician, no matter what therapeutic modality is employed.

The following principles of management, with their accompanying rationale, will help establish a patient–physician context in which the hypochondriacal patient may find a hospitable setting and the physician will find opportunities for workable alliances with otherwise "difficult" patients.

**1.** *Respect the patient's symptoms and acknowledge their validity.* Rationale: This is not merely an appropriate stance for physicians with all patients, but is especially relevant for those patients whose style of interacting may easily trigger doubt, annoyance, and rejection. Physicians generally respond most positively to symptoms that can be rapidly understood, clearly diagnosed, and effectively treated, with a corresponding diminution in the patient's level of complaining. Physicians have a low tolerance for uncertainty, subjectivity, and refractoriness to treatment. It is helpful to accept symptoms as they are expressed, to assume that they have meaning that may require time to understand. While the patients may have "no physical findings," they almost certainly have "something" that triggers their visit to a physician.

**2.** *Avoid the temptation to label patients when diagnosis is uncertain.* Rationale: This is especially antitherapeutic for the patient who tends to feel misunderstood, not listened to, and generally devalued, characteristics of the hypochondriacal patient whose deficient self-esteem fosters the search for an accepting relationship more than alleviation of the manifest symptom (Kasl, 1975).

**3.** *Perform a standard workup even with patients whose "reputation" as "difficult" has been handed on from doctor to doctor.* Rationale: Many hypochondriacal patients are, in fact, tarred with a broad brush of negative reports from previous physicians. This diminishes opportunities for such patients to identify and form an alliance with a potentially accepting physician but also heightens the possibility of other missed diagnoses. Hypochondriacal patients can also have organic disease!

**4.** *Know when to limit a workup.* Rationale: Discomfort with uncertainty and doubt may prompt physicians to engage in limitless studies and procedures, largely out of anxiety about a "missed diagnosis." A perspective on the "total patient" rather than a single symptom will help inform the physician when "enough is enough" (see also Chapter 13).

**5.** *Follow-up appointments are not merely useful, they are essential.* Rationale: No matter how warm, empathic, and desirous of helping a physician may be in a first visit, hypochondriacal patients will not be convinced of the physician's interest without subsequent appointments. Interest in the patient is persuasive only when it does not depend upon a continuation or worsening of symptoms to warrant another appointment. Appointments should be given (not asked for) at regular (if wide) intervals of time, not dependent upon symptom intensity. The interval should be adjusted to permit development of the patient's "safe" dependence upon the physician, without depriving the patient of the important sense of self-control and independence. Delicate management of this aspect of the relationship will encourage trust and alliance, without the hazards of regressing to more symptomatic levels. Some investigators assert that it is the relationship itself that is the crucial element, not the exchange of information that is therapeutic (Kasl, 1975).

**6.** *Reassure sparingly.* Rationale: It has been amply recorded that the symptoms of hypochondriacal patients serve many purposes: expiation of guilt, justified dependence, binding of anxiety, and so on. It is not so easy to abandon that which has become essential to adaptation, no matter how painful it may be. Premature or excessive reassurance may instill in these patients a need to intensify or cling to symptoms out of a fear of something more terrible and frightening. Furthermore, one cannot reassure about something that is not yet understood (see also Chapter 13).

**7.** *Restrain the impulse to translate physical symptoms into psychological explanations.* Rationale: It is difficult for physicians to treat patients "as if" they had physical problems when they know the most likely cause is emotional. But hypochondriacal patients do not speak the language of emotion. Efforts of the physician in this direction will be a foreign language, even gobbledygook, to the hypochondriacal patient's ears. Furthermore, it will heighten the patient's conviction that he or she is not listened to or understood.

**8.** *Explore psychosocial history slowly.* Rationale: Hypochondriacal patients remain intensely focused on somatic complaints until they experience trust, dependability, receptivity, and acceptance in the patient–physician relationship. They will "test out" their perception of these dimensions of the relationship and only begin to detach themselves from their symptoms when they achieve a degree of security in the relationship to their physician. At such a moment, there may be a spontaneous "breakthrough" of historical data about family relationships, losses, disappointments, and fears. This is the physician's clue to readiness for gentle exploration of psychosocial history.

**9.** *If you do encourage patients to try to remain healthy, advise them to do it not so much for themselves, but for those who depend upon them.* Rationale: Because hypochondriacal patients harbor so much unconscious guilt, it is difficult for them to accept anything "good" for themselves. Doing for others fits with their characteristic self-sacrifice, suffering for others, and using symptoms defensively for expiation (Kahana and Bibring, 1964).

**10.** *Do not pursue the vanishing symptom.* Rationale: When hypochondriacal patients begin to relinquish symptoms in favor of a broader orientation to their story, asking patients about the whereabouts of the lessening symptom persuades them of the physician's greater interest in the symptom than in them as individuals. This defeats the purpose of trying to bolster self-esteem.

**11.** *Try to avoid the wish to rescue the hypochondriacal patient.* Rationale: For some, the "physicianly" trait of wanting to be helpful, even to cure, is preeminent in the doctor's repertoire of valued skills. Because many hypochondriacal patients manifest remarkable suffering, a first visit can elicit a marked response in physicians of empathy, pity, and an urgency to help. Physicians sometimes rise to the challenge to "cure" those who have failed with so many of one's colleagues. Implicit or explicit promises of improvement that cannot be realized will worsen the patient's condition. Hypochondriacal patients develop marked ambivalence for the "omnipotent," authoritarian physician who elicits both idealization and aggressive tendencies in the patient.

**12.** *Referral for specialty consultation should be rare.* Rationale: Referral is most often made out of frustration or fear of "missing" a diagnosis. It signals to the hypochondriacal patient not greater interest and attention but the threat of loss of the primary physician in the belief that he or she cannot tolerate the patient. The result is often increased symptom intensity and anxiety, and sometimes reluctance or failure to follow through with the referral.

**13.** *Exercise restraint in writing prescriptions.* Rationale: Unless there is clear and persuasive evidence that a patient's hypochondriasis is secondary to treatable conditions (e.g., depression, panic disorder, obsessive-compulsive disorder), then searching for a pharmacologic solution to the patient's problems often signals a wish to avoid the "personal" aspects of the relationship by displacing interest onto inanimate substitutes. Furthermore, all patients know that physicians consider drugs the "big guns" of medical treatment, intended to shortcut deeper interest in the patient's total being. It has been observed that hypochondriacal patients, "threatened" with symptom removal by these powerful agents, usually complain of side effects from medication, or comply poorly with recommendations. Judicious use of medication is always an option, but the physician should assess the quality of the patient–physician relationship for timing the most propitious opportunity for a drug trial, keeping in mind that somatizing patients generally are high placebo-responders (both positive and negative). Until a trusting alliance is established, psychopharmacologic treatment has a low likelihood of benefit (see also Chapter 15).

**14.** *Strengthening commitment to the relationship rather than zealous treatment of the hypochondriacal patient will result in more effective management.* Rationale: Rather than seeking the individual treatments, the hypochondriacal patients' quest is primarily for a meaningful connection to another individual who will be supportive, accepting, nonjudgmental, and "loving" in ways which no one else in their experience has likely ever been. This cannot happen quickly and may take months or years. It is the kind of relationship that can only be found within the context of an understanding patient–physician relationship that does not respond to masochistic "invitations" with sadistic responses.

## Conclusion

It would appear that the physician who does not take account of the unique aspects of the patient–physician relationship with hypochondriacal patients is destined to have an unhappy experience. These patients do not fit the mold of the traditional "sick role," but nonetheless suffer greatly. But before they can engage with a physician in a therapeutic relationship, their shaky sense of self-worth, their exquisite vulnerability to feelings of incompleteness, and their propensity for unwittingly engaging physicians in repeated cycles of sadomasochistic interactions must be recognized. Any attempts to dismiss these features in pursuit of other aspects of the encounter will engage patient and physician in a "corrupt bargain" that will disappoint both (Balint, 1957).

Adler (1981), describing the physician and the hypochondriacal patient in the *New England Journal of Medicine*, emphasizes that if the physician is to help restore the patient's sense of worth, often compromised by poor object relations and significant losses, the physician must be able to tolerate the patient's negative features, resentment, anger, and manipulativeness so as to provide a trustworthy setting in which the patient's anxiety, vulnerability, and fear of death can be contained. If the anger, helplessness, and fear are mirrored in the physician, the greatest risk of rupturing the relationship exists. The hypochondriacal patient's atypical responses to attempts at treatment—which in other patients would be regarded as effective interventions—often puzzle and vex the physician (Garcia-Campayo et al., 1998; Kaplan et al., 1988).

For many years, treatment of hypochondriasis has been shrouded in a mantle of pessimism (Barsky, 1996; Ladee, 1966; Pilowsky, 1968), but more recently it has begun to show greater promise, as highlighted in several chapters of this book. It is not only the advances in diagnostic clarity and pharmaceutical discoveries that have improved the prognosis of patients with hypochondriasis; greater understanding of patient–physician transactions through such concepts as transference, countertransference, working or therapeutic alliance, and empathy have enlightened physicians about the sometimes complex nuances of medical encounters. Physicians can often perform very effectively without insight into the psychodynamic complexities of a positive therapeutic alliance, but they can be rendered virtually helpless by a negative relationship. When a misalliance occurs, it is in the best interests of both patient and physician to be able to reframe the relationship in terms that both can comprehend and tolerate.

Although the primary-care physician is inevitably the "gatekeeper" for these patients, the psychiatrist consultant has been shown to be helpful in the patient's management without breaking the essential connection the patient has with his or her personal physician (Barsky, 1996; Barsky *et al.*, 1991; Lowy, 1975; Smith *et al.*, 1986). Calling patients "borderline," or "narcissistic," or "hypochondriac," even when reflective of legitimate diagnosis, seldom helps to cement a relationship. Jargon, pejorative labeling, despair, cynicism, empathic failure, and therapeutic nihilism are sure to worsen it.

With failure to "translate" vague and puzzling symptoms into comprehensible and familiar modalities, the physician is faced with his or her own feelings of helplessness, ineptitude, and diminished self-regard; such compromising feelings in the physician may cause him or her to miss treatable illnesses and underidentify conditions that do not require extensive physical workups but rather supportive approaches that help maintain the patient at optimal functioning capacity. When psychiatrist and primary care physician collaborate to render otherwise "troublesome" (and troubled) patients less puzzling or burdensome, discordant or dysfunctional relations can be made more harmonious, with enhanced opportunities for patient well-being and physician interest and gratification (Lipsitt, 1996).

While studies of the hypochondriacal patient exist in large number, research studies of the patient–physician relationship in which both patient and physician are studied simultaneously are few because of the complexity of the relationship. Nonetheless, some efforts have been made and will continue to clarify the essential nature of medical encounters (Cassidy, 1992; Farmer, 1994; Gore and Ogden, 1998; Hulka and Roberts, 1975; Kaplan *et al.*, 1989; Kertesz, 1970; McGaghie and Whiteneck, 1982; Peveler *et al.*, 1997; Werner and Schneider, 1974). Better understanding will enhance not only patient and physician satisfaction, but will have major economic implications for the future of medicine (Johnson *et al.*, 1997).

**References**

Adler G. 1972. Helplessness in the helpers. *British Journal of Medical Psychology* 45: 314–326.
Adler G. 1981. The physician and the hypochondriacal patient. *New England Journal of Medicine* 304: 1394–1396.
American Psychiatric Association. 1994. *Diagnostic and Statistical Manual of Mental Disorders, Fourth Edition (DSM-IV)*. Washington, DC: American Psychiatric Association.

Anstett R. 1980. The difficult patient and the physician–patient relationship. *Journal of Family Practice* 11: 281–286.

Balint M. 1957. *The Doctor, His Patient, and the Illness.* New York: International Universities Press.

Barsky A.J. 1979. Patients who amplify bodily sensations. *Annals of Internal Medicine* 91: 63–69.

Barsky A.J. 1996. Hypochondriasis. Medical management and psychiatric treatment. *Psychosomatics* 37: 48–56.

Barsky A.J., Borus J.F. 1995. Somatization and medicalization in the era of managed care. *Journal of the American Medical Association* 274: 1931–1934.

Barsky A.J., Wyshak G., Latham K., Klerman G. 1991. Hypochondriacal patients, their physicians and their medical care. *Journal of General Internal Medicine* 6: 413–419.

Barsky A.J., Ahern D.K., Bailey E.D., Delamater B.A. 1996. Predictors of persistent palpitations and continued medical utilization. *Journal of Family Practice* 42: 465–472.

Becker H.S., Geer B. 1958. The fate of idealism in medical school. *American Sociological Review* 23: 50–56.

Bennett A.E. 1976. *Communication Between Doctors and Patients.* Oxford: Oxford University Press.

Bloom S.W. 1963. *The Doctor and His Patient.* New York: The Free Press.

Bloom S.W. 1979. Socialization for the physician's role: a review of some contributions of research to theory. In *Becoming a Physician: Development of Values in Medicine* (eds. Shapiro E.C., Lowenstein L.M.), Cambridge: Ballinger.

Bloom S.W., Wilson R.N. 1972. Patient–practitioner relationships. In *Handbook of Medical Sociology* (eds. Freeman H.L., Levine S., Reeder L.G.), Englewood Cliffs, NJ: Prentice-Hall.

Bosc C. 1979. *Forgive and Remember: Managing Medical Failure.* Chicago: University of Chicago Press.

Brandt C.C., Kutner B. 1957. Physician–patient relationship in a teaching hospital. *Journal of Medical Education* 32: 703–707.

Brenner C. 1979. Working alliance, therapeutic alliance and transference. *Journal of the American Psychoanalytic Association* 27: 137–157.

Cassidy J. 1992. Outcomes data: rational utilization, better doctor-patient relations. *Health Progress* 73: 36.

Coombs R.N., Goldman L.J. 1973. Maintenance and discontinuity of coping mechanisms in an intensive care unit. *Social Problems* 20: 342–355.

Cousins N. 1981. Internship: preparation or hazing? *Journal of the American Medical Association* 246: 377.

Daniels M.J. 1960. Affect and its control in the medical intern. *American Journal of Sociology* 16: 259–267.

Davis M. 1968. Attitudinal and behavioral aspects of the doctor–patient relationship as expressed and exhibited by medical students and their mentors. *Journal of Medical Education* 43: 337–343.

Docherty J.P., Fiester S.J. 1985. The therapeutic alliance and compliance with psychopharmacology. In *APA Annual Review, Vol. 4* (eds. Hales R.E., Frances A.J.), Washington, DC: American Psychiatric Association.

Drossman D.A. 1978. The problem patient. Evaluation and care of medical patients with psychosocial disturbances. *Annals of Internal Medicine* 88: 366–372.

Engel G.L. 1977. The need for a new medical model: a challenge for biomedicine. *Science* 196: 129–136.

Epstein R.M., Campbell T.L., Cohen-Cole S.A., McWhinney I.R., Smilkstein G. 1993. Perspectives on patient–doctor communication. *Journal of Family Practice* 37: 377–388.

Eron L.D. 1955. Effect of medical education on medical students. *Journal of Medical Education* 10: 559–566.

Escobar J.L., Golding J.M., Hough R.L., Karno M., Burnham M.A., Wells K.B. 1987. Somatization in the community. Relationship to disability and use of services. *American Journal of Public Health* 77: 837–840.

Farmer R.G. 1994. The doctor–patient relationship: quantification of the interaction. *Annual of the New York Academy of Science* 729: 27 35.

Ford C.V. 1983. *The Somatizing Disorders. Illness as a Way of Life.* New York: Elsevier Biomedical.

Fox R. 1957. Training for uncertainty. In *The Student-Physician: Introductory Studies in the Sociology of Medical Education* (eds. Merton R., Reader G.C., Kendall P.), Cambridge, MA: Harvard University Press.

Fredericks M.A., Mundy P. 1976. *The Making of a Physician.* Chicago: Loyola University Press.

Freud S. 1910. Future prospects of psycho-analysis. In *Standard Edition, Vol. 11*: 141–151. London: Hogarth Press, 1957.

Freud S. 1912a. The dynamics of transference. In *Standard Edition, Vol. 12*: 99–108. London: Hogarth Press, 1958.

Freud S. 1912b. Recommendations to physicians practising psychoanalysis. In *Standard Edition, Vol. 12*: 111–120. London: Hogarth Press, 1958.

Freud S. 1912c. On beginning the treatment. In *Standard Edition Vol. 12*: 123–144. London: Hogarth Press, 1958.

Gallagher E.B. 1978. *The Doctor–Patient Relationship in the Changing Health Scene.* Washington, DC: U.S. Department of Health, Education and Welfare.

Garcia-Campayo J., Sanz-Carrillo C., Yoldi-Elcid A., Lopez-Aylon R., Monton C. 1998. Management of somatisers in primary care: are family doctors motivated? *Australian and New Zealand Journal of Psychiatry* 32: 528–533.

George V., Dundes A. 1978. The gomer: a figure of American hospital folk speech. *Journal of American Folklore* 91: 568– 581.

Glauber P.I. 1953. A deterrent in the study and practice of medicine. *Psychoanalytic Quarterly* 22: 381–412.

Gore J., Ogden J. 1998. Developing, validating and consolidating the doctor–patient relationship: the patients' views of a dynamic process. *British Journal of General Practice* 48: 1391–1394.

Gorlin R., Zucker H.D. 1983. Physicians' reactions to patients. A key to teaching humanistic medicine. *New England Journal of Medicine* 308: 1059–1063.

Goodwin J.M., Goodwin J.S., Kellner R. 1979. Psychiatric symptoms in disliked medical patients. *Journal of the American Medical Association* 241: 1117–1120.

Grant W.B. 1980. The hated patient and his hating attendants. *Medical Journal of Australia* 2: 727–729.

Groves J.E. 1978. Taking care of the hateful patient. *New England Journal of Medicine* 298: 883–887.

Gutwinski-Jeggle J. 1997. Hypochondria versus the relation to the object. *International Journal of Psycho-Analysis* 78: 53–68.

Hahn S.R., Thompson K.S., Wills T.A., Stern V., Budner N.S. 1994. The difficult doctor–patient relationship: somatization, personality and psychopathology. *Journal of Clinical Epidemiology* 47: 647–657.

Hahn S.R., Kroenke K., Spitzer R.L., Brody D., Williams J.B., Linzer M., deGruy F.V. 1996. The difficult patient: prevalence, psychopathology, and functional impairment. *Journal of General Internal Medicine* 11: 1–8.

Hall J.A., Roter D.L., Rand C.S. 1981. Communication of affect between patient and physician. *Journal of Health and Social Behavior* 22: 18–30.

Hall J.A., Epstein A.M., DeCiantis M.L., McNeil B.C. 1993. Physicians' liking for their patients: more evidence for the role of affect in medical care. *Health Psychology* 12: 140–146.

Hellstrom O., Lindqvist P., Mattsson B. 1998. A phenomenological analysis of doctor–patient interactions: a case study. *Patient Education and Counseling* 33: 83–89.

Henderson L.F. 1935. Illness and the role of the physician: a sociological perspective. *New England Journal of Medicine* 212: 819–823.

Hooper E.M., Comstock L.M., Goodwin J.M., Goodwin J.S. 1982. Patient characteristics that influence physician behavior. *Medical Care* 20: 630–638.

Horowitz M., Marmar C. 1985. The therapeutic alliance with difficult patients. In *American Psychiatric Association Annual Review, Vol. 4* (eds. Hales R.E., Frances A.J.), Washington, DC: American Psychiatric Press.

Hulka B., Roberts A.B. 1975. Practice characteristics and quality of primary medical care: the doctor–patient relationship. *Medical Care* 13: 808–820.

Jeffery R. 1979. Normal rubbish: deviant patients in casualty departments. *Sociology of Health and Illness* 1: 90–107.

John C., Schwenk T.L., Roi L.D., Cohen M. 1987. Medical care and demographic characteristics of "difficult" patients. *Journal of Family Practice* 24: 607–610.

Johnson P.B., Staubach J.B., Millar A.P. 1997. High utilizers of health services: the purchaser perspective and experience with the personal health improvement program (PHIP). In *Primary Care Meets Mental Health: Tools for the 21st Century* (eds. Haber J.D., Mitchell G.E.), Tiburon, CA: CentraLink Publications.

Kahana R.F., Bibring G.L. 1964. Personality types in medical management. In *Psychiatry and Medical Practice in a General Hospital* (ed. Zinberg N.E.), New York: International Universities Press.

Kaplan C., Lipkin M., Jr., Gordon G.H. 1988. Somatization in primary care: patients with unexplained and vexing medical complaints. *Journal of General Internal Medicine* 3: 177–190.

Kaplan S.H., Greenfield S., Ware J.E., Jr. 1989. Assessing the effects of physician–patient interactions on the outcomes of chronic disease. *Medical Care* 27 (Suppl. 3): S110–S127.

Kasl S.V. 1975. Issues in patient adherence to health care regimens. *Journal of Human Stress* 1: 5–17.

Katon W., Von Korff M., Lin E., Lipscomb P., Russo J., Wagner J., Polk E. 1990. Distressed high utilizers of medical care. *DSM-III-R* diagnoses and treatment needs. *General Hospital Psychiatry* 12: 355–362.

Kertesz R. 1970. Research on doctor/patient relationship in a general hospital. *Psychotherapy and Psychosomatics* 18: 50–55.

Kleinman A. 1978. Culture, illness and care. *Annals of Internal Medicine* 88: 251–258.

Knight J.A. 1973. *Medical Student*. New York: Appleton-Century-Crofts.

Konner M. 1987. *Becoming a Doctor: A Journey of Initiation in Medical School*. New York: Viking.

Ladee G.A. 1966. *Hypochondriacal Syndromes*. Amsterdam: Elsevier.

Leiderman D.B., Grisso J. 1985. The GOMER phenomenon. *Journal of Health and Social Behavior* 26: 222–232.

Lewin B.D. 1946. Counter-transference in the technique of medical practice. *Psychosomatic Medicine* 8: 195–199.

Light D. 1980. *Becoming Psychiatrists: The Professional Transformation of Self*. New York: Norton.

Lin E.H., Katon W.J., Von Korff M., Bush T., Lipscomb P., Russo J., Wagner E. 1991. Frustrating patients: physician and patient perspectives among distressed high users of medical services. *Journal of General Internal Medicine* 6: 241–246.

Lipp M.R. 1977. *Respectful Treatment: The Human Side of Medical Care*. Hagerstown, MD: Harper & Row.

Lipsitt D.R. 1970. Medical and psychological characteristics of "crocks." *Psychiatry in Medicine* 1: 15–25.

Lipsitt D.R. 1973. Psychodynamic considerations of hypochondriasis. *Psychotherapy and Psychosomatics* 25: 201–206.

Lipsitt D.R. 1983. The influence of dualistic thinking on the role of psychiatry in medicine. In *General Hospital Psychiatry* (eds. Lopez-Ibor J.J., Saiz J., Lopez-Ibor J.M.), Amsterdam: Excerpta Medica.

Lipsitt D.R. 1986. Therapeutic alliance in psychiatric consultation. In *Psychiatry, Vol. 2* (eds. Michels R., Cavenar J.O., Brodie H.K.H.), Philadelphia: Lippincott.

Lipsitt D.R. 1996. Primary care of the somatizing patient: a collaborative model. *Hospital Practice* 31: 77–88.

Longhurst M.F. 1980. Angry patient, angry doctor. *Canadian Medical Association Journal* 123: 597–598.

Lorber J. 1975. Good patients and problem patients: conformity and deviance in a general hospital. *Journal of Health and Social Behavior* 16: 213–225.

Lowy F.H. 1975. Management of the persistent somatizer. *International Journal of Psychiatry in Medicine* 6. 227–239.

Mally M.A., Ogston W.D. 1964. Treatment of the "untreatables." *International Journal of Group Psychotherapy* 14: 369–374.

Martin P.A. 1955. The obnoxious patient. In *Tactics and Techniques in Psychotherapy: Vol. 2, Countertransference*. New York: Jason Aronson.

Martin W. 1957. Preference for types of patients. In *The Student-Physician* (eds. Merton R.K., Reader G.G., Kendall P.L.), Cambridge, MA: Harvard University Press.

Mathers N., Jones N., Hannay D. 1995. Heartsink patients: a study of their general practitioners. *British Journal of General Practice* 45: 293–296.

McGaghie W.C., Whiteneck D.C. 1982. A scale for measurement of the problem patient labeling process. *Journal of Nervous and Mental Disease* 170: 598–604.

Mechanic D. 1972. Social psychologic factors affecting the presentation of bodily complaints. *New England Journal of Medicine* 286: 1132–1139.

Menninger K.A. 1957. Psychological factors in the choice of medicine as a profession. Parts I and II. *Bulletin of the Menninger Clinic* 21: 51–58, 99–106.

Merton R.K., Bloom S., Rogoff N. 1956. Studies in the sociology of medical education. *Journal of Medical Education* 31: 552–565.

Merton R.K., Reader G.G., Kendall P.L. 1957. *The Student-Physician*. Cambridge, MA: Harvard University Press.

Mizrahi T. 1986. *Getting Rid of Patients: Contradictions in the Socialization of Physicians*. New Brunswick, NJ: Rutgers University Press.

Moos R.H., Yalom I.D. 1966. Medical students' attitudes toward psychiatry and psychiatrists. *Mental Hygiene* 50: 246–256.

Mumford E. 1970. *Interns: From Students to Physicians*. Cambridge, MA: Harvard University Press.

Myerson P. 1979. Issues of technique where patients relate with difficulty. *International Review of Psycho-Analysis* 6: 363–375.

Nunberg H. 1938. Psychological interrelations between physician and patient. *Psychoanalytic Quarterly* 25: 197–308.

O'Malley C.D. 1970. *The History of Medical Education*. Berkeley and Los Angeles: University of California Press.

Ort R.S., Ford A.B., Liske R.E. 1964. The doctor–patient relationship as described by physicians and medical students. *Journal of Health and Human Behavior* 5: 25–34.

Ort R.S., Ford A.B., Liske R.E., Pattishall E.G. 1965. Reactions to chronic illness. *Journal of Medical Education* 40: 840–849.

Papper S. 1970. The undesirable patient. *Journal of Chronic Disease* 22: 777–779.

Parets A.D. 1967. Emotional reactions to chronic physical illness. Implications for the internist. *Medical Clinics of North America* 51: 1399–1408.

Parsons T. 1951a. *The Social System*. Glencoe, IL: The Free Press.

Parsons T. 1951b. Illness and the role of the physician: a sociological perspective. *American Journal of Orthopsychiatry* 21: 452–460.

Peabody F.W. 1927. The care of the patient. *Journal of the American Medical Association* 88: 877–882.

Peters S., Stanley I., Rose M., Salmon P. 1998. Patients with medically unexplained symptoms: sources of patients' authority and implications for demands on medical care. *Social Science and Medicine* 46: 559–604.

Peveler R., Kilkenny L., Kinmonth A.L. 1997. Medically unexplained symptoms in primary care: a comparison of self-report screening questionnaires and clinical opinion. *Journal of Psychosomatic Research* 42: 245–252.

Pilowsky I. 1968. The response to treatment in hypochondriacal disorders. *Australian and New Zealand Journal of Psychiatry* 2: 88–94.

Reynolds R., Brice T. 1971. Attitudes of medical interns toward patients and health professionals. *Journal of Health and Social Behavior* 12: 307–311.

Rezler A.G. 1974. Attitude changes during medical school: a review of the literature. *Journal of Medical Education* 49: 1023–1030.

Ries R.K., Bokan J.A., Katon W.J., Kleinman A. 1981. The medical care abuser: differential diagnosis and management. *Journal of Family Practice* 13: 257–265.

Rogoff N. 1957. The decision to study medicine. In *The Student-Physician* (eds. Merton R.K., Reader G.G., Kendall P.L.), Cambridge, MA: Harvard University Press.

Roter D.L., Hall J.A. 1992. *Doctors Talking With Patients/Patients Talking With Doctors: Improving Communication in Medical Visits*. Westport, CT: Auburn House.

Schwenk T.L., Parquez J.T., Lefever R.D., Cohen M. 1989. Physician and patient determinants of difficult physician–patient relationships. *Journal of Family Practice* 28: 59–63.

Schwenk T.L., Romano S.E. 1992. Managing the difficult physician–patient relationship. *American Family Physician* 46: 1503–1509.

Shapiro E.C., Lowenstein L.M. 1979. *Becoming a Physician: Development of Values in Medicine*. Cambridge: Ballinger.

Sharpe M., Mayou R., Seagroatt V., Surawy C., Warwick H., Bulstrade C., Dawber R., Lane D. 1994. Why do doctors find some patients difficult to help? *Quarterly Journal of Medicine* 87: 187–193.

Shem S. 1978. *The House of God*. New York: Marek.

Siegler M., Osmond H. 1974. *Models of Madness, Models of Medicine*. New York: Macmillan.

Simmel E. 1938. The "doctor game": illness and the profession in medicine. *International Journal of Psycho-Analysis* 7: 470–483.

Smith G.R., Mouson R.A., Ray D.C. 1986. Psychiatric consultation in somatization disorder: a randomized controlled study. *New England Journal of Medicine* 314: 1407–1413.

Smith R.C., Zimny G.H. 1988. Physicians' emotional reactions to patients. *Psychosomatics* 29: 92–97.

Starcevic V. 1990. Role of reassurance and psychopathology in hypochondriasis. *Psychiatry* 53: 383–395.

Starcevic V. 1991. Reassurance and treatment of hypochondriasis. *General Hospital Psychiatry* 13: 122–127.

Starr P. 1982. *The Social Transformation of American Medicine*. New York: Basic Books.

Stern E.M. 1984. *Psychotherapy and the Abrasive Patient*. New York: Haworth Press.

Stoeckle J. 1987. *Encounters Between Patients and Doctors*. Cambridge, MA: MIT Press.

Strauss R. 1978. Medical education and the doctor–patient relationship. In *The Doctor–Patient Relationship in the Changing Health Scene* (ed. Gallagher E.B.), Washington, DC: U.S. Department of Health, Education and Welfare.

Szasz T.S., Hollender M.H. 1956. A contribution to the philosophy of medicine: the basic models of the doctor–patient relationship. *Archives of Internal Medicine* 97: 585–597.

Thomasma D.C. 1983. Beyond medical paternalism and patient autonomy: a model of physician conscience for the physician-patient relationship. *Annals of Internal Medicine* 98: 243–248.

Tucker G.J., Reinhardt R.F. 1968. Psychiatric attitudes of young physicians: implications for teaching. *American Journal of Psychiatry* 124: 146–150.

Vaillant G.E. 1972. Some psychological vulnerabilities of physicians. *New England Journal of Medicine* 287: 372–375.

Valenstein A.F. 1973. On attachment to painful feelings and the negative therapeutic reaction. *Psychoanalytic Study of the Child* 28: 365–391.

Wahl C.W. 1963. Unconscious factors in the psychodynamics of the hypochondriacal patient. *Psychosomatics* 4: 9–14.

Waitzkin H., Stoeckle J. 1972. The communication of information about illness. *Advances in Psychosomatic Medicine* 8: 180–215.

Walker E.A., Katon W.J., Keegan D., Gardner G., Sullivan M. 1997. Predictors of physician frustration in the care of patients with rheumatological complaints. *General Hospital Psychiatry* 19: 315–323.

Werner A., Schneider J.M. 1974. Teaching medical students interactional skills. A research-based course in the doctor–patient relationship. *New England Journal of Medicine* 290: 1232–1237.

Zabarenko R.N., Zabarenko L.M. 1978. *The Doctor Tree: Developmental Stages in the Growth of Physicians*. Pittsburgh: University of Pittsburgh Press.

# 13

# Reassurance in the Treatment of Hypochondriasis

## VLADAN STARCEVIC

The use of reassurance in the treatment of hypochondriasis may depend on how closely we follow current diagnostic manuals, because manuals such as the *DSM-IV* tell us that hypochondriasis persists despite "appropriate medical reassurance" (American Psychiatric Association, 1994). Contrary to the experience of many physicians who work with hypochondriacal patients and use reassurance in their treatment, this diagnostic conceptualization of hypochondriasis implies that provision of reassurance is not likely to be effective for hypochondriasis, and that attempts to use it will probably be futile. In short, why reassure if, by definition, reassurance is not effective?

This is a paradoxical situation because a disorder is defined by a lack of response to a particular type of treatment, whereby it is not clearly spelled out what that treatment ("appropriate medical reassurance") consists of. It is difficult to find an analogy in medicine—for example, defining tuberculosis as an infectious disease not responsive to penicillin. But be that as it may, the "official," negative position about therapeutic use of reassurance in hypochondriasis, even when couched in implicit terms, is influential. That may explain why some physicians feel very uncomfortable while attempting to reassure hypochondriacal patients. Another problem is that there are so few guidelines on how to reassure properly and effectively.

Complicating matters further, another influential position states that a repeated provision of reassurance to hypochondriacal patients maintains this condition and that it should not be used at all in the treatment of such patients (Warwick and Salkovskis, 1990) (see also Chapters 9 and 14). As argued persuasively by Salkovskis and Warwick (1986), "the unrealistic fear or belief [of having a disease] persists *because* of repeated medical reassurance" (p. 601), and not *despite* receiving medical reassurance, as the diagnostic manuals suggest. Incidentally, the classical psychoanalytic school (Greenson, 1967) is also opposed to the provision of reassurance, although for a different reason: Because all symptoms are determined by unconscious factors, reassurance that does not take account of them cannot be effective.

Finally, one view (Kellner, 1982, 1992; Pilowsky, 1983; Starcevic, 1991) holds that repeated and carefully planned and provided reassurance can be helpful in the treatment of hypochondriasis. For example, in an uncontrolled study of the treatment of hypochondriasis with a "package" that included repeated provision of reassurance and repeated physical examinations, Kellner (1982) reported that 64% of 36 patients with hypochondriasis either recovered or improved, and that this improvement was largely maintained on follow-up.

Some confusion about the role of reassurance in hypochondriasis stems from the fact that provision of reassurance is considered as a treatment technique by some (e.g., Kellner, 1992), and as the main aim in the treatment of hypochondriasis by others (e.g., Warwick, 1992). However, most of the confusion surrounding the role of reassurance in hypochondriasis can be attributed to a failure to conceptualize reassurance in more detail, particularly reassurance that could be used for treatment purposes. To address these issues, an attempt will be made first to define medical reassurance, followed by an illustration of a careful, well-planned provision of medical reassurance in the treatment of hypochondriasis. This chapter will also critically review the most salient issues in the provision of reassurance to hypochondriacal patients.

## Definition of Reassurance

Warwick and Salkovskis (1985) have aptly observed that it is the meaning of the symptom to the patient that determines the need for reassurance. As virtually all human beings are interested in or curious about the meaning of the symptoms they experience, there is thus little disagreement about the importance and benefit of reassurance in general. Provision of reassurance is an essential part of good medical practice and consultation (Cooper, 1996; Howard and Wessely, 1996; Kessel, 1979), a therapeutic skill (Cooper, 1996), "one of the main treatment methods used in primary care" (Howard and Wessely, 1996, p. 309), and even "the most widely used psychotherapeutic maneuver in medical practice" (Warwick and Salkovskis, 1985, p. 1028). Barr (1965) has stated that providing reassurance is "the very basis of the whole art of medicine" (p. 356), and Ingram (1997) went even further by proclaiming reassurance as a "kind of art form" (p. 232). Among the many roles of reassurance are: alleviation of patients' anxieties (Howard and Wessely, 1996; Warwick and Salkovskis, 1985); enabling "patients to tolerate or endure the dysphoria associated with threats, losses, conflicts, and other inner psychic turmoil" (Glucksman, 1997, p. 245); encouragement of hope, promotion of patients' well-being, enhancement of the doctor–patient relationship (Kessel, 1979); and "giving of insight" (Barr, 1965). Schwartz (1966) has observed that reassurance is usually linked with the future because of the "promise of better things" (p. 291).

Beyond this general acknowledgment of the importance of reassurance, few have examined what it consists of and how it works. Both Kessel (1979) and Warwick (1992) draw on the dictionary definition of reassurance, as "restoring to confidence" (*Oxford English Dictionary*), and they emphasize the implications of this definition. Kessel (1979) suggests that, in a broad sense, "what is restored in the medical context is a former state of health" (p. 1128), Warwick (1992) states more specifically that "successful reassurance must be our aim of treatment of all patients, especially those with hypochondriasis" (p. 77). How the latter is to be achieved is a matter of controversy. A first step in attempting to resolve that controversy is defining medical reassurance and specifying its constituents.

Howard and Wessely (1996) suggest that reassurance may consist of "explanation of symptoms, informing the patient of current medical knowledge, and telling the patient there is nothing to worry about" (p. 307). These authors also add that reassurance can include "performing investigations" (p. 307). In a similar vein, Starcevic (1991) defines medical reassurance as a "process of providing a patient with information about and explanation of the benign and/or innocuous nature and origin of his symptoms and complaints, after an adequate medical examination has been performed and/or after all the relevant medical data about the patient have been collected and examined" (p. 123). On the other hand, Warwick and Salkovskis (1985) give a more restricted definition of "appropriate reassurance" as the "provision of new information that is relevant to the patient's clinical condition" (p. 1028).

The difference between these two approaches to the conceptualization of reassurance reflects for the most part differences between the recipients of reassurance. The definitions given by Howard and Wessely (1996) and Starcevic (1991) refer more to general medical patients, whereas the definition offered by Warwick and Salkovskis (1985) is "geared" more to patients with hypochondriasis. Can these two views on medical reassurance be reconciled when reassurance is used in patients with hypochondriasis? This chapter will explore the possibility of such an integration after examining the specific aspects of reassurance in the psychopathology and treatment of hypochondriasis.

## Reassurance and Hypochondriasis

Reassurance takes on a special role in hypochondriasis for several reasons. First, current definitions of hypochondriasis emphasize that one of its essential fea-

tures (and also, one of its diagnostic criteria) is resistance to "appropriate medical reassurance" (American Psychiatric Association, 1994). Some (Fava and
Grandi, 1991) consider this particular characteristic crucial for distinguishing hypochondriasis from related conditions and phenomena, such as disease phobia
and health anxiety.

Second, it is not clear what "appropriate medical reassurance" exactly refers
to, which paves the way for arbitrary interpretations of this term. More funda-
mentally, is "appropriate medical reassurance" in the context of hypochondriasis
an elaborate process that consists of giving explanations to patients, performing
additional physical examinations if necessary, and persuading patients that their
worries about health are groundless—or is it the provision of carefully selected,
new information to which the patient had not been previously exposed? Is there
yet another meaning of "appropriate medical reassurance?"

Third, how does "appropriate medical reassurance" differ from ordinary,
standard, or routine reassurance? What are the criteria for "appropriate medical
reassurance?"

Fourth, reassuring hypochondriacal patients entails more than telling them that
"everything is all right" and that "there is no reason to worry about health." The
fact that these patients are obviously not satisfied with such simple, reassuring
statements leads some to suggest that they are resistant to *any* reassurance. However, it is not surprising that hypochondriacal patients do not respond to such reassurance, as they usually seek an explanation of what *does* account for their
symptoms (House, 1989).

It appears that clinical observation and research have resolved some of these
issues. Patients with hypochondriasis usually do not respond to the kind of medical reassurance that many patients would consider sufficient or appropriate
("Don't worry, you are in a very good state of health"). Such reassurance, whether
it is termed ordinary, standard, or routine, rarely includes more than a very basic suggestion that the patient's health is good, very good, or excellent. Relatively
few patients are interested in a detailed explanation of the basis for such a suggestion. They accept it at face value, usually because they trust their physicians
and do not question their medical authority. Clearly, this approach does not work
with hypochondriacal patients, for they often perceive routine reassurance as inappropriate. Why? Appleby (1987) believes it is because reassurance is not provided properly and does not take into consideration the patient's needs: "The
sufferer from hypochondriacal neurosis sees perfunctory or ill directed reassurance as dismissal, as failure to take him seriously. He does not want to be told
that there is nothing wrong; he needs to understand his symptoms as a first step
to overcoming them" (p. 857).

It can also be hypothesized that routine medical reassurance has no effect in
hypochondriasis because its prerequisite is interpersonal trust in general and trust

in physicians in particular—"something" that hypochondriacal patients usually lack (Avia, 1999; Kellner *et al.*, 1987; Starcevic, 1988, 1990a). Others (Haenen *et al.*, 1997) have found that hypochondriacal patients are less suggestible than are healthy control subjects; therefore, it is not easy to reassure them in an ordinary manner.

What may be an "appropriate" medical reassurance for some, or for most patients, certainly does not appear so for those with hypochondriasis. As a result, it can be proposed that hypochondriacal patients usually do not respond to *routine* medical reassurance. But do they respond to other "types" of reassurance, and especially to a more elaborate and process-like reassurance, which might indeed be considered "appropriate?" If the answer to this question is basically affirmative, there seems to be little reason *not* to use such reassurance in the treatment of hypochondriasis.

## Use of Reassurance and Goals of Treatment in Hypochondriasis

The use of reassurance in the treatment of hypochondriasis is naturally linked to the goals of treatment of this condition. It appears logical to use reassurance if the "hypochondriacal patient needs to be converted to the new belief that the symptoms can be unpleasant, distressing and terrifying but are caused by benign processes and that the patient is in excellent health" (Kellner, 1992, p. 74). In other words, if one of the main aims of treatment is to persuade patients that they are wrong (Kellner, 1982, 1983), persuasion can be attempted through reassurance. Of course, it is another matter how such reassurance should be "delivered" to hypochondriacal patients so that they would feel persuaded that there is no reason to suspect the presence of a serious disease.

The goal of persuading hypochondriacal patients that their fears and suspicions are unfounded is very similar to the treatment goal in hypochondriasis, as formulated by cognitive therapists: "to help the patients realize that their problem was worrying about illness, rather than illness *per se*" (Clark *et al.*, 1998, p. 219). But instead of using reassurance, cognitive therapists directly challenge patients' specific illness beliefs to reach that goal (by means of cognitive procedures), and they demonstrate that such an approach is effective in the treatment of hypochondriasis (Clark *et al.*, 1998; Warwick *et al.*, 1996). Although that may not be readily apparent, there appears to be some overlap between challenging and modifying patients' erroneous illness beliefs and persuading them through a complex process of reassurance that there is no reason to worry about illness.

Medical reassurance can also be used to achieve other goals of treatment of hypochondriasis, such as improved coping with and better control of symptoms

(Barsky, 1996), alleviation of fear about having a disease, and helping patients to understand the nature of their symptoms (Kellner, 1982, 1983). As for understanding the symptoms, some authors emphasize that this might be achieved through patient education; they propose that the main goals of treatment in hypochondriasis pertain to learning about the "nature, perception, and reporting of physical symptoms, and about the psychological factors that amplify somatic distress" as in "cognitive-educational therapy" (Barsky, 1996, pp. 51–52).

In treatments that are less focused on the psychophysiology of symptoms (e.g., "illness adaptation program," Kirmayer and Robbins, 1991), the goal of the treatment is set so that patients learn that symptoms themselves are not as disabling as the worry that accompanies them, and therefore patients are taught to adapt to their illness. In such an approach, patients are taught through reassurance that their symptoms are not life-threatening and that the symptoms will "almost certainly not shorten their lives" (p. 218) despite the fact that the cause of the symptoms is not known.

Regardless of the goals of treatment in hypochondriasis, steps in the *process* of providing appropriate and effective medical reassurance need to be taken, leading to the acceptance of reassurance by the patients and their "deliverance" from disease fears and suspicions. These steps will now be described within the framework of the proposed criteria for appropriate and effective medical reassurance.

## Criteria for Appropriate and Effective Medical Reassurance

Both the "appropriateness" and effectiveness of medical reassurance in hypochondriasis depend on who provides reassurance, when, to whom, and how. Each of these four aspects of the reassurance process will be considered in more detail.

### Who Provides Reassurance?

Reassurance, to be effective, should be provided by a single physician, who can be easily contacted by the patient (Barsky, 1996; Kessel, 1979; Starcevic, 1991). This physician need not be a psychiatrist; in fact, in many settings it is a well-trained primary care physician who is in a better position to provide appropriate and effective reassurance. Multiple reassurance-providing physicians can give contradictory or confusing information to patients, a situation that is particularly difficult for hypochondriacal patients. In addition, having a single, accessible physician enhances a therapeutic relationship and the patient's sense of confidence and security. A single reassuring figure also provides a framework of consistency and continuity of care, so important in the process of reassurance.

The physician should become accessible by clarifying to patients that access to the physician is not "contingent on continued symptoms and suffering" (Barsky, 1996, p. 50). Of course, this accessibility should not be construed as an unlimited availability of the physician. Rather, it is in the service of fostering more confidence in the physician.

For a physician's reassurance to be effective, he or she must be perceived by the patients as a benevolent medical authority who can be trusted. Ingram (1997) is right in pointing to the contemporary "flattening of hierarchies" and "diffusion of authority" as contributing to the weaker impact of reassurance nowadays. However, it still holds true that "patients require the doctor to be an expert" (Kessel, 1979, p. 1129), although this may not be sufficient for hypochondriacal patients. They might have seen several medical experts who failed to reassure them. In such cases, a failure to reassure is usually not a result of the patients' questioning of these physicians' knowledge, but has to do with physicians' attitudes. "They treated me like just another case" is a frequent complaint made by hypochondriacal patients, for whom medical authority dissipates if the physicians fail to display a genuine interest in their patients' overall well-being. It is a combination of sensitivity to a particular patient and firmness and authority based on medical knowledge that make it possible for a hypochondriacal patient to *begin* to trust physicians and accept their reassurance with a measure of credibility.

In addition to professional experience and knowledge, as well as sensitivity and ability to relate to patients, several factors contribute to the perception of the physician as a trustworthy figure by hypochondriacal patients (Kellner, 1982; Schwartz, 1966; Starcevic, 1990a): the physician's level of general self-confidence; means of communicating knowledge, which also reveals the physician's own attitude to the content of reassurance (that is, the extent to which the physician is "comfortable with" and believes in the reassuring information he or she is providing); and his or her own patience in dealing with these patients. The latter is particularly important in view of the frequent lack of an obvious, expected response to reassurance and hypochondriacal patients' frequent testing of their physicians' patience by sending them the following message: "I will trust you insofar as you are able to withstand my doubts, accept me and understand what I'm going through."

## When Should Reassurance Be Provided?

Proper "timing" for providing reassurance has often been mentioned (Cooper, 1996; Kellner, 1982, 1992; Kessel, 1979; Schwartz, 1966; Starcevic, 1991), but rarely explained and elaborated. It may refer to several considerations in the sequencing of the provision of reassurance. One is to first elicit and identify the underlying fears (e.g., fears of disease, bodily decay, or death), and then provide the targetted reassuring, anxiety-decreasing information (Kessel, 1979). Another consideration is to provide reassurance only after the physician has understood the nature of the problem, as reflected in Lipsitt's words: "One cannot really reassure until one knows what is wrong" (Lipsitt, 1995, p. 1797). This position echoes Kohut's postulation of the sequence of "events" in the course of analytic therapy in general: The first task is understanding the patient, which is followed by giving explanations or interpretations to the patient (Kohut, 1984).

Finally, establishing a dependable, trusting relationship between the patient and the physician is a "prerequisite" for the provision of reassurance (Starcevic, 1991) (see also Chapter 12). While establishing such a relationship between the patient and the physician is a "prerequisite" for provision of reassurance, the successful provision of reassurance itself reciprocally strengthens that relationship in a mutually enhancing interaction.

An important component of the patient–physician relationship is the physician's ability to empathize with the patient and to understand him or her. Schwartz (1966) considers "empathetic reassurance" valuable because it "presupposes both an identification with the patient's distress and a simultaneous unwillingness to topple regressively as a result of that identification" (p. 293). Kessel (1979) explicitly states that the patient "will not be reassured unless he believes that the doctor is sensitive to, and understands, that [what the patient is going through]" (p. 1131). Indeed, it can be suggested that one cannot reassure patients adequately and successfully without understanding them empathically. This means that to reassure hypochondriacal patients effectively, some of the same components in the process of empathic understanding may need to be present: A physician should be sensitive and receptive to the patient's feelings, he or she should listen to patients empathically, be able to project himself or herself into the self of the patients (and thus "be in their shoes"), and also be able to be emotionally affected by them (Starcevic and Piontek, 1997). Glucksman (1997) has identified three components of successful reassurance: communicating to the patient that the therapist knows and understands the reasons for the patient's fears; being continuously available to the patient to allay any fear that the patient may have of being abandoned; and showing that the therapist feels confident about the patient's ability to "make it through."

Reassuring hypochondriacal patients early in the course of their treatment would generally not be recommended, although this is not spelled out clearly and unequivocally. Some authors (e.g., Warwick, 1992) state that "in the initial stages of treatment of some cases of hypochondriasis, *more* reassurance is necessary" (p. 78), whereas others (e.g., Kellner, 1992) suggest that "attempts to reassure these [hypochondriacal] patients directly in the early stages of the therapeutic encounter are likely to fail" (p. 73). Obviously, there is no absolute rule for dealing with this issue, and it is very much up to the physician to assess empathically when the patients are "ready" to accept reassurance. This is likely to vary from one patient to another and to depend, to a large extent, on the quality of the previously established therapeutic relationship. In any case, it seems almost like a "crowning achievement" of a longer, rather than a shorter therapy, that hypochondriacal patients feel fully reassured that their fears and suspicions are unfounded.

## Who Should Be Provided With Reassurance?

Elaborate medical reassurance is not likely to be effective for all patients with hypochondriasis. Some hypochondriacal patients, especially those with an associated or underlying severe character pathology, may react to reassurance with inordinate anger and rupture of the relationship with the physician (Starcevic, 1990a); this usually occurs when reassurance is attempted early and in a tactless manner. Although it does not mean that hypochondriacal patients with severe personality disturbance should never be reassured, the physician must be very cautious when attempting to provide reassurance to such patients, because reassurance is perceived by them as aggressive undermining of their defenses, to which they may therefore respond with rage. As a result, an important step in the process of reassurance is identification of those hypochondriacal patients who may be receptive to reassurance and are likely to benefit from it. Usually, these are patients with associated features of depression and anxiety, for whom reassurance has additional meanings and significance within a framework of a stable, secure, and continuous therapeutic relationship with their physicians (Starcevic, 1990a, 1991). These meanings often pertain to the patients' unmet needs for acceptance and dependence and their sense of low self-esteem.

## How Should Reassurance Be Provided?

**Examining medical records.** The first step in the provision of medical reassurance to hypochondriacal patients is examination of their medical documents (House, 1989; Starcevic, 1991). Such an approach is understandable in view of the importance that hypochondriacal patients attach to their medical "papers." The "record" is a crucial aspect of their identity and a feature through which they are easily recognized, so that it is no wonder that they often carry unflattering labels such as "thick chart patients" (Lipsitt, 1974). Some authors (House, 1989) also suggest bypassing the record and retaking a full medical (physical) history.

Reviewing the patients' complaints and details of their health problems, and examining carefully the results of all previous physical examinations and medical investigations, demonstrates to patients that they are being taken seriously. It also helps the physician become better acquainted with the patients' condition. A thorough review of the patients' case notes, as recommended by House (1989), has the purpose of making sure that the necessary diagnostic evaluation has been performed. In addition, it is important to ascertain whether anything has been omitted in the course of previous medical workup (Warwick, 1992).

**Showing acceptance of the patient.** Although it is often stated that it is very important, or indeed crucial, to accept hypochondriacal patients "unconditionally" (Barsky, 1993, 1996; Brown and Vaillant, 1981; Kellner, 1982; Kessel, 1979; Kirmayer and Robbins, 1991; Starcevic, 1990a, 1991), it is relatively rarely explained in more detail just how such acceptance is communicated to patients.

Unconditional acceptance of the patients initially means that they are accepted through their symptoms, and that the physician has accepted the somatic "mode" of communication used by these patients. In practice, this means that the physician has several tasks:

- Taking patients' complaints seriously (Adler, 1981; Kellner, 1990; Kessel, 1979; Starcevic, 1991)
- Allowing, and even encouraging, patients to talk about their symptoms (Adler, 1981; Kellner, 1990)
- Specifically telling patients that their symptoms are not "imaginary" or "only in your mind" (Kessel, 1979; Starcevic, 1991; Wahl, 1963)
- Acknowledging the reality, genuineness, importance, and intensity of the patients' symptoms and distress (Barsky, 1993; Brown and Vaillant, 1981; Kessel, 1979; Warwick, 1992)
- Refraining from asking patients to relinquish their physical complaints (Barsky, 1996; Brown and Vaillant, 1981)
- Communicating to the patients that it is reasonable and legitimate to worry about symptoms (Kessel, 1979)

**Scheduling regular visits.** Several authors consider regular scheduling of appointments important in the treatment of hypochondriasis (Barsky, 1996; Brown and Vaillant, 1981; Kirmayer and Robbins, 1991; Starcevic, 1991). Several reasons account for this. First, it is in the service of better accessibility of the physician, and signals to patients that there will be a dependable continuity in their relationship with the physician. Hypochondriacal patients need to know, often in explicit terms, that their physician is available for help and that he or she is genuinely interested in their well-being. Second, regular physician visits contribute to greater confidence of patients in their physicians and a better therapeutic relationship, which would help "neutralize" the patients' previous, disappointing experiences with physicians. Third, the message given to the patients is that they do not have to "feel sick" in order to be "entitled" to see their physician. Patients should also enjoy the "privilege" of having additional (unscheduled) visits should the physician judge that under the given circumstances such visits are justified.

**Using clear and simple language.** Medical reassurance can be effective only if it is provided in unambiguous terms, using clear and simple language, and avoiding complex terminology (Barr, 1965; Kellner, 1982; Kirmayer and Robbins, 1991; Starcevic, 1991; Wahl, 1963; Warwick, 1992). Barr (1965) is right in calling reassurance the "art of simplification."

Conflicting or "mixed" messages to patients with hypochondriasis must be carefully avoided, and any discrepancy with previously received information explained to them. Hypochondriacal patients are particularly prone to misinterpreting ambiguous information; they are often disturbed if the medical reports are not identical, and even minor disagreements between physicians may elicit inordinate anxiety or even confusion. Therefore, a "straightforward" and unequivocal communication with hypochondriacal patients is of paramount importance.

**Providing relevant information and explanation.** Provision of relevant information and explanation to patients is the key component of the process of reassurance. Its aim is the patients' understanding of the origin and nature of their symptoms. Many authors (Barr, 1965; Barsky, 1996; Cooper, 1996; House, 1989; Kellner, 1982; Kirmayer and Robbins, 1991; Starcevic, 1991; Wahl, 1963; Warwick, 1992; Wise, 1992) emphasize the importance of this cognitive aspect of reassurance, although they have expressed it in different ways. Wise (1992) suggests that hypochondriacal patients have a "distorted understanding" of their condition, so that it is the physician's task to help such patients understand their symptoms through explanation.

Reassurance through understanding and knowledge is considered crucial, as seen in one patient's quote: "The doctor keeps telling me what I *don't* have, but he never tells me what I *do* have" (Barsky, 1996, p. 50). Likewise, House (1989) suggests a two-step process in the provision of reassurance: The first step, which he refers to as "reassurance" (proper), consists of a statement that symptoms are "not based on any detectable and serious physical pathology" (p. 160), which the second step involves "an explanation of the physiologic basis for the patient's symptoms" (p. 160).

As for the explanations, they may vary from giving simple "anatomical and physiological explanations" to patients as to "how muscle spasm itself can produce the symptoms that frighten and concern them" (Wahl, 1963, p. 13) to a complex provision of "complete and unambiguous medical information, and systematic education in the normal psychology of bodily symptoms" (Kirmayer and Robbins, 1991, p. 218). In the course of what Kellner (1982) refers to as "explanatory therapy," he emphasizes provision of "accurate information" about the interactions between emotional states and reactivity of the autonomic nervous system, which often accounts for the nature of the patients' symptoms. In addition, Kellner (1982) suggests educating patients about selective perception, which is, in his opinion, often responsible for closing the "vicious circle" in the development of hypochondriasis.

There is some controversy about the nature of information to be given to patients. According to some authors (Salkovskis and Warwick, 1986; Warwick, 1992), only new information should be offered as part of reassurance. Others do not consider it harmful to repeat previously discussed information, and they emphasize that whatever new information is given must not contradict information provided previously (Starcevic, 1991). In other words, provision of any information, new or "old," should be consistent, so as to avoid confusing the patients. Kellner (1990) also advocates repeating the reassuring information because patients often forget or distort information.

Warwick (1992) considers it essential to check whether patients feel reassured with the information and explanation provided to them, and Starcevic (1991) states that the "process of reassurance is completed when the patient obtains an explanation of what accounts for his symptoms, and even more so, of what accounts for his reactions to them" (p. 124). Cooper (1996) notes that "when patients feel reassured they will usually make it obvious in what they say and do" (p. 697). However, the latter is not always the case, and the effects of reassurance may become apparent only later.

"Checking" and "making sure" that hypochondriacal patients do indeed understand their symptoms and thus feel reassured entails a physician's capacity for empathy and must not be reduced to simple "questioning" of the patients. Because every test of the efficacy of a therapeutic technique ultimately rests on a change in behavior, the efficacy of the process of reassurance will be reflected not only in patients' better understanding of their condition, but even more in the cessation of the reassurance-seeking behavior.

**Fostering the patient's responsibility.** It is particularly important for hypochondriacal patients not to be passive "recipients" of medical knowledge and not to "surrender" the responsibility for the outcome of their treatment to the physician. It would be a mistake for the physician to "do the whole job for the patient" and thus encourage greater dependence and regressive trends. This is implied in the cautionary statement made by Schwartz (1966) that "reassurance should not be aimed at reducing psychologic suffering to zero" (p. 293). Likewise, the provision of reassurance should not be in the service of giving hypochondriacal patients a false sense of complete invulnerability.

Some hypochondriacal patients are prone to interpret the physician's provision of reassurance as an indication that the physician is responsible for the course and outcome of their treatment (Kessel, 1979). This attitude may denote a resistance to treatment, particularly in patients with passive-aggressive features. When this becomes an obvious problem, it is the physician's task to confront patients with their self-defeating and even health risk-taking behaviors (e.g., smoking cigarettes; Pilowsky, 1997, p. 116)—and also encourage patients to assume greater responsibility by facing their problems, making relevant decisions, rearranging their own priorities, and setting their goals more clearly.

**Shifting attention to the underlying issues and to patients' assets.** Provision of reassurance must not be perceived as a dull educational exercise. In addition to providing hypochondriacal patients with information and explanation, the physician should also shift the patients' attention from the somatic "realm" to the underlying emotions and problems, encourage them to express their feelings and difficulties openly, and point to their assets (Kessel, 1979; Wahl, 1963). This "desomatizing" process can be a powerful means of accessing the underlying psychological issues, and should accompany the provision of the reassuring information. In addition, hypochondriacal patients often focus on their presumed deficits and weaknesses and tend to perceive themselves in negative terms. A successful provision of reassurance also includes counteracting such self-perception. This is accomplished through consistent emphasis on patients' strengths and achievements, which leads to their more realistic self-appraisal.

**Adjusting a "reassuring style" to the patient.** Ultimately, a provision of reassurance may be effective insofar as it takes into account the personality of the hypochondriacal patient. Therefore, it is important for the physician to adjust his or her "reassuring style" to the individual patient. In doing so, the physician can realize that, indeed, indirect rather than direct reassurance might be more effective (Brewin, 1991). Although most patients with hypochondriasis are usually considered explanation-driven (Starcevic *et al.*, 1992), with a "surplus" of obsessional features (Starcevic, 1990b), that does not mean that they should be reassured in the same (obsessional) manner. What is reassuring to one person may be anxiety-inducing, harmful, or humiliating to another. Some patients need more information, while others seem to be satisfied with fewer details. Among the factors that need to be considered when deciding *how* to reassure patients are their intelligence and degree of medical sophistication (Kessel, 1979).

Kessel (1979) and Starcevic (1991) give examples of different "reassuring styles" adapted for different patients. These "styles" make use of an essential distinction between the need of certain patients to be "unique" and the need of others to be told that their plight is commonly encountered in medical practice and similar to that of other people. Hence, patients with a dominance of narcissistic traits may be well served if they are told that their illness is "special," "unusual,"

"peculiar," or "very difficult to understand" (Kessel, 1979; Starcevic, 1991), because only such a perception of their illness can be incorporated into their character structure and accepted by them.

Other patients are better reassured if they are told that they suffer from a "common" condition, and that their physician is not puzzled by it, having seen many
cases like that (Cooper, 1996; Kessel, 1979; Starcevic, 1991). This approach usually "works" with patients with anxious character structure and/or prominent
pathological anxiety, because their comfort is derived from a congruence of the
reassuring message with a cognitive scheme that "no threat comes from the simple, common, and well-known."

Between these two somewhat extreme "reassuring styles," many approaches
can also be used in accordance with the specific character structure of hypochondriacal patients and their particular needs. Indeed, it is very much a reflection of
the physician's creativity as to how he or she will use reassurance. For example,
a physician can produce a reassuring effect by unexpectedly and paradoxically
agreeing with a passive-aggressive patient that it is most reasonable to worry
about a disease and to distrust doctors: This approach may have an effect of neu-
tralizing oppositional tendencies in these patients. They may find themselves in
an unusual situation that they have nothing to complain about, because their physician agrees with them!

Likewise, paradoxical maneuvers may be effective for patients who cannot tolerate uncertainty and who may therefore insist on "perfect" evidence that they
are not ill. Typical questions posed by such patients are "What makes you so sure
that my heart won't stop beating suddenly?" or "How do you know that I don't
have a brain tumor?" The physician must avoid the "trap" of trying to prove the
negative, and of arguing with the patients about the validity of such proofs. Instead, it is the physician's task to help patients learn to accept and tolerate the
uncertainty of everyday life (Starcevic, 1991). If hypochondriacal patients ask
for a "guarantee" that there is no disease, they can be reassured by a suggestion
that the next examination will surely "uncover" something, so that performing it
to feel more secure makes no sense. This paradoxical "praise of the ignorance
because of the unpleasant certainty" instead of "quest for absolute certainty" may
have a profoundly reassuring effect, leading such patients to abandon their search
for ultimate perfection and certainty.

A paradoxical approach can be used with the goal of demonstrating to
hypochondriacal patients the absurdity of their preoccupations and concerns. In
many instances, the effectiveness of such an approach depends on the patient's
intelligence, sense of humor, and ability to withstand direct confrontations. Kleinman (1988) has observed that hypochondriacal patients may be "extremely hu-
morous" (p. 195) behind a rigid and overly serious mask, and Pilowsky (1997,
p. 153) has noted how greeting a patient with "Well, what [disease] have you had

this week?" might lead to a productive examination of the basis for hypochondriacal concerns.

In a case report, Slavney (1987) described how a paradoxical approach, based on Murphy's *The Logic of Medicine* (Murphy, 1976), helped an intelligent hypochondriacal patient realize that the fewer examinations and investigations that he undergoes, the greater are his chances to have a reassuring, negative finding. A mathematical model of reasoning led to a logically "unbeatable" conclusion that "a normal person is anyone who has not been sufficiently investigated" (Slavney, 1987, p. 303).

Paradoxical interventions in hypochondriasis make sense whenever repeated and disabling reassurance-seeking is conceptualized as akin to a "neurotic paradox," which consists of two components. Patients first dismiss previous, reassuring experience, consider it irrelevant ("It does not matter") or interpret it as a matter of sheer luck. Then, as a consequence, they believe it is "reasonable" to continue worrying about disease and to continue checking their health, as well as asking for reassurance, because "the next time may be different," that is, they may not feel reassured again.

Discussing details of the differential diagnosis of the hypochondriacal patient's symptoms *with* the patient must be avoided, especially if the patient is overly suspicious and obsessive. The idea of an illness that patients have not thought about previously may only enter their minds after the physician has mentioned it in the course of such a discussion, and at that point it might be too late to apply the "rule" that patients should never be reassured about something that they have not already worried about (Brewin, 1991).

**Providing reassurance repeatedly.** Repeated provision of reassurance is a matter of considerable controversy. On one side, there are authors who state that repeated provision of reassurance should generally be avoided: "Repeated discussion of information that is already known to and understood by the patient should be avoided, and reassurance restricted to areas of doubt which have not previously been addressed" (Warwick, 1992, p. 80). Moreover, repeated provision of reassurance to hypochondriacal patients may contribute to the maintenance of hypochondriasis in the same way that compulsions maintain obsessive-compulsive disorder: According to Warwick and Salkovskis (1985) and Salkovskis and Warwick (1986), both provision of reassurance and compulsions reduce anxiety in the short-term, while increasing it in the long-term. Provision of reassurance in such cases, "when it consists of repeated discussion of the nature of symptoms and repeated attempts to allay improbable fears" (Warwick and Salkovskis, 1985, p. 1028), is considered antitherapeutic, because it increases anxiety in the long-term.

On the other side, Kellner (1992) states that "there is no convincing evidence to suggest that appropriate reassurance in the course of psychotherapy prolongs hypochondriacal concerns" (p. 74), and he suggests that "persuasion" is the crucial component in his treatment "package" for disease conviction. Although it is not explicitly stated here, "persuasion" can hardly be imagined without a repetition of the information used initially to reassure patients. Elsewhere, Kellner (1990) makes it very clear that he believes that reassurance should be provided repeatedly (with small rather than with large amounts of information), because with repetition, reassurances "tend to have longer effects, appear to be more frequently recalled, and when recalled, carry more conviction than at the beginning of treatment" (p. 2140).

A repeated but careful provision of reassurance may be considered akin to a "working through" in the process of psychotherapy (Starcevic, 1991). Similar to the insight acquired in the course of psychotherapy, the information that patients have received and the knowledge that they have gained need to be reconsidered in order to be used for therapeutic purposes. This reconsideration takes place within the framework of repeated provision of reassurance, whereby the "material" with which the patients are reassured may be completely new or contain information that had been given previously. According to Kessel (1979), "reassuring information can bear repetition" (p. 1130). He quotes one patient as saying, "Once isn't enough" (p. 1130), and Kathryn Small (1977) who concludes that "repetition of facts will be needed" (p. 1130). It must be emphasized that such repetition must never be stereotyped and reassurance never given in such a way that patients believe their physician has nothing else to offer. Therefore, repeated provision of reassurance does *not* consist of repeated statements that "everything is all right with your health."

In addition to decreasing anxiety, repeated provision of reassurance can counteract hypochondriacal patients' sense of low self-esteem and their feelings of being unworthy and unlovable, and it can reverse their attitude of negative expectancy (Starcevic, 1991). It also strongly reinforces, in these patients, an emerging sense of being accepted the way they are.

**Performing additional physical examinations and medical investigations.** The issue of whether hypochondriacal patients should undergo additional physical examinations and investigations is also highly controversial. Most authors do not recommend them, but some do (Brown and Vaillant, 1981; Kellner, 1982). Kellner (1982) justifies his attitude on the basis of observations that "patients did not develop new fears because the physician chose to reexamine them" (p. 148), and that, therefore, patients "did not suspect that the physician was unsure of his diagnosis" (p. 148). Furthermore, according to Kellner (1982), patients "perceived their repeated examinations as an evidence of thoroughness and care and that their physician took their complaints seriously" (p. 148).

Other authors (House, 1989; Mayou, 1991; Warwick and Salkovskis, 1985) disagree with this line of reasoning. Indeed, there is almost a consensus that hypochondriacal patients should not undergo additional physical examinations and medical investigations, except under rare and clearly specified circumstances. The rationale for such an attitude is expressed clearly by House (1989): "However carefully it [repeated physical examination] was explained, it was always construed as a check on previous findings and therefore as confirmation of the patient's suspicions about those findings" (p. 158). In a similar vein, Warwick and Salkovskis (1985) argue that "if unnecessary investigations are carried out to allay fears the fact that there is apparently enough doubt in the mind of the doctor that he may have 'missed something' confirms for the patient the validity of his fears" (p. 1028). In other words, repeated and unnecessary physical examinations could be seen as contributing to the maintenance of hypochondriasis (Warwick and Salkovskis, 1990) and reinforcing this disorder iatrogenically.

House (1989) offers additional, compelling reasons for considering repeated physical examinations unnecessary and even harmful. First, physical examinations are perceived as "invalidating the physical experience of the patient rather than explaining it," because they indicate what is *not* present (p. 158). Second, multiple investigations are often confusing "because they bring to attention trivial or irrelevant findings upon which doctors disagree" (p. 158). Third, repeated examinations are not seen as reassuring because they constantly raise "the possibility that something *might* be found" (p. 158).

However, are there situations when additional physical examinations and medical investigations might be justified or considered appropriate? This is obviously a matter of "clinical judgment," as reflected in a suggestion to perform a diagnostic workup if "new symptoms appear" (House, 1989; Kellner, 1982). But while some take "new symptoms" at face value (Kellner, 1982), others justify additional physical examinations and investigations only if "new symptoms" suggest *to the physician* a possibility of an underlying organic pathology (House, 1989).

Performing numerous physical examinations and diagnostic investigations "just" to reassure hypochondriacal patients would certainly not be a recommended course. If the physician has any dilemma in a situation like that, the question that needs to be asked—and answered—is whether the physician is in fact trying to reassure himself or herself. For some physicians—especially for those who are preoccupied with the fear of missing a somatic disease or those who cannot tolerate diagnostic uncertainty (Kassirer, 1989; Todd, 1984)—this is not easy to deal with.

If hypochondriacal patients insist on another "check" of their health status, and the physician does not see any need for that at the moment, a reasonable course is to not go along with such requests. In some cases, it may be wise to do that also because patients may be "checking" how sure their physicians are that there is no organic pathology. Instead of being involved in making a decision about patients' further examinations, it is the physician's task to communicate to a patient that the latter should take responsibility for making such a decision. It is also important to stress that if patients were not to follow physician recommendations and if they were to undergo additional examinations, they would not be "punished" or rejected by their physicians. In other words, the relationship with their physicians is not contingent upon the patients' "obedience."

## Can Reassurance Be Harmful in Hypochondriasis?

A debate (Kellner, 1992; Starcevic, 1991; Warwick, 1992) between those who favor reassurance in the treatment of hypochondriasis and those who are apparently opposed to it and consider it antitherapeutic, for the most part appears to be resolved. In retrospect, it seems that this debate resulted largely from different meanings attached to the key concepts, including "reassurance," and from the consequent misunderstanding of the treatment techniques and processes involved in therapy. It is also true that there are now more areas of agreement between the two positions and that the gap between them has narrowed somewhat.

Although Warwick and Salkovskis state that repeated provision of reassurance contributes to the maintenance of hypochondriasis (Salkovskis and Warwick 1986; Warwick, 1992; Warwick and Salkovskis, 1990), they clearly refer to inappropriate reassurance, which has the effects of "nurturing" hypochondriacal fears and suspicions and rejecting hypochondriacal patients. Therefore, it is not difficult to agree with them that reassurance should not be used indiscriminately (Warwick and Salkovskis, 1985). In addition, routine reassurance should not be attempted with hypochondriacal patients, and provision of such reassurance may even contribute to the persistence of hypochondriasis and may therefore be positively harmful.

Warwick (1992) does not suggest a "ban" on provision of reassurance in any absolute way, but rather calls for a more careful conceptualization of reassurance that might be effective and considers that such reassurance be "restricted to areas of doubt which have not previously been addressed" (p. 80). Furthermore, Warwick (1992) states explicitly that the "main aim in treatment of primary hypochondriasis is to provide successful reassurance" (p. 80). So, the question might not be "To reassure or not to reassure," but how to reassure effectively and avoid inappropriate, and indeed, futile reassurance. Appleby (1987) offers the following suggestion, based on Kessel's paper (Kessel, 1979): "To be effective, reassurance must be credible, educative and specific, and directed at both expressed and concealed fears" (p. 857). It would be difficult to find a physician who would disagree that provision of such reassurance might be helpful in the treatment of hypochondriasis.

## Research Considerations

We live in an era of "empirically validated treatments" and consumerism in medicine, which demands that physicians provide "guaranteed services" to patients and deliver treatments with proven efficacy. Under such social circumstances, is there room for treatment that emphasizes provision of reassurance as a relatively nonspecific, context-dependent "art of improvisation" performed by individual physicians? The "art" component of any medical procedure is difficult to assess rigorously and scientifically, but some evidence of efficacy needs to be demonstrated if reassurance is to "survive" as an acceptable treatment modality for hypochondriasis.

Therefore, the efficacy of a "reassurance program" in the treatment of hypochondriasis remains to be established in controlled studies, using the "waiting list" groups of patients as controls for comparison. Essentially, two steps need to be made to set the stage for conducting such studies. First, the treatment procedures should be described in more detail and standardized inasmuch as possible to ensure that different physicians provide reassurance in a manner that approaches *technical* uniformity. Stages of treatment need to be outlined and a time limit set for its duration. In this regard, it would be helpful to develop a manual for the use of reassurance in hypochondriasis.

The second step is to develop an instrument that would be used to monitor changes in the course of the "reassurance therapy." Such an instrument would be administered on a weekly basis to assess the attainment of the reassurance-related goals of treatment. These goals pertain to (*1*) the degree to which the patient understands his or her symptoms and his or her condition in general and (*2*) the degree to which the patient feels that he or she is threatened by a serious disease, whereby both the extent of suspicion and the extent of fear about the presence of the disease are assessed. These ratings should be accompanied by a patient's weekly rating of the overall quality of the patient–physician relationship, and in particular, a rating of the perceived ability of the physician to empathize. A good example of the latter instrument is the Empathy Scale (Burns, 1989; Burns and Auerbach, 1996).

## Conclusion

The provision of reassurance to hypochondriacal patients can be regarded in a similar way to the combined use of psychotherapy and pharmacotherapy: Although many endorse negative attitudes toward them, it seems that both are widespread in clinical practice. It is argued here that there is a crucial distinction between routine and complex, process-like reassurance, and that hypochondriacal patients usually do not respond only to the former. If response to medical reassurance is to remain one of the diagnostic criteria for hypochondriasis in future diagnostic manuals, this distinction must be taken into consideration, and it should be clarified what is meant by "appropriate medical reassurance." Such reassurance, conceptualized as a process, in which it is more clear who should provide medical reassurance, to whom, when, and how, has been described in this chapter.

A successful provision of reassurance results in a disappearance of the repeated reassurance-seeking behavior, one of the most conspicuous and disabling features of hypochondriasis. Other consequences of the successful provision of reassurance would be better understanding of the symptoms, alleviation of hypochondriacal fears and suspicions, freedom from excessive bodily preoccupation, counteracting a sense of low self-esteem and excessive perception of personal vulnerability, and improved coping and functioning.

It appears that we have come a long way from the previous controversy "To reassure or not to reassure?" Today, few would argue that an *absolute* ban on the provision of reassurance is a treatment of choice for patients with hypochondriasis, and it is easy to agree with Kellner (1992) that "the question is which is the most effective strategy of reassurance—which is the best method to convince them [the hypochondriacal patients] that they are in fact healthy" (p. 74). Several such strategies or methods have been proposed: Some can be seen as a combination of the provision of reassurance and techniques of cognitive therapy (House, 1989), others use reassurance within a framework of psychodynamically oriented psychotherapy (Starcevic, 1991), and still others have evolved into a more specific and more elaborate form of treatment (for example, "cognitive-educational therapy"; Barsky, 1996; Barsky *et al.*, 1988). This chapter has outlined "ingredients" of an appropriate and successful reassurance, common to all

**Table 13.1.** Areas of controversy in the therapeutic use of reassurance in hypochondriasis

|  | "Flexible" position | "Strict" position |
|---|---|---|
| 1. What information is given? | Various, as required by the situation, and as determined by the physician | Only new (not discussed previously) |
| 2. Should reassurance be provided repeatedly? | In principle, yes | No |
| 3. Should additional physical examinations and medical investigations be encouraged/ allowed? | Yes, if judged necessary and appropriate by the physician | In principle, no |

these forms of treatment. They include selecting patients who are most likely to benefit from reassurance; "timing" reassurance properly; establishing a dependable and trusting relationship between the patient and the physician; showing acceptance of the patient by a single, accessible, and empathic physician; scheduling regular visits; providing relevant information and explanation; adjusting a "reassuring style" to a particular patient; fostering patient's responsibility; and shifting attention to the underlying issues and to the patient's assets.

The contemporary debate about reassurance in the treatment of hypochondriasis revolves around the content of reassurance and the question of whether it is to be provided repeatedly (Table 13.1). Opinions seem to differ most on the nature of the information given to the patients in the process of reassurance. Thus, identification of the information with the most reassuring "power" remains firmly on the research agenda for reassurance. Shedding more light on this issue would also contribute to a better assessment of the efficacy of reassurance in the treatment of hypochondriasis.

**References**

Adler G. 1981. The physician and the hypochondriacal patient. *New England Journal of Medicine* 304: 1394–1396.

American Psychiatric Association. 1994. *Diagnostic and Statistical Manual of Mental Disorders, Fourth Edition* (*DSM-IV*). Washington, DC: American Psychiatric Association.

Appleby L. 1987. Hypochondriasis: an acceptable diagnosis? *British Medical Journal* 294: 857.

Avia M.D. 1999. The development of illness beliefs. *Journal of Psychosomatic Research* 47: 199–204.

Barr G. 1965. Reassurance. *Scottish Medical Journal* 10: 356–360.

Barsky A.J. 1993. The diagnosis and management of hypochondriacal concerns in the elderly. *Journal of Geriatric Psychiatry* 26: 129–141.

Barsky A.J. 1996. Hypochondriasis: medical management and psychiatric treatment. *Psychosomatics* 37: 48–56.

Barsky A.J., Geringer E., Wool C.A. 1988. A cognitive-educational treatment for hypochondriasis. *General Hospital Psychiatry* 10: 322–327.

Brewin T.B. 1991. Three ways of giving bad news. *Lancet* 337: 1207–1209.

Brown H.N., Vaillant G.E. 1981. Hypochondriasis. *Archives of Internal Medicine* 141: 723–726.

Burns D.D. 1989. *The Feeling Good Handbook.* New York: William Morrow.

Burns D.D., Auerbach A. 1996. Therapeutic empathy in cognitive-behavioral therapy: does it really make a difference? In *Frontiers of Cognitive Therapy* (ed. Salkovskis P.M.), New York: Guilford Press.

Clark D.M., Salkovskis P.M., Hackmann A., Wells A., Fennell M., Ludgate J., Ahmad S., Richards H.C., Gelder M. 1998. Two psychological treatments for hypochondriasis: a randomised controlled trial. *British Journal of Psychiatry* 173: 218–225.

Cooper C. 1996. The art of reassurance. *Australian Family Physician* 25: 695–698.

Fava G.A., Grandi S. 1991. Differential diagnosis of hypochondriacal fears and beliefs. *Psychotherapy and Psychosomatics* 55: 114–119.

Glucksman M.L. 1997. Discussions of "Reassurance in analytic therapy," by Douglas H. Ingram. *American Journal of Psychoanalysis* 57: 243–251.

Greenson R.R. 1967. *The Technique and Practice of Psychoanalysis, Vol. 1*. New York: International Universities Press.

Haenen M-A., Schmidt A.J.M., Schoenmakers M., van den Hout M.A. 1997. Suggestibility in hypochondriacal patients and healthy control subjects: an experimental case-control study. *Psychosomatics* 38: 543–547.

House A. 1989. Hypochondriasis and related disorders: assessment and management of patients referred for a psychiatric opinion. *General Hospital Psychiatry* 11: 156–165.

Howard L.M., Wessely S. 1996. Reappraising reassurance—The role of investigations. *Journal of Psychosomatic Research* 41: 307–311.

Ingram D.H. 1997. Reassurance in analytic therapy. *American Journal of Psychoanalysis* 57: 221–241.

Kassirer J.P. 1989. Our stubborn quest for diagnostic certainty. *New England Journal of Medicine* 320: 1489–1491.

Kellner R. 1982. Psychotherapeutic strategies in hypochondriasis. *American Journal of Psychotherapy* 34: 146–157.

Kellner R. 1983. Prognosis of treated hypochondriasis: a clinical study. *Acta Psychiatrica Scandinavica* 67: 69–79.

Kellner R. 1990. Hypochondriasis and body dysmorphic disorder. In *Treatments of Psychiatric Disorders* (ed. Karasu T.B.), Washington, DC: American Psychiatric Press.

Kellner R. 1992. The treatment of hypochondriasis: to reassure or not to reassure? The case for reassurance. *International Review of Psychiatry* 4: 71–75.

Kellner R., Abbott P., Winslow W.W., Pathak D. 1987. Fears, beliefs, and attitudes in DSM-III hypochondriasis. *Journal of Nervous and Mental Disease* 175: 20–25.

Kessel N. 1979. Reassurance. *Lancet* I: 1128–1133.

Kirmayer L.J., Robbins J.M. 1991. Conclusion: prospects for research and clinical practice. In *Current Concepts of Somatization: Research and Clinical Perspectives* (eds. Kirmayer L.J., Robbins J.M.), Washington, DC: American Psychiatric Press.

Kleinman A. 1988. *The Illness Narratives*. New York: Basic Books.

Kohut H. 1984. *How Does Analysis Cure?* Chicago: University of Chicago Press.

Lipsitt D.R. 1974. Psychodynamic considerations of hypochondriasis. *Psychotherapy and Psychosomatics* 23: 132–141.

Lipsitt D.R. 1995. Hypochondriasis and body dysmorphic disorder. In *Treatments of Psychiatric Disorders: Second Edition* (ed. Gabbard G.O.), Washington, DC: American Psychiatric Press.

Mayou R.A. 1991. Medically unexplained physical symptoms. *British Medical Journal* 303: 534–535.

Murphy E.A. 1976. *The Logic of Medicine*. Baltimore: The Johns Hopkins University Press.

Pilowsky I. 1983. Hypochondriasis. In *Handbook of Psychiatry, Vol. 4* (eds. Russell G.E., Hersov L.), Cambridge: Cambridge University Press.

Pilowsky I. 1997. *Abnormal Illness Behaviour*. Chichester: John Wiley.

Salkovskis P.M., Warwick H.M.C. 1986. Morbid preoccupations, health anxiety and reassurance: a cognitive-behavioural approach to hypochondriasis. *Behaviour Research and Therapy* 24: 597–602.

Schwartz L. 1966. Some notes on reassurance in medical practice. *Psychosomatics* 7: 290–294.

Slavney P.R. 1987. The hypochondriacal patient and Murphy's "law." *General Hospital Psychiatry* 9: 302–303.

Small K. 1977. *Elective Dissertation*. Manchester, England: Manchester University Medical School.

Starcevic V. 1988. Diagnosis of hypochondriasis: a promenade through the psychiatric nosology. *American Journal of Psychotherapy* 42: 197–211.

Starcevic V. 1990a. Role of reassurance and psychopathology in hypochondriasis. *Psychiatry* 53: 383–395.

Starcevic V. 1990b. Relationship between hypochondriasis and obsessive-compulsive personality disorder: close relatives separated by nosological schemes? *American Journal of Psychotherapy* 44: 340–347.

Starcevic V. 1991. Reassurance and treatment of hypochondriasis. *General Hospital Psychiatry* 13: 122–127.

Starcevic V., Piontek C.M. 1997. Empathic understanding revisited: conceptualization, controversies and limitations. *American Journal of Psychotherapy* 51: 317–328.

Starcevic V., Kellner R., Uhlenhuth E.H., Pathak D. 1992. Panic disorder and hypochondriacal fears and beliefs. *Journal of Affective Disorders* 24: 73–85.

Todd J.W. 1984. Investigations. *Lancet* II: 1146–1147.

Wahl C.W. 1963. Unconscious factors in the psychodynamics of the hypochondriacal patient. *Psychosomatics* 4: 9–14.

Warwick H. 1992. The treatment of hypochondriasis: to reassure or not to reassure? Provision of appropriate and effective reassurance. *International Review of Psychiatry* 4: 76–80.

Warwick H.M.C., Salkovskis P.M. 1985. Reassurance. *British Medical Journal* 290: 1028.

Warwick H.M.C., Salkovskis P.M. 1990. Hypochondriasis. *Behaviour Research and Therapy* 28: 105–117.

Warwick H.M.C., Clark D.M., Cobb A.M., Salkovskis P.M. 1996. A controlled trial of cognitive-behavioural treatment of hypochondriasis. *British Journal of Psychiatry* 169: 189–195.

Wise T.N. 1992. The somatizing patient: "perspectivism" in use. *Annals of Clinical Psychiatry* 4: 9–17.

# 14

# Cognitive-Behavioral Treatment of Hypochondriasis

HILARY M. C. WARWICK
PAUL M. SALKOVSKIS

Although medicine has been aware of the problem of severe health anxiety and hypochondriasis for centuries, treatment attempts have been largely futile. Most commonly, doctors have resorted to reassurance as the primary approach. By modern definitions (such as the one found in the *DSM-IV*; American Psychiatric Association, 1994), such strategies are doomed to failure, given that hypochondriasis is only identified in individuals in whom preoccupation persists despite medical reassurance. Until recently, attempts to understand the nature of hypochondriasis were confined to theories derived from basic psychoanalytic and quasi-neurological approaches such as so-called *alexithymia* (Kellner, 1986). However, the last few years have seen the application and validation of cognitive-behavioral approaches in the understanding and treatment of health anxiety. Most importantly, randomized controlled trials of cognitively based treatment have established such approaches as both effective and economical.

The cognitive-behavioral theory of hypochondriasis was described in Chapter 9. As described there, the theory provides a comprehensive account of the psychological processes involved in the disorder, including etiological and maintaining factors. Treatment strategies derived from this formulation have been found to be effective in clinical cases of hypochondriasis. Effective therapy therefore involves modification of both the central threat-related appraisals that form the core of the experience of health anxiety, and the specific factors involved in the maintenance of the misinterpretations (and therefore anxiety) in each case. The main targets of cognitive-behavioral treatment are the patient's false beliefs that he or she is physically ill, based on the misinterpretation of innocuous physical symptoms and/or signs, and the responses that are motivated by such misinterpretations.

This chapter describes cognitive-behavioral treatment strategies derived from this formulation, and their clinical applications. Difficulties in applying cognitive-behavioral treatments, which are specific to patients with hypochondriasis, are described, along with some solutions. The importance of evaluating previous medical interventions is discussed, and emphasis is placed on developing a comprehensive psychological formulation in each case, so that health anxiety is a positive diagnosis, rather than being identified by exclusion. Studies investigating the efficacy of this treatment are critically discussed, along with suggestions for future directions of cognitive-behavioral research and treatment.

## The Concept of Hypochondriasis

The term "hypochondriasis" was first coined over 2,000 years ago to describe a physical illness afflicting the *hypochondrium*. It was used for a variety of physical illnesses until the seventeenth century when Robert Burton and Thomas Sydenham described hypochondriasis as a form of melancholia. Subsequently, various behaviors and psychiatric disorders, ranging from malingering to a form of schizophrenia, have been given the term "hypochondriasis" (see Kellner, 1986).

Hypochondriasis is now accepted as a false belief in illness. The most recent debate surrounding the disorder is whether such false beliefs are the center of a *primary* condition. Kenyon's (1964) influential study of patients with hypochondriacal beliefs suggested that hypochondriasis is always secondary to another primary psychiatric disorder, usually an affective disorder. It has also been suggested that hypochondriacal beliefs occurring in the absence of affective symptoms were due to "masked depression" (Lesse, 1967). Subsequent studies have identified a primary disorder in which false beliefs about health are the central problem, to which affective symptoms are secondary (Bianchi, 1971). Primary hypochondriasis is included in both the ICD-10 (World Health Organization, 1992) and the *DSM-IV* (American Psychiatric Association, 1994).

## Previous Treatment Approaches

Despite the considerable health-care resources utilized by patients with hypochondriasis, neither physical medicine nor psychiatry have previously established an effective treatment. Hypochondriasis has long been regarded as an intractable disorder, with supportive therapy the best that can be offered. In response to the view that hypochondriasis could be secondary to "masked depression," antidepressant medication was used in the absence of a primary affective disturbance. This approach has not been successful in treatment of hypochondriasis (Kellner,

1983). Some recent studies have used fluoxetine in a small number of cases and claim promising results (Fallon *et al.*, 1993). However, the efficacy of antidepressants has yet to be clearly established, and there are indications that treatment acceptance and adherence are poor (Fallon, personal communication, 1998).

Some authors have suggested that health concerns are not central to the problem and it is not uncommon for secondary gain to be suggested as an important motivating factor in these cases (see Warwick and Salkovskis, 1990, for a more detailed critique of this view). No evidence has been found to support any role of secondary gain, and incautious attempts to find hidden motives for their presentation can make hypochondriacal patients worse or can lead them to drop out of treatment. Patients may feel that their health concerns are not being given proper consideration and are then likely to seek further physical investigations and other sources of help. Patients are angered by such approaches and may become hostile to future attempts at psychological treatment.

To reassure a patient successfully is one of the most common aims in medicine and indeed the diagnosis of hypochondriasis can only be made when this basic medical intervention has failed. Some authors (e.g., Kellner, 1983) suggest that repeated reassurance should be a component of psychological treatment for hypochondriasis. Conversely, it has also been suggested (Salkovskis and Warwick, 1986; Warwick and Salkovskis, 1985) that repeated reassurance, containing no new information, may serve to reinforce the patient's fears, leading to short-term decrease in health anxiety but a longer-term *increase* in anxiety and need for reassurance. Therapists who repeatedly carry out discussions, examinations, and investigations in response to the patient's anxiety rather than as a result of the clinical indications may inadvertently be maintaining the hypochondriacal concerns.

Lucock *et al.* (1997) examined the time course and prediction of effectiveness of responses to oral reassurance in 60 patients after gastroscopy showing no serious illness. Physician and patient rated the extent of reassurance at the time of the consultation, and patients rated their anxiety about their health and their illness belief at the time of consultation, and at follow-up at 24 hours, 1 week, 1 month, and 1 year. While health anxiety and illness belief decreased markedly after reassurance, patients with high health anxiety showed a significant resurgence in their worry and illness belief at 24 hours and 1 week, maintained at 1 month and 1 year later. Those with low levels of preexisting health anxiety maintained low health worry and illness belief throughout. The authors conclude that reduction in worry and illness belief after reassurance may be very short-term, and that measurable individual differences in health anxiety predict response to reassurance. Similar findings have been obtained in our group examining the impact of population-based health screening procedures (Rimes and Salkovskis, 1999).

## Cognitive-Behavioral Treatment of Hypochondriasis

There have been some uncontrolled case series in which behavioral treatment of hypochondriasis has had promising results (e.g., Warwick and Marks, 1988). Salkovskis and Warwick (1986), reporting two cases of hypochondriasis successfully treated with cognitive-behavioral treatment, went on to describe a comprehensive cognitive-behavioral formulation of hypochondriasis.

## The Importance of Providing a Psychological Explanation as a Noncatastrophic Alternative

In Chapter 9, it was described how patients suffering from anxiety disorders overestimate the threat associated with ambiguous situations. Hence, in hypochondriasis innocuous symptoms are misinterpreted as serious threats to health. Successful therapy must lead the patients to an alternative, less threatening explanation of their symptoms (Salkovskis, 1989, 1996). One of the reasons for the persistence of hypochondriacal concerns despite medical reassurance may be the frequent lack of an alternative explanation; reassurance seeks to tell patients what is *not* wrong with them, despite the fact that what patients want is a clear account of what *is* wrong with them. Most hypochondriacal patients will have already been referred to several specialists for exclusion of relevant pathology. The specialist will be able to find no evidence of serious illness, but may not be capable of offering an alternative more general explanation. Exclusion of particular illnesses alone is clearly not sufficient to alleviate hypochondriacal concerns.

If an alternative explanation for the patient's symptoms is offered, it must appear valid and credible. It must not diverge from the patient's previous experience and, with time, must survive his or her future experience. For example, patients may be told that their symptoms are due to stress, but they are unable to fit their symptoms and signs with their understanding of stress. This discordant experience will lead to rapid disconfirmation of the explanation and to persistence of the health concerns in the patient. It may also lead to feelings of distrust in medical opinions.

The cognitive-behavioral treatment of hypochondriasis offers a positive account of what is going on, an alternative, comprehensive explanation for the patient's concerns, reactions, and, in some instances, symptoms. Patients are encouraged to discuss aspects of their problems that do not fit with the cognitive-behavioral formulation. The new explanation will lead patients to reinterpret their innocuous symptoms and attribute them to a less threatening cause. It will also demonstrate to patients that behaviors such as bodily checking and other maintaining factors serve to make their problems worse and should be terminated.

It is reasonable to suggest that any treatment which convinces patients of a valid alternative explanation for their symptoms should lead to improvement in hypochondriasis. Examples of such a treatment include cognitive-behavioral treatment (Warwick *et al.*, 1996) and behavioral stress management, specifically adapted as a highly credible control modality in the recent outcome trial of two psychological treatments for hypochondriasis (Clark *et al.*, 1998).

## Treatment Strategies Derived From the Cognitive-Behavioral Formulation

If the cognitive-behavioral formulation is correct, then treatment strategies derived from the formulation should be successful in the treatment of hypochondriasis. The enduring tendency to misinterpret physical symptoms must be rectified by direct examination of the patient's cognitive errors. Factors that maintain anxiety must also be addressed. For long-term improvement to be achieved, particularly if new symptoms develop, other etiological factors, such as dysfunctional beliefs, must be corrected.

The cognitive-behavioral therapist should clearly establish, from discussion and medical records, whether adequate physical investigations have been carried out and all possible underlying physical illness has been excluded. It may be necessary to speak directly with the physicians involved to help verify this. One of the aims of assessment is to obtain a thorough description of the patient's problems and psychopathology, which can then be expressed as the patient's own version of the cognitive-behavioral formulation. This formulation must be able to identify the etiologic and maintaining factors of the patient's health anxiety, and it must be able to account for all the symptoms that the patient is experiencing. Development of a satisfactory psychological formulation that clearly describes the psychological processes occurring confirms to the therapist that there is a *positive* psychological diagnosis. If the symptoms do not fit such a formulation, then the possibility of a physical illness should be reconsidered.

For example, a 30-year old man was referred for psychological treatment of his health anxiety, which centered on fears of stomach cancer. He described epigastric pain that was worst when he was hungry and was relieved by certain foods such as milk. The pain was exacerbated by eating spicy foods. No other triggers for his symptoms were established and few psychological maintaining factors were established. The psychopathology could not be made to fit the cognitive-behavioral formulation of hypochondriasis, and he was referred back to the physicians, who discovered a peptic ulcer.

The main components of cognitive-behavioral treatment for hypochondriasis are as follows:

1. Assessment and engagement
2. Formulation; reaching a shared understanding
3. Self-monitoring
4. Identification and reattribution of negative automatic thoughts
5. Modification of maintaining factors
6. Identification and reattribution of dysfunctional assumptions
7. Relapse prevention

These will be considered separately, below.

## 1. Assessment and Engagement

Assessment has the following aims:

- Establishing a satisfactory relationship with the patient.
- Completing a thorough and comprehensive cognitive-behavioral analysis of the patient's problems, including symptoms, beliefs, behaviors, and consequences.
- Establishing the psychological processes involved in each case, and deciding if a positive diagnosis of hypochondriasis can be made.
- Constructing a psychological formulation as an alternative, less threatening account of the person's symptoms.
- Enabling the patient to consider and systematically evaluate this alternative psychological explanation for his or her problems; listening to the physician's or therapist's explanation of the suggested treatment rationale and treatment strategies derived from it.

Specific Problems Assessing Hypochondriacal Patients

**1.** *Distrust of psychological treatments due to belief in physical illness.* Hypochondriacal patients are often extremely reluctant to engage in any psychological treatment, fearing a delay in further physical investigations. They may have been brought along under protest by relatives or sent by physicians who refuse any further physical investigations until a psychological assessment has been made. The patients, however, often feel that psychological treatment is of no relevance to their case and that it may be harmful, as it prevents them from getting the physical treatment they believe they need. Patients often set out to use the consultation solely for the purpose of proving that they are not "mad."

**2.** *Previous experience of medical consultations.* Cases of hypochondriasis may have had many previous consultations. Many of these will have been unsatisfactory. Patients may have been left feeling that their concerns have not been adequately considered and that doctors are angry with them for wasting their time. They may have been told that the physical problems that concern them are "not real" or are they "all in the mind."

**3.** *Habitual reassurance-seeking.* Reassurance-seeking may begin even in the assessment interview, before a proper formulation of the problems can be established. The therapist knows this will be detrimental and should not give in. However, explanation of such refusal can be difficult before the treatment rationale has been given.

**4.** *Embarrassment about concerns.* Some patients may be too embarrassed to describe the illnesses that concern them or to reveal the extent of their reassurance-seeking behaviors.

## Ways of Overcoming Problems Associated with Assessment and Engagement

Two main tactics are employed to deal with such problems, enabling the therapist to engage the patient in psychological treatment. First, the *style* of the therapist is crucial. The interview should be conducted without rushing, in a sympathetic manner, and must culminate in the patient's conviction that all his or her concerns have been properly considered. The therapist should acknowledge that the patient's physical concerns are real and are taken seriously. Such patients may well have been told previously that their symptoms are "all in the mind," and thus they will be watching for evidence of similar attitudes in their therapists. When discussing the diagnosis and treatment, it should be stated that the therapist has seen similar cases in the past, as patients often feel extremely isolated, believing that no one can help them with their problems. Second, the assessment should be used to construct a comprehensive psychological formulation of the patient's concerns. A version using actual examples from the patient is drawn up, explaining each step. Figure 14.1 shows an example of a formulation.

### 2. Formulation: Reaching a Shared Understanding

Following a construction of their formulation, patients are then asked to explain their own hypothesis of their problems, which is usually that they have an undiagnosed serious physical illness requiring further investigations and treatment. Patients will usually accept that following this approach in the past has not re-

Previous attitudes to health

↓

Stomach pains

↓

"This must be stomach cancer"

↓↑

Anxiety

Focusing on stomach pains

Reading about cancer

Repeatedly weighing self

Repeatedly demanding endoscopy

Asking wife for reassurance

**Figure 14.1.** Simplified example of cognitive-behavioral formulation.

solved their problems. The psychological formulation is then discussed as a competing hypothesis. If patients accept the possibility that their problems could be explained by the psychological formulation, then they are offered a brief course of treatment using psychological techniques derived from the formulation. It is stressed that if, after this treatment, they are still convinced they are physically ill, then they will be able to seek further physical treatment.

Throughout the treatment the therapist must continue to show understanding of his or her patient's situation and distress. Socratic questioning is very important when trying to establish the nature of the patient's beliefs and the evidence supporting these beliefs. For example, a patient with hypochondriacal concerns about stomach pain was describing a recent episode of severe pain. The therapist asked the patient what was going through his mind when the stomach pain was present. The patient replied, "This pain is so severe it must be cancer; nothing else could hurt this much."

In this way patients know their concerns have been heard and a faulty belief about the nature of pain elicited, which is then corrected during treatment.

Hypochondriacal patients will often have a tendency, particularly early in treatment, to try repeatedly to extract reassurance from the therapist. The therapist must be on the alert for such attempts and, by referring back to the formulation, explain to the patient why giving such reassurance would be detrimental to treatment. Summaries should be made at regular intervals by both

therapist and patient to ensure correct understanding of information and homework instructions.

## 3. Self-Monitoring

Patients are asked to keep a diary and to monitor episodes of health concern, noting triggering symptoms, level of anxiety, and negative thoughts about health and
action taken. This provides the therapist with further information and examples
to work within initial cognitive restructuring. It also helps to confirm to the patient that the psychological formulation is correct, and that the suggested sequence of events is actually occurring. Using the above example of a patient with
stomach pain, an entry in a diary record is shown below:

- Situation—reading in bed
- Trigger—severe stomach pain
- Thoughts—"I've got such a bad pain it must be cancer" (belief = 90%)
- Emotion—Severe anxiety, rating 90 (visual analog rating 0–100)
- Action taken—Repeatedly prodded my stomach for lumps and woke my
  wife to ask if she thought that I have cancer. Rang for appointment with
  GP next day.

A record of a week's activities is kept, along with notes of physical symptoms
and anxiety, providing the therapist with information about triggers of health
anxiety.

## 4. Identification and Reattribution of Negative Automatic Thoughts

Patients are asked to give a full list of all their "evidence" for being physically
ill, along with any evidence that there may be nothing wrong with them. Much
of their evidence might be idiosyncratic and obviously faulty, but it must all be
considered and reevaluated during the course of treatment. The therapist points
out the errors apparent in cognitions. The next step is for patients to recognize
these errors as they occur and to construct more rational responses to symp-
toms/signs. The therapist must work in collaboration with the patients to enable
them to construct their own rational responses, rather than giving prescriptive explanations for their symptoms. Behavioral experiments are constructed wherever
possible, to test out the rational responses.

For example, the patient who was 90% convinced that his stomach pain means
he has stomach cancer was asked to construct a list of causes of stomach pain.
He came up with a lengthy list containing a number of illnesses, but also a number of innocuous causes, such as indigestion or "wind." He was asked to choose

the most common cause and suggested indigestion. A brief behavioral experiment was carried out in which patient and therapist concentrated on their stomachs for several minutes. The patient developed a pain, with some similarities to the one troubling him and was surprised to see that attention could have an effect on his symptoms. His belief that he had stomach cancer fell to 70%.

Patients learn to reattribute their automatic thoughts between treatment sessions and are encouraged to devise their own behavioral experiments to check the accuracy of their rational responses. Patients may need considerable help to reattribute their false beliefs about symptoms, and examples are given below of particular strategies that may be of use.

**1.** *Discussion of all evidence, for and against illness, however idiosyncratic.* A list of evidence for and against the illness is compiled with the patient, and the items gradually worked through during treatment. Simple education may solve many of the patient's misunderstandings. It is important to check the patient's understanding of previous medical interventions, and to correct any inaccuracies. The therapist must be careful that this does not lapse into repetition of old information, thus providing reassurance.

**2.** *Discussion of probabilities.* "If you take a million stomach aches, how many will be stomach cancer?" This will help patients to increase their range of rational alternatives accounting for innocuous symptoms, instead of considering only serious illness. A "pie-chart" can be a useful method of examining this issue.

**3.** *Discussion of the "100% certainty issue."* Hypochondriacal patients often exhibit a strong need to know 100% that they are not ill, which is an unrealistic aim. What is required is the reattribution of thoughts and assumptions of this nature.

**4.** *Role-play using "Convince the judge and jury that you have stomach cancer."* This exercise can help patients to consider with care the evidence they have that they are ill. Not infrequently, the evidence is reduced to the argument that the patients are ill because they feel they must be—and they can be encouraged to reflect on this emotional reasoning.

**5.** *Induction of symptoms in session, such as muscle tension or overbreathing.* The demonstration that physical symptoms can be induced by simple innocuous procedures can be helpful. In some cases it may be possible to reproduce the exact or similar sensations to those involved in patients' concerns, helping to increase belief in an alternative innocuous explanation.

## 5. Modification of Maintaining Factors

*Exposure and response prevention.* Abnormal illness-related behaviors have a crucial role in the maintenance of hypochondriasis. Appropriate graded exposure is used if avoidance is present, along with response prevention for checking. In addition, it is important to carry out *reassurance-prevention* by referring the patient to the formulation and explaining the importance of the cessation of reassurance-seeking. It is often necessary to instruct families how to respond to repeated requests for reassurance. They are taught to reply as follows: "Hospital instructions are that I should not answer such questions." Others involved in the patient's care should be contacted and asked to carry out no further investigations or examinations which are prompted by anxiety rather than by clinical indications.

*Rumination and reattribution.* *Cognitive factors* that maintain health anxiety are identified and modified. *Preoccupation* with health anxiety often improves when patients learn successful reattribution of their negative automatic thoughts, but training patients to postpone their worries to a short period of the day can also be helpful, particularly during the early stages of treatment. Distraction techniques may be used to decrease bodily focussing.

*Addressing and modifying other maintaining factors.* *Physiological* maintaining factors are usually the result of the misinterpretation of the autonomic nervous system symptoms of anxiety, and can be dealt with by education and reattribution.

*Secondary affective* symptoms must be carefully monitored. Some cases of primary hypochondriasis may have severe secondary depressive symptoms, including hopelessness and suicidal ideation. Such symptoms may need appropriate direct clinical attention prior to or along with the cognitive-behavioral intervention for hypochondriasis.

### 6. Identification and Reattribution of Dysfunctional Assumptions

To prevent future relapse, it is important to identify dysfunctional core and intermediate beliefs, and to correct them using reattribution and behavioral experiments.

For example, the "stomachache" patient believed that "A physical symptom is always caused by physical illness." As a homework exercise he was asked to construct with his wife a list of examples of situations where this belief is false. He was surprised on his return to find himself armed with a thorough, extensive list of everyday examples such as tension headache, resulting in a marked drop in the strength of his faulty belief.

Simple exercises of this nature can be very successful in helping with reattribution of dysfunctional assumptions, although some may prove resistant to change and require prolonged painstaking reattribution. It is important to be aware that dysfunctional assumptions may not be restricted to health, illness and medical interventions. While these occur in nearly all cases of hypochondriasis, there may be further dysfunctional assumptions of a more general negative nature. For example, a patient firmly believed that "I'm Mrs. Jinx, anything bad is going to happen to me." Different situations activated this assumption, leading to numerous episodes of anxiety. If the situation happened to be a physical symptom, then her anxieties centered around her health. For treatment to be successful, particularly in the longterm, such general negative assumptions must also be identified and modified.

## 7. Relapse Prevention

Successfully treated hypochondriacal patients will continue to be faced with physical symptoms and with a barrage of information about health, illness and medical treatments. They must therefore be given careful instructions regarding relapse prevention towards the end of their treatment.


## Treatment Studies

Warwick *et al.* (1996) reported a controlled trial of cognitive-behavioral treatment for hypochondriasis. In that study, 32 patients were randomly assigned to either cognitive-behavioral therapy or a "no treatment" waiting list control. Cognitive-behavioral treatment consisted of sixteen individual treatment sessions over a 4-month period. The waiting list control lasted for 4 months and was followed by sixteen sessions of cognitive-behavioral treatment. Assessments were made before allocation and after treatment or waiting list control. Patients who had cognitive-behavioral treatment were reassessed 3 months after completion of treatment. Paired comparisons on posttreatment/waiting scores indicated that the cognitive-behavioral group showed significantly greater improvements than did the waiting list on all but one patient rating, all therapist ratings, and all assessor ratings. After 3 months the benefits of therapy were maintained.

Although this study suggests that cognitive-behavioral treatment is an effective therapy for hypochondriasis, the study has limitations. There was only one therapist, and it is necessary to establish that similar results can be obtained by other suitably trained therapists. The waiting list group did not control for the effects of attention, although it is unlikely that attention alone could have brought about the improvements seen in the treated group.

In a second controlled study (Clark *et al.*, 1998), a number of therapists carried out cognitive-behavioral treatment. This treatment was compared with a high credibility stress-management package and a waiting list control. Both active treatments did significantly better than the waiting list condition, which the authors claim is not surprising as behavioral stress management provides patients with a detailed alternative explanation for their symptoms and comprehensive treatment based on this alternative explanation.

In an uncontrolled study, Stern and Fernandez (1991) treated a group of patients with hypochondriasis with cognitive-behavioral treatment. This study had promising results and demonstrated that group cognitive-behavioral treatment is feasible in a general hospital setting. A controlled trial of group treatment has been reported, using the cognitive-educational approach put forward by Barsky *et al.* (1988), compared with a waiting list control (Avia *et al.*, 1996). Experimental subjects showed significant reduction in illness fears and attitudes, reported fewer somatic symptoms, and dysfunctional beliefs, while waiting list controls also changed some illness attitudes, but showed no change in somatic symptoms, and increased their visits to doctors.

In a crossover design (Visser and Bouman, 1992), 3 patients with hypochondriasis received exposure and response prevention followed by a block of cognitive therapy. Three more patients were treated with cognitive therapy followed by behavioral treatment. The use of the crossover design and the small numbers treated render this study uninterpretable. Furthermore, the description of cognitive therapy in this study suggests that it was an idiosyncratic version, lacking the emphases and many of the techniques used by the Oxford group.


## Future Research

Further controlled evaluations of cognitive-behavioral treatment of hypochondriasis are required to clearly establish its efficacy. Follow-up studies are in progress to examine the longer-term efficacy of the approach. In an effort to make the treatment briefer and more easily accessible, future studies should attempt to discover which of the components of cognitive-behavioral treatment are most effective. Similarly, further controlled trials in a group setting are needed, as this method of delivery should be more cost-effective.

Future studies are also required to examine the efficacy of cognitive-behavioral treatment in cases of hypochondriasis occurring in medical settings. It may be that such cases are more difficult to treat, as they may be more reluctant to consider psychological treatment. It is also necessary to see whether the approach can be modified for use for those with a number of related concerns—for example, for patients with physical illnesses whose anxieties are thought to be excessive, and for those presenting in general practice settings with somatic complaints and associated features that are not yet as severe as in hypochondriasis.

## Conclusion

Cognitive-behavioral therapy has been shown to be effective in the treatment of severe hypochondriasis. There is evidence that the effects of therapy are not solely due to nonspecific factors, and that gains obtained in treatment are relatively enduring. Treatment is brief (8 to 16 sessions) and there are good theoretical and empirical reasons to suppose that it may be effective in less severe health anxiety, probably with even shorter duration of treatment. The available data suggest that the provision of a convincing and easily applied alternative explanation may be a crucial element of any effective treatment.

## Acknowledgments

Paul Salkovskis is a Wellcome Trust Senior Research Fellow in Basic Biomedical Science.

### References

American Psychiatric Association. 1994. *Diagnostic and Statistical Manual of Mental Disorders, Fourth Edition (DSM-IV)*. Washington, DC: American Psychiatric Association.

Avia M.D., Ruiz M.A., Olivares M.E., Crespo M., Guisado A.B., Sanchez A., Varela A. 1996. The meaning of psychological symptoms: effectiveness of a group intervention with hypochondriacal patients. *Behaviour Research and Therapy* 34: 23–31.

Barsky A., Geringer E., Wool C. 1988. A cognitive-educational treatment for hypochondriasis. *General Hospital Psychiatry* 10: 322–327.

Bianchi G.N. 1971. The origins of disease phobia. *Australian and New Zealand Journal of Psychiatry* 5: 241–257.

Clark D.M., Salkovskis P.M., Hackmann A., Wells A., Fennell M., Ludgate J., Ahmad S., Richards H.C., Gelder M. 1998. Two psychological treatments for hypochondriasis: a randomised controlled trial. *British Journal of Psychiatry* 173: 218–225.

Fallon B.A., Liebowitz M.R., Salman E., Schneier F.R., Jusino C., Hollander E., Klein D.F. 1993. Fluoxetine for hypochondriacal patients without major depression. *Journal of Clinical Psychopharmacology* 13: 438–441.

Kellner R. 1983. Prognosis of treated hypochondriasis: a clinical study. *Acta Psychiatrica Scandinavica* 67: 69–79.

Kellner R. 1986. *Somatization and Hypochondriasis*. New York: Praeger.

Kenyon F.E. 1964. Hypochondriasis: a clinical study. *British Journal of Psychiatry* 110: 478–488.

Lesse S. 1967. Hypochondriasis and psychosomatic disorders masking depression. *American Journal of Psychotherapy* 21: 607–620.

Lucock M.P., Morley S., White C., Peake M.D. 1997. Responses of consecutive patients to reassurance after gastroscopy: results of self administered questionnaire survey. *British Medical Journal* 315: 572–575.

Rimes K.A., Salkovskis P.M. (1999) *Psychological factors predict the reaction to health screening: a prospective study.* (Manuscript submitted for publication.)

Salkovskis P.M. 1989. Somatic problems. In *Cognitive-Behavioural Approaches to Adult Psychiatric Disorder: A Practical Guide* (eds. Hawton K., Salkovskis P.M., Kirk J.W., Clark D.M.), Oxford: Oxford University Press.

Salkovskis P.M. 1996. The cognitive approach to anxiety: threat beliefs, safety seeking behaviour, and the special case of health anxiety and obsessions. In *Frontiers of Cognitive Therapy* (ed. Salkovskis P.M.), New York: Guilford Press.

Salkovskis P.M., Warwick H.M.C. 1986. Morbid preoccupations, health anxiety and reassurance: a cognitive-behavioural approach to hypochondriasis. *Behaviour Research and Therapy* 24: 597–602.

Stern R., Fernandez M. 1991. Group cognitive and behavioural treatment for hypochondriasis. *British Medical Journal* 303: 1229–1231.

Visser S., Bouman T.K. 1992. Cognitive-behavioural approaches in the treatment of hypochondriasis: six single case cross-over studies. *Behaviour Research and Therapy* 30: 301–306.

Warwick H.M.C., Marks I.M. 1988. Behavioural treatment of illness phobia and hypochondriasis. *British Journal of Psychiatry* 152: 239–241.

Warwick H.M.C., Salkovskis P.M. 1985. Reassurance. *British Medical Journal* 290: 1028.

Warwick H.M.C., Salkovskis P.M. 1990. Hypochondriasis. *Behaviour Research and Therapy* 28: 105–117.

Warwick H.M.C., Clark D.M., Cobb A.M., Salkovskis P.M. 1996. A controlled trial of cognitive-behavioural treatment of hypochondriasis. *British Journal of Psychiatry* 169: 189–195.

World Health Organization. 1992. *The ICD-10 Classification of Mental and Behavioural Disorders: Clinical Descriptions and Diagnostic Guidelines.* Geneva: World Health Organization.

# 15

# Pharmacologic Strategies for Hypochondriasis

## BRIAN A. FALLON

Very little controlled research has been conducted on the pharmacotherapy of hypochondriasis as a primary disorder. However, the therapeutic nihilism regarding the pharmacotherapy of hypochondriasis that characterized so much of the pre-1990s has now been replaced by cautious optimism that specific pharmacologic agents may be particularly helpful. Given the paucity of information about the pharmacotherapy of hypochondriasis, this chapter will present what is known, reviewing the extant literature using case reports, small series, and controlled studies. The pharmacotherapy of other disorders that may be concurrent with hypochondriasis will also be examined, for which agents are helpful, as well as for what can be learned about how to enhance the design of clinical trials.

## Pharmacotherapy of Secondary Hypochondriasis

Studies dating back to the 1980s have reported that when hypochondriasis is a secondary manifestation of another disorder such as major depression, panic disorder, obsessive-compulsive disorder, or chronic pain, treatment of the primary disorder results in a diminution of the hypochondriasis as well.

### Major Depression

"Masked depression" refers to depressive states that are hidden behind other facades to such an extent that the physician and psychotherapist may be unaware that a serious psychiatric disorder is present. In a seminal descriptive paper, Lesse (1967) reviewed the clinical characteristics of 100 adults with masked depression, finding that hypochondriacal or psychosomatic symptoms and signs were the most common presenting features. Corroborating the concept of "masked depression," Kellner *et al.* (1986) in a study evaluating the effectiveness of amitriptyline among 20 consecutive nonpsychotic inpatients with *DSM-III* melancholic major depression found that one-third of the 20 patients had scores on the Illness Attitude Scales (IAS; Kellner *et al.*, 1983–84) that were characteristic of patients with hypochondriasis. After treatment, no differences were seen in the frequency of hypochondriacal responses between the 20 patients and 20 matched controls.

## Panic Disorder

Noyes *et al.* (1986) reported that 60 patients with panic disorder and agoraphobia had responses on the hypochondriasis scale of the Illness Behaviour Questionnaire (Pilowsky and Spence, 1975) that were as high as had been reported previously among hypochondriacal psychiatric patients. After pharmacologic treatment, a significant decrease occurred in all three dimensions of hypochondriasis (disease fear, disease conviction, bodily preoccupation), paralleling the decrease in panic attacks.

## Obsessive-Compulsive Disorder (OCD)

In a case report describing a patient with obsessive-compulsive disorder (OCD) who also had the hypochondriacal fear that he had AIDS despite medical reassurance, Bodkin and White (1989) reported that clonazepam was very helpful in ameliorating both the OCD and the hypochondriasis. In another case, Fallon *et al.* (1991) reported on the successful use of fluoxetine to treat a patient with *DSM-III-R* hypochondriasis and OCD, noting that the hypochondriasis returned each time the dose of fluoxetine was lower than 60 mg/day. This raised the question of whether, at least in those patients whose hypochondriasis was accompanied by marked obsessionality, the higher doses of fluoxetine often needed to treat OCD would also be needed to treat hypochondriasis.

## Delusional Disorder, Somatic Type, and Major Depression with Psychotic Features

Also referred to as "atypical psychosis" or "monosymptomatic hypochondriacal psychosis," delusional disorder, somatic subtype, is applied to hypochondriasis when the conviction of illness is delusional in intensity. Patients with this condition typically have a long-standing delusion that they are dying, often from a bizarre or rare illness, such as rabies or spongiform encephalitis ("mad cow disease"). Several case reports suggest that delusions about illness can be reduced to nonpsychotic dimensions by antipsychotic medications, such as haloperidol (Fishbain *et al.*, 1992), pimozide (Lippert, 1986; Scarone and Gambini, 1991), or thioridazine (Scarone and Gambini, 1991). Whether illness delusions represent a truly distinct diagnostic disorder or simply the extreme end of a hypochondriasis spectrum of insight is unclear. Such delusional intensity about illness may also be seen among patients with major depression with psychotic features. Typically, these patients would have a preceding major depression that develops into a delusion of destruction from within by an illness.

## Pharmacotherapy of Primary Hypochondriasis

### Early Reports of Somatic Therapies for Primary Hypochondriasis

In 1968, Pilowsky conducted a retrospective chart review of hospitalized psychiatric patients and identified 66 thought to have "primary hypochondriasis" (Pilowsky, 1968). Half of the patients were given either electroconvulsive therapy or antidepressants. It was not stated what the other half received. At 2-year follow-up, 50% of the 66 patients were improved, with good outcome being associated with short duration of illness and no personality disorder. To my knowledge, this is the first large study that attempted to examine biological treatment of patients with primary hypochondriasis. However, results of the study are difficult to interpret given the retrospective design, the lack of structured diagnostic criteria to differentiate primary hypochondriasis from other disorders, the lack of standardized instruments of change, and the limited information about the actual treatments received by patients.

### Serotonin Reuptake Inhibitors

Clomipramine. Clomipramine has been reported as helpful in several case reports. Prior to hepatic metabolism to its more noradrenergic metabolite desmethylclomipramine, clomipramine has primarily serotonin reuptake blockade properties. Kamlana and Gray (1988) found low-dose (25 mg/day) clomipramine to be helpful in treating a man who had developed fears of having AIDS and of transmitting it to his pregnant wife and unborn baby; the improvement was sustained for 8 months. Stone (1993) found 200 mg/day of clomipramine to be helpful in treating a 31-year old man with a 10-year history of hypochondriasis and no Axis I comorbidity. Noteworthy is that this man previously had failed to respond to numerous pharmacologic agents, including benzodiazepines, mood stabilizers, beta-blockers, antipsychotics, and tricyclic antidepressants.

Fluvoxamine. Fluvoxamine may also be particularly beneficial, as was demonstrated in a case report and one open trial.

---

### Case Report

Fallon *et al.* (1996) presented a case of a 38-year-old woman without OCD or major depression who had a 3-year history of recurrent obsessional fears that she had contracted breast cancer; this fear resulted in repeated self-checking and doctor visits. Although no improvement was noted after a 12-week trial of fluoxetine up to 80 mg/day, marked improvement was noted after 8 weeks on fluvoxamine, 300 mg/day, and continued over the ensuing 2 years.

### Open Trial with a Blinded Placebo Run-In

In a 12-week treatment study (Fallon, unpublished data) of fluvoxamine among patients with *DSM-IV* hypochondriasis, all patients first received placebo for 2 weeks during a single-blind placebo run-in phase, followed by 10 weeks of open treatment with fluvoxamine. Patients were told that at some point during their 12-week treatment they would be given placebo for 2 weeks. The goal was to eliminate patients from the 10-week open trial who would show an initial immediate resolution of symptoms during the first 2 weeks simply by starting the study and receiving a pill.

Prior to study entry, all patients had a comprehensive evaluation including physical exam, electrocardiogram, blood tests, and diagnostic interviews including Structured Clinical Interview for *DSM-IV* Axis I Disorders (SCID-I; First *et al.*, 1997a) and Structured Clinical Interview for *DSM-IV* Axis II Personality Disorders (SCID-II; First *et al.*, 1997b). Patients were asked to complete a daily diary self-rating form (Table 15.1), which would allow the physician each week to more accurately assess the patients' status (Table 15.2). (Mean scores on the Heightened Illness Concern Diary among a group of 30 patients with *DSM-IV* hypochondriasis are presented in Table 15.3.) Rating scales included physician and patient measures of clinical global improvement (Clinical Global Improvement [CGI] scale; Guy, 1976); patient-rated measures of improvement in hypochondriasis (Analogue scale, Whiteley Index [Pilowsky, 1967], IAS); physician-rated measures of severity of hypochondriasis (Heightened Illness Concern Severity Scale [see Table 15.4]; a Yale–Brown Obsessive-Compulsive Scale [Goodman *et al.*, 1989] modified to focus on dimensions of hypochondriasis); and a patient-rated measure of functional status (Short-Form 36; Ware and Sherbourne, 1992). Responder status was defined by the physician-rated CGI improvement of at least "much improved." Minimum treatment required at least 6 weeks of medicine.

Among the 18 patients who enrolled in the study, 4 patients were dropped during the 2-week placebo run-in phase owing to either marked improvement or noncompliance with medication or study visits. Among the 14 patients who entered the 10-week open treatment phase, 3 dropped out before 6 weeks of treatment. Of the 11 patients who completed at least 6 weeks, 8 (72.7%) were responders, 1 was a

**Table 15.1.** Heightened Illness Concern Diary *(Patient completes at end of each day)*

Name: _____

Date:   /   /        Day of Week:  Mon   Tues   Wed   Thurs   Fri   Sat   Sun

- Today, did you worry that you *might have a physical illness* - or - that your illness is worsening?    Yes   No

a) Which physical illness did you worry about? _____

b) How many times did this fear of having a physical illness *last longer than 5 minutes*?
   ___ None   ___ Once   ___ Twice   ___ 3 or more than three times

c) How long did your *longest episode* of physical illness fear last today?
   ___ No time      ___ Less than 5 minutes   ___ 5 minutes to 1 hour
   ___ 1–3 hours   ___ 3–5 hours          ___ >5 hours to all day

d) Adding up *all* your episodes, how much time did you spend today worrying about having an illness?
   ___ No time      ___ Less than 5 minutes   ___ 5 minutes to 1 hour
   ___ 1–3 hours   ___ 3–5 hours          ___ >5 hours to all day

e) During your *worst episode* today, how severe was your anxiety or fear about having an illness?
   ___ No distress   ___ Mild         ___ Moderate
   ___ Severe        ___ Very severe distress

- Today, did you worry that you *might get a physical illness?*    Yes   No

- Did you have any *physical symptoms* that bothered you?    Yes   No
    If yes, which ones? _____
    How much discomfort or distress did your physical symptoms cause today?
    ___ None   ___ Mild   ___ Moderate   ___ Severe   ___ Very severe

- Did you *seek reassurance* from anybody or from medical sources (e.g., books, Internet)?    Yes   No
    If yes, describe: _____

- Did you *avoid* any illness-related situations today?    Yes    No
    If yes, describe: _____

minimal responder, and 2 were nonresponders. One of the nonresponders was dropped from the study after week 6 because of a progressive worsening of symptoms. New blood tests in this man revealed a previously undiagnosed Lyme disease, which, when treated with antibiotics, led to a complete resolution of his severe hypochondriacal preoccupations. More detailed results of this fluvoxamine study will be published elsewhere. The excellent CGI responder rate from this fluvoxamine trial (72.7% for the minimum treatment analysis and 57.1% for the intent-to-treat analysis) was comparable to the results reported below for fluoxetine in both the open and double-blind trials.

**Table 15.2.** Heightened Illness Concern (HIC) Diary scoring summary sheet.

Name:_____          Date:    /   /
1. # of days since last visit for which patient returned completed diaries (#dslv): _____
2. # of days from completed diaries that patient feared *having* an illness or feared a stable illness worsening (#dhic): _____
3. HIC Frequency Ratio (HICFR) since last visit: _____#dhic/ _____#dslv = _____

*Instructions to rater: Complete at appointment. Mark the frequency, duration, or severity for each day of the interval, then multiply # marks during interval by value indicated, sum weighted value for all days (interval sum), and calculate ratio.*

1. HIC Daily Frequency: How many times during the day did the fear of *having* an illness last longer than 5 minutes?

|                | #days        |               |
| Once           | _____     | × 1 = _____ |
| 2×             | _____     | × 2 = _____ |
| 3× or more     | _____     | × 3 = _____ |
|                | Interval sum = _____ |    |

HIC Daily Frequency Ratio (HDFR) = _____ sum/ _____ #dhic = _____

2. HIC Duration of Worst Episode: How long did the worst episode of illness fears last for each day?

|                        | #days        |               |
| >0 and ×5 minutes      | _____     | × 1 = _____ |
| 5 minutes–1 hour       | _____     | × 2 = _____ |
| 1–3 hours              | _____     | × 3 = _____ |
| 3–5 hours              | _____     | × 4 = _____ |
| >5 hours to all day    | _____     | × 5 = _____ |
|                        | Interval sum = _____ |    |

HIC Daily Duration Worst Ratio (HDDWR) = _____ sum/ _____ #dhic = _____

3. HIC Duration Total: What was the cumulative duration of illness worries for each day?

|                        | #days        |               |
| >0 and < 5 minutes     | _____     | × 1 = _____ |
| 5 minutes–1 hour       | _____     | × 2 = _____ |
| 1–3 hours              | _____     | × 3 = _____ |
| 3–5 hours              | _____     | × 4 = _____ |
| >5 hours to all day    | _____     | × 5 = _____ |
|                        | Interval sum = _____ |    |

HIC Daily Duration Total Ratio (HDDTR) = _____ sum/ _____ #dhic = _____

4. HIC Severity of Distress: During the worst episode, how severe was the patient's fear?

| Mild        | _____ | × 1 = _____ |
| Moderate    | _____ | × 2 = _____ |
| Severe      | _____ | × 3 = _____ |
| Very Severe | _____ | × 4 = _____ |
|             | Interval sum = _____ |    |

HIC Daily Severity Worst Ratio (HDSWR) = _____ sum/ _____ #dhic = _____

**Table 15.2.** Heightened Illness Concern (HIC) Diary scoring summary sheet (*continued*).

5. Illness Fear: # of days patient worried about *getting* an illness: _____
   Getting Ill Frequency Ratio (GIFR) = _____ sum/ _____ #dslv = _____

6. Physical Symptoms: # of days patient had troubling physical symptoms (#dphs): _____
   Physical Symptom Frequency Ratio (PSFR) = _____ sum/ _____ #dslv = _____
   How severe were the physical symptoms?
   Mild          _____ × 1 = _____
   Moderate      _____ × 2 = _____
   Severe        _____ × 3 = _____
   Very Severe   _____ × 4 = _____
                 Interval sum = _____
   Physical Symptoms Daily Severity Ratio (PSDSR) = _____ sum/ _____ #dphs = _____

7. Reassurance: # of days patient sought reassurance? _____
   Reassurance Frequency Ratio (ReFR) = _____ sum/ _____ #dslv = _____

8. Avoidance: # of days patient avoided illness-related situations? _____
   Avoidance Frequency Ratio (AvFR) = _____ sum/ _____ #dslv = _____

Fluoxetine. The efficacy of fluoxetine in hypochondriasis has been examined in studies with various designs.

### Case Reports

Viswanathan and Paradis (1991) described a 41-year-old woman with a 17-year history of treatment-refractory hypochondriasis (having failed behavior therapy, desipramine, and buspirone) who was treated with fluoxetine, 40 mg/day, and responded well for over one year. Fallon *et al.* (1991) similarly noted 2 patients whose hypochondriasis largely remitted after treatment with fluoxetine (60–80 mg/day), with one of these patients having had no benefit previously from years of psychotherapy, tricyclic antidepressants, antianxiety agents, and antipsychotics.

### Open Trial

A 12-week open trial of fluoxetine for 16 patients with hypochondriasis without major depression was reported by Fallon *et al.* (1993). Doses of fluoxetine starting at 20 mg/day were increased every 2 weeks by 20 mg as tolerated and needed to 80 mg/day. Standardized rating scales were used (Whiteley Index, Hamilton Depression Scale [HAM-D; Hamilton, 1960], Hamilton Anxiety Scale [HAM-A; Hamilton, 1959], and CGI). The minimum treatment period was 6 weeks and the full course 12 weeks. Two patients dropped out during the first 2 weeks, and 14 patients completed all 12 weeks. Noteworthy is that although the mean duration of illness was 11 years (*SD* = 12) and that these patients made frequent doctor visits (a mean of

**Table 15.3.** Scores on the Heightened Illness Concern (HIC) Diary for 30 patients with *DSM-IV* hypochondriasis.

Patient sample:
• Gender distribution: 16 males/14 females
• Age: mean = 35.9 (*SD* = 10.6) years; range: 19–62 years

|                                                                                          | Mean | (*SD*) |
|------------------------------------------------------------------------------------------|------|--------|
| Frequency ratio of # of days with fears of having illness since last visit (HICFR):       | 0.79 | (0.29) |
| Frequency ratio of # of days with fears of getting ill since last visit (GIFR):           | 0.27 | (0.37) |
| Frequency ratio of # of days with physical symptoms since last visit (PSFR):              | 0.74 | (0.34) |
| Frequency ratio of # of days patient sought reassurance for HIC since last visit (ReFR):  | 0.18 | (0.27) |
| Frequency ratio of # of days of HIC-related avoidance since last visit (AvFR):            | 0.16 | (0.31) |
| HIC characteristics: Daily frequency of 5 minute or longer episodes of HIC (HDFR):        | 2.51 | (2.84) |
| Daily duration of worst episode of HIC (HDDWR):                                           | 3.08 | (3.83) |
| Daily duration total of HIC (HDDTR):                                                      | 3.59 | (4.56) |
| Daily severity of worst distress due to HIC (HDSWR):                                      | 2.83 | (3.67) |
| Physical symptom characteristics: Daily severity of physical symptoms (PSDSR):            | 2.82 | (3.75) |

6 visits during the prior year), 10 of the 14 completers had never before seen a psychiatrist and 9 had never before taken psychotropic medications.

After 6 weeks of treatment, 5 of 14 patients were responders. By 12 weeks, the responder rate had doubled, such that 10 of 14 (70%) were responders: 4 were rated "very much improved" and 6 "much improved." The larger responder rate after 12 weeks of treatment suggested that either longer treatment confers greater benefit or that higher doses of fluoxetine are more beneficial (the maximum dose of 80 mg/day would not have been reached until week 7). In fact, at 6 weeks the mean fluoxetine dosage was 39 ± 16 mg/day, whereas at 12 weeks the mean dose was 52 ± 28 mg/day.

Hypochondriacal patients without a comorbid major Axis I disorder appeared more likely to respond to treatment (6 of 7 patients) than did hypochondriacal patients with a comorbid major Axis I disorder (4 of 7 patients responded), a nonsignificant

**Table 15.4.** Heightened Illness Concern (HIC) Severity Scale *(Completed by clinician).*

Severity of Illness Concerns

Considering your total experience with this particular population, how *troubled by illness concerns* has this patient been over the last week?

| | |
|---|---|
| 0 = Not assessed | 4 = Moderate HIC |
| 1 = No HIC | 5 = Marked HIC |
| 2 = Minimal fleeting HIC | 6 = Severe HIC |
| 3 = Mild HIC | 7 = Extreme HIC |

Severity of HIC Illness Guidelines

1 = No HIC

2 = Minimal HIC. Occasional illness concerns that are fleeting, not distressing, and do not require reassurance seeking or avoidance.

3 = Mild HIC. Illness concerns that are occasional (<3 episodes per week) and mildly distressing. Patient may spend up to 1 hour worrying about illness per episode, but may not need to check with others or avoid illness cues.

4 = Moderate HIC. Illness concerns may be occasional and moderately distressing—or—more frequent and mildly distressing. Patient may spend more than 1 hour worrying. Patient may have a moderate urge to check with friends, family, or health professionals for reassurance—or—avoid illness-related situations.

5 = Marked HIC. Illness concerns are occasional and very distressing—or—frequent and moderately distressing. The distress may last more than 1 hour per episode. Patient may have a marked urge to check with others for reassurance—or—markedly avoid illness cues.

6 = Severe HIC. Illness concerns are frequent, very distressing, and prolonged. This must lead to an overwhelming urge to check with others for reassurance or intense avoidance of illness-related situations. This must be associated with social and/or occupational impairment.

7 = Extreme HIC. Among the most ill of all HIC patients, causing extreme distress and significant social and occupational impairment.

difference in this small sample. A statistically significant improvement between week 12 and baseline was noted on the scales of anxiety (HAM-A), depression (HAM-D), and hypochondriasis (Heightened Illness Concern Severity Scale, Whiteley Index). On the subscales of the Whiteley Index, significant improvement was noted in disease conviction and disease fear, but not in bodily preoccupation.

**Double-Blind Study**

In a mid-phase analysis of an ongoing randomized, double-blind, placebo-controlled 12-week study of fluoxetine for patients with hypochondriasis, Fallon *et al.* (1996) reported on the first 25 patients to sign consent. In this study, all patients received 2 weeks of placebo followed by randomization to either drug or placebo at which time they received either 20 mg of fluoxetine or a matching placebo. The physician had the option of starting the patient on a lower dose of 10 mg if the patient appeared to be highly anxious or had a history of marked intolerance of psychotropic medication. The physician was also advised to increase the dose by 1 pill every 2 weeks to a maximum of 4 pills (80 mg/day), with dosage increases governed by patient response and side effects.

Among the 25 patients who entered the study, 5 were excluded from randomization during the initial 2-week placebo run-in phase, either because of a placebo response or noncompliance with medication. Among the 20 randomized patients, 4 dropped out during the first few weeks, 16 completed a minimum treatment of at least 6 weeks, and 15 completed the full 12 weeks. Among the 16 patients who completed at least 6 weeks, 8 of 10 patients randomized to fluoxetine were rated "much improved" or "very much improved" on the clinician CGI Scale (at 6 and 12 weeks) versus 3 of 6 patients randomized to placebo at 6 weeks and 3 of 5 patients on placebo at 12 weeks.

These response rates for fluoxetine versus placebo (at 6 weeks, 80% for fluoxetine and 50% for placebo; at 12 weeks, 80% for fluoxetine and 60% for placebo), although not statistically significantly different given the small sample size, suggest a preferential benefit for fluoxetine and quite a high placebo-response rate among hypochondriacal patients. If one examined this data in a more stringent way by redefining response to include only those patients rated "very much improved" (the equivalent of being virtually symptom free), among those who completed at least 6 weeks of treatment, 5 of the 10 fluoxetine-randomized patients were very much improved versus only 1 of 6 placebo-randomized patients: 50% versus 16%. This double-blind, placebo-controlled study therefore raises critical questions about the nonspecific therapeutic effects of placebo and of patient–clinician encounters. The implications of these nonspecific effects will be discussed in the section below on research design questions.

## Tricyclic Antidepressants

Imipramine has been reported as helpful for patients with hypochondriasis.

### Case Reports

At least three case reports describe the successful use of imipramine (100–200 mg/day) to treat the fear of having AIDS (Freed, 1983; Jenike and Pato, 1986; Lippert, 1986), with one case being a 40-year-old man who did not have any major Axis I comorbidity.

### Open Trial

An 8-week prospective, open trial of imipramine for *DSM-III-R* hypochondriasis with good insight ("illness phobia") was conducted by Wesner and Noyes (1991), using structured and self-report ratings. Patients with comorbid major depression were excluded. Ten patients signed consent, 2 dropped out after 1 week owing to side effects, and 8 patients completed at least 4 weeks of treatment. Imipramine was increased as tolerated to 150 mg/day, with a mean final dose at 8 weeks of 144 mg/day. Among the eight patients who completed at least 4 weeks, all showed at least moderate improvement, with 1 patient being free of symptoms. Comparing the results of this open trial with imipramine to the placebo-controlled trial of fluoxetine, the percentage of patients virtually without symptoms differed considerably depending on the treatment: 50% symptom free for fluoxetine, 16% for placebo, and 12.5% for imipramine. This comparison, although limited by the small sample sizes and differing study design, suggests that the efficacy of imipramine appears to be more modest than that of the serotonin reuptake inhibitor fluoxetine.

## Lessons from the Pharmacologic Treatment of Related Disorders

"Misinterpretation of bodily symptoms" is a component of criterion A for hypochondriasis in *DSM-IV* (American Psychiatric Association, 1994). Because patients who are hypochondriacal will hyperfocus on any bodily symptom, therapeutic interventions that diminish the bodily symptoms themselves may also be helpful. An examination of studies of chronic pain, somatization, chronic fatigue syndrome, and fibromyalgia may shed light on additional strategies for the treatment of hypochondriasis, particularly if the bodily symptoms include pain or fatigue.

### Chronic Pain

Onghena and Van Houdenhove (1992) performed a meta-analysis on 39 placebo-controlled studies and concluded that antidepressants have demonstrated efficacy in providing analgesia in chronic nonmalignant pain. The mean size of the analgesic effect was 0.64. Greater analgesia was associated with (a) tricyclic drugs (imipramine, amitriptyline, doxepin, dothiepin, desipramine, clomipramine, trimipramine, dibenzepine) rather than heterocyclic drugs (mianserin, maprotiline, nomifensine, zimelidine, femoxetine, trazodone); with (b) medicines having a mixed serotonergic and noradrenergic profile (amitriptyline, imipramine, doxepin, dothiepin, trimipramine) rather than medicines that are either primarily serotonergic (zimelidine, trazodone, femoxetine, clomipramine) or noradrenergic (maprotiline, desipramine, dibenzepine, mianserin); and with (c) pain in the head region (migraine, tension headache, central pain, atypical facial pain) rather than pain in other parts of the body. Medicines with at least two placebo-controlled comparisons revealed the following analgesic effect sizes: doxepin (0.96), amitriptyline (0.73), imipramine (0.57), zimelidine (0.45), mianserin (0.35), clomipramine (0.29), and trazodone (0.29).

Only one placebo-controlled study of a monoamine oxidase inhibitor (phenelzine) was included in Onghena and Van Houdenhove's (1992) meta-analysis, with a remarkable effect size of 1.30, but the numerous methodologic problems within that study make interpretation difficult. Another controlled study (Davidson et al., 1987), not included in Onghena and Van Houdenhove's report, found phenelzine (median dose 75 mg/day) to be superior to imipramine (median dose 150 mg/day) and placebo in managing pain/depression syndromes. More recent, controlled studies indicate that selective serotonin reuptake inhibitors (SSRIs) as single therapy and neuroleptic treatment as an adjunct to tricyclic drugs are most likely not effective for pain relief (Krishnan, 1995; Max et al., 1992; Tollefson, 1995; Zitman et al., 1991).

The anticonvulsant gabapentin has been reported to be effective for peripheral and central neuropathic pain syndromes at doses between 2400 mg/day and 3600 mg/day (Attal et al., 1998), with preferential antihyperalgesic and/or antiallodynic effects. Randomized controlled studies confirm the efficacy of gabapentin for pain resulting from postherpetic neuralgia (Rowbotham et al., 1998) and diabetes mellitus (Backonja et al., 1998).

## Somatoform Disorders

Noyes et al. (1998) conducted an 8-week open trial of fluvoxamine in a sample of 29 patients with *DSM-IV* somatoform disorders recruited from a general medicine clinic. Eighteen had one somatoform disorder and 11 had two. In this uncontrolled study, 61% of the 23 patients who completed at least 2 weeks of treatment with fluvoxamine were at least moderately improved on global psychiatric and functional status measures. Of note, patients with and without major depressive disorder responded equally well to fluvoxamine. Further, although measures of anxiety, depression, and insomnia revealed improvement after fluvoxamine treatment, pain was relatively less responsive. This finding is similar to the open fluoxetine trial in treatment of hypochondriasis (Fallon et al., 1993) in which disease fear and conviction improved but not bodily preoccupation.

## Bodily Waste Obsessions

Jenike et al. (1987) presented four cases of patients with primary bowel obsessions characterized by an overwhelming fear of losing bowel control in public. Each patient spent over an hour on the toilet to ensure a complete cleansing of the bowel and each patient planned his or her travels to ensure he or she would not be far from a bathroom. These patients did not have other features of OCD nor did they have irritable bowel syndrome. Two of the 4 patients developed panic attacks after the onset of the bowel obsessions. Treatment with imipramine (dose range: 50–100 mg/day) led to a resolution of the bowel obsessions in 3 patients, and doxepin (150 mg/day) was helpful for the fourth.

Fishbain and Goldberg (1991) reported on a significant improvement after an 8-week treatment with fluoxetine (30 mg/day) of a 28-year-old man who had been obsessively preoccupied with gaseousness and flatulence for about 3 years. The patient received a *DSM-III-R* diagnosis of undifferentiated somatoform disorder, not having qualified for diagnoses of OCD, delusional disorder, and major depression. The preoccupation with the fear of the production and loss of control of malodorous flatulence was considered an overvalued idea, and previously did not respond to various medications, including antipsychotic agents, lithium, a tricyclic antidepressant, and buspirone.

Epstein and Jenike (1990) reported on 2 patients without other OCD features who had primary urinary obsessions characterized by fear of urinary incontinence without organic pathology and extreme efforts to always be near a bathroom. One patient's symptoms markedly diminished after a 6-week treatment with imipramine, 100 mg/day, with improvement sustained over 8 months. The second patient's urinary obsessions failed to improve with an 8-week trial of buspirone (up to 60 mg/day) or diazepam (up to 8 mg/day). He was never treated with imipramine or an SSRI.

## Fibromyalgia

Criteria for fibromyalgia include the major criteria of "generalized aches or stiffness involving three or more anatomic sites for at least three months," not explained by an inflammatory or degenerative musculoskeletal disorder, and "at least six typical and reproducible tender points" (Komaroff and Goldenberg, 1989). Minor criteria symptoms include fatigue, headache, sleep disturbance, neuropsychiatric symptoms, subjective joint swelling, numbness, irritable bowel syndrome, and modulation of symptoms by activity, weather, and stress. A greater number of tender points has been shown to correlate with depression, fatigue, anxiety, and somatic symptoms (Croft *et al.*, 1994; Wolfe *et al.*, 1995). Patients with fibromyalgia have a generalized hypervigilance to both pain and auditory stimuli, now considered to be a reflection of altered central nervous system processing of nociceptive stimuli (Kosek *et al.*, 1995, 1996; McDermid *et al.*, 1996).

Given strong evidence to suggest an association between fibromyalgia and major depression based on overlapping symptoms, patterns of comorbidity, and family history studies, antidepressants have been tested and shown to be helpful at low doses for patients with fibromyalgia. Gruber *et al.* (1996) reviewed thirteen double-blind, placebo-controlled studies and found that drug was statistically significantly superior to placebo on at least one measure in nine of the thirteen studies.

By drug group, a statistically significant improvement in tender point and in other features was noted using the following: tricyclic-type antidepressants (predominantly amitriptyline, 25–50 mg/day; 5 of 7 studies on tender point and 4 of 7 on other features); SSRIs (fluoxetine, 20 mg/day; 0 of 1 study on tender point and 1 of 1 on other features); atypical antidepressants (maprotiline, 75 mg/day; 0 of 1 study on tender point and 0 of 1 on other features); benzodiazepines (0 of 2 studies on tender point and 1 of 2 on other features); and other agents (S-adenosylmethionine, 200–800 mg/day; 0 of 2 studies on tender point and 1 of 2 on other features). A controlled study of citalopram, an SSRI, failed to find a beneficial effect in fibromyalgia (Norregaard et al., 1995). A study published more recently (Goldenberg et al., 1996), not included in the review by Gruber et al. (1996), used a randomized, double-blind, crossover design to examine the efficacy of fluoxetine and amitriptyline for fibromyalgia; it found that the combination of fluoxetine and amitriptyline was more effective than either drug alone.

In a critical analysis of twenty double-blinded controlled drug trials of fibromyalgia, White and Harth (1996) demonstrated that the degree of responsiveness to drug was largely influenced by the way response was measured. Drugs assessed in two or more controlled studies included: amitriptyline, cyclobenzaprine, ibuprofen, S-adenosylmethionine, and zopiclone. On a physician-reported global assessment ordinal or visual analogue scale, drug was more effective than placebo in eight of eleven trials (73%). When response was examined by focusing on specific symptoms, the response rate diminished to 38% for pain, 18% for stiffness, 39% for sleep, and 47% for fatigue. When measures of functional status were used as the outcome measure, the responder rate dropped to 13%. Studies that relied on physician-reported global assessments revealed higher responder rates than did studies using self-reported global assessments (73% versus 41%). White and Harth (1996) conclude by recommending that future studies add outcome measures that are frequently overlooked, such as measures of functional status and psychological distress.

## Chronic Fatigue Syndrome (CFS)

In an 8-week placebo-controlled trial, Vercoulen et al. (1996) examined the efficacy of fluoxetine, 20 mg/day, in a sample of 96 patients with rigorously diagnosed chronic fatigue syndrome (CFS), half with comorbid depression and half without depression. Because no beneficial effect of fluoxetine was observed using self-report measures of depression, physical symptom intensity and functional activity, it seems unlikely that CFS simply represents "masked depression." In a brief placebo-controlled trial of the monoamine oxidase inhibitor phenelzine among 20 patients with CFS without comorbid depression or major Axis I disorder, Natelson *et al.* (1996) found that 15 mg/day was modestly but significantly better than placebo on ratings of functional status, severity of somatic symptoms, and nonaffective components in the Profile of Mood States (McNair *et al.*, 1971).

More recently, based on the observation that many patients with CFS appear to have mild hypocortisolism, Cleare *et al.* (1999) conducted a 4-week placebo-controlled trial of oral hydrocortisone therapy. The results indicated that 5–10 mg/day of hydrocortisone was significantly better than placebo in reducing fatigue and CFS-related disability, with responder rates of 62% for drug-randomized patients versus 22% for placebo-randomized patients.

## Thoughts on the Design and Analysis of Clinical Trials for Hypochondriasis

### Assessing a Disorder with Considerable Flux

Hypochondriasis is a disorder that, while often stable in being present over a long time, also waxes and wanes in severity. Patients come to the physician or researcher when symptomatic, making it likely that time alone would result in a regression to the mean and consequent improvement in symptoms. In a 1-year follow-up study of 50 patients with hypochondriasis, Noyes *et al.* (1994a) found that one-third of the patients no longer met criteria for the diagnosis. The 50 patients as a group reported a substantial (nearly 30%) reduction in hypochondriasis on self-report measures such as the Whiteley Index and the Somatic Symptom Inventory (the Minnesota Multiphasic Personality Inventory [MMPI; Greene, 1991] hypochondriasis scale plus Symptom Checklist-90 [Lipman *et al.*, 1979] somatization scale). These results may be attributed to the fact that patients often seek treatment when symptoms are more severe or that the medical examination and subsequent reassurance were responsible for the symptomatic improvement. Patients with more severe hypochondriasis or longer duration of illness at baseline had a worse outcome.

Because patients with more severe hypochondriasis or longer duration of illness at baseline would be less likely to have a placebo response or a natural improvement over time, future research on hypochondriasis should consider either restricting study to patients with more severe hypochondriasis or randomizing patients with severe hypochondriasis separately from those with less severe hypochondriasis, thereby ensuring a comparable level of severity in the treatment arms. In addition, studies of chronic pain indicate that duration of illness should be examined both in terms of the mean and the minimum duration of illness. Although mean duration of illness may not be associated with outcome, studies of chronic pain have shown that when patients with shorter duration of pain are included in placebo-controlled studies, the effect size is lessened. These duration variables should be examined in hypochondriasis as well.

## Assessing a Disorder in Which Nonspecific Therapeutic Support May Be Helpful

Placebo-controlled drug trials have the design advantage that all patients have the same number of meetings with the clinical and evaluative staff. Psychotherapy or medication studies that employ an active treatment compared to a waitlist control have the disadvantage that at the end of the study the question will still remain whether there was anything specific about the treatment intervention itself rather than simply the supportive effect of regularly scheduled visits with a clinician. The nonspecific therapeutic effects of regularly scheduled meetings may account for the observation in studies of chronic pain that controlled trials where the comparison treatment was "no treatment" yielded larger effect sizes than controlled trials that employed placebo.

## Assessing Global States versus Specific Aspects

Hypochondriasis is a disorder with several dimensions, including the fear of illness, the conviction of illness, awareness of bodily symptoms, avoidance of or attraction to environmental cues that trigger new illness obsessions, and checking for reassurance that one is not ill. Depression and anxiety are common comorbid features. If one measures response solely on the rater's global impression of improvement, one may be unable to distinguish between improvement of mood from improvement of hypochondriasis. Studies therefore need to include separate measures of depression and anxiety. Even if one asks specifically about global improvement in hypochondriasis, one might miss aspects of hypochondriasis that are not improving.

In our open fluoxetine study (Fallon *et al.*, 1993), a statistically significant improvement was noted over 12 weeks in illness fear and illness conviction but not in bodily symptoms, as measured by the subscales of the Whiteley Index. The treatment of somatic preoccupation therefore may require a different approach than the treatment of illness fear or conviction. Supporting the need for assessment that includes global and specific aspects, the review of fibromyalgia studies demonstrates far different responder rates, depending on whether global rating or symptom-specific scales are used.

## Assessing Comorbidity

Studies of hypochondriasis often include very different populations. Regarding psychiatric comorbidity, some studies allow for concurrent depression or panic disorder, whereas others may exclude patients with major Axis I comorbidity (Fallon *et al.*, 1993; Wesner and Noyes, 1991). Regarding medical comorbidity, some studies include a large percentage of patients with comorbid medical illness or functional somatic disorders (Noyes *et al.*, 1994a, 1994b); other studies have excluded these patients (Fallon *et al.*, 1993). The determination of the diagnosis of hypochondriasis is considerably more difficult when a patient has a comorbid medical diagnosis or functional somatic syndrome because of the difficulty in determining whether a patient is worrying excessively and inappropriately about illness.

Some physicians dismiss patients with functional somatic syndromes as having hypochondriasis, a dismissal that ignores the growing body of evidence supporting physiological and biochemical abnormalities among patients with these disorders. For example, SPECT scans indicated heterogeneous hypoperfusion in the brains of patients with CFS (Ichise *et al.*, 1992; Schwartz *et al.*, 1994), and abnormally elevated levels of substance P and antinociceptive peptides were found in the cerebrospinal fluid among patients with fibromyalgia (Russell *et al.*, 1992, 1994).

Given that patients with multiple unexplained medical symptoms may be misdiagnosed as having hypochondriasis, any research study of hypochondriacal patients needs to have a physician independently and carefully review the medical history to ensure that all known medical diseases or syndromes have been ruled out. In a series of 10 patients referred consecutively for the treatment of hypochondriasis by primary care providers, 4 of the 10 patients were not hypochondriacal but had either a medical illness that the referring physician had missed, a functional somatic syndrome as the cause of the patient's symptoms, or excessive concern about a stable medical illness due to physician–patient miscommunication (Fallon, 1999). Reports of treatment studies should include a detailed description of the psychiatric and medical comorbidity of the sample with an analysis to determine whether the presence of significant psychiatric or medical comorbidity was associated with treatment response.

## Creating a Treatment Alliance (see also Chapter 12)

Patients with somatoform disorders may be hard to engage in treatment, and patients with hypochondriasis may be the most reluctant, as Noyes and colleagues (1998) observed in one of their treatment trials. The following clinical recommendations might be helpful. First, a patient with hypochondriasis needs to know that the clinician believes that he or she is ill. Hypochondriacal patients have often been shamed or angered through invalidation by the medical establishment, resulting in a suspicion of any new clinicians. Acknowledgment of the patient's very real distress can be helpful in itself. For our hypochondriasis studies at Columbia University, we use the term "Heightened Illness Concern" to refer to the disorder rather than "hypochondriasis," as the latter term has taken on pejorative connotations and is also inaccurate: Patients are not suffering from a disorder that emanates from below the ribs. Not uncommonly, patients will say: "I'm not a hypochondriac but I do worry about illness."

Second, an initial medical evaluation including physical exam and blood tests can be very helpful to patients by demonstrating that the clinical team is taking their symptoms seriously and can be helpful to the clinician by confirming that the patients do not in fact have a real undetected medical illness. Third, reviewing the patients' Heightened Illness Concern Diary (Table 15.1) at each visit gives patients a sense that their experience is valuable and provides the clinician with a better understanding of the daily vicissitudes of hypochondriasis from which precipitating triggers might be sought. Fourth, if the treatment is a medication trial, patients often respond well to a careful explanation of how the medicine might reduce illness obsessions and distress over bodily symptoms by acting on the neurochemistry of the brain and correcting an imbalance. Equally important is an explanation that the medicine generally takes 4 to 8 weeks before an effect is seen and that initial side effects often abate after the first 2 weeks.

## Data Analyses

Data analyses need to take into account not only outcome analyses based on minimum treatment but also intent-to-treat analyses, particularly because large dropout rates have clinical significance and may reintroduce selection bias into the study despite randomization. Given that medications often have revealing side effects, studies should include ways to determine the effectiveness of blinding by asking both subjects and independent raters to guess to which treatment group the subject was assigned.

## Outcomes

Because there is considerable flux to the natural course of hypochondriasis, clinical trials should include measures over multiple time-points so that the analyses can evaluate improvement over an extended time-interval rather than at just one point in time. Second, outcome should be reassessed 6 months to a year later to determine whether the initial improvement is sustained. Third, outcome measures should include clinically significant measures, such as functional capacity, frequency of health care visits, expenditures, and amount of sick leave and/or hospital days.

## Conclusion

This review leads to the following conclusions. First, secondary hypochondriasis responds well to pharmacologic treatment of the primary disorder. Second, serotonin reuptake inhibitors may be particularly helpful for primary hypochondriasis, and tricyclic antidepressants such as imipramine might be modestly beneficial for patients with hypochondriasis accompanied by good insight. Third, although pharmacotherapy can be helpful for syndromes that might accompany patients with hypochondriasis, such as chronic pain and fibromyalgia, the pharmacologic strategies are by no means identical. For example, for chronic pain or fibromyalgia, lower doses of medicine can be as effective as higher doses, and serotonin reuptake inhibitors appear less effective than tricyclic antidepressants. The role of monoamine oxidase inhibitors for patients with hypochondriasis is unknown, although in chronic pain and CFS this category of medicine might be particularly helpful. Fourth, treatment studies of hypochondriasis should take into consideration severity of hypochondriasis, minimum and mean duration of illness, the hazards of relying upon a wait-list as the control group, the importance of measuring both global and more specific responses to treatment, and the importance of detailed reporting of medical and psychiatric morbidity in the study sample with an assessment of the impact of comorbidity on treatment response.

While there is data to support the recommendation of pharmacologic therapy for patients with hypochondriasis, much of the data is uncontrolled. The one controlled study (Fallon *et al.*, 1996) reported high rates of response after 6 weeks of treatment for both fluoxetine (80%) and placebo (50%). These results, while reflecting only a preliminary analysis of a small number of patients enrolled in an ongoing study, should raise considerable concern about the nonspecific effects that accompany any treatment intervention for patients with hypochondriasis. The common behavioral medicine recommendation that primary care physicians schedule regular supportive care and focused office visits may in fact be a very helpful strategy for patients with hypochondriasis, much as this strategy has been shown to be helpful for patients with somatization disorder (Smith *et al.*, 1986). Whether pharmacologic therapy is actually conferring an additional significant benefit is a question that requires well-designed controlled investigation.

**References**

American Psychiatric Association. 1994. *Diagnostic and Statistical Manual of Mental Disorders, Fourth Edition (DSM-IV)*. Washington, DC: American Psychiatric Association.

Attal N., Brasseur L., Parker F., Chauvin M., Bouhassira D. 1998. Effects of gabapentin on the different components of peripheral and central neuropathic pain syndromes: a pilot study. *European Neurology* 40: 191–200.

Backonja M., Beydoun A., Edwards K.R., Schwartz S.L., Fonseca V., Hes M., LaMoreaux L., Garofalo E. 1998. Gabapentin for the symptomatic treatment of painful neuropathy in patients with diabetes mellitus: a randomized controlled trial. *Journal of the American Medical Association* 280: 1831–1836.

Bodkin J.A., White K. 1989. Clonazepam in the treatment of OCD associated with panic disorder in one patient. *Journal of Clinical Psychiatry* 50: 265–266.

Cleare A.J., Heap E., Malhi G.S., Wessely S., O'Keane V., Miell J. 1999. Low-dose hydrocortisone in chronic fatigue syndrome: a randomized crossover trial. *Lancet* 353: 455–458.

Croft P., Schollum J., Silman A. 1994. Population study of tender point counts and pain as evidence of fibromyalgia. *British Medical Journal* 309: 696–699.

Davidson J., Raft D., Pelton J. 1987. An outpatient evaluation of phenelzine and imipramine. *Journal of Clinical Psychiatry* 48: 143–146.

Epstein S., Jenike M.A. 1990. Disabling urinary obsessions: an uncommon variant of obsessive-compulsive disorder. *Psychosomatics* 31: 450–452.

Fallon B.A. 1999. Somatoform disorders. In *Primary Care Psychiatry and Behavioral Medicine: Brief Office Treatment and Management Pathways.* (eds. Feinstein R.E., Brewer A.A.), New York: Springer Publishing.

Fallon B.A., Javitch J.A., Hollander E., Liebowitz M.R. 1991. Hypochondriasis and obsessive compulsive disorder: overlaps in diagnosis and treatment. *Journal of Clinical Psychiatry* 52: 457–460.

Fallon B.A., Liebowitz M.R., Salman E., Schneier F.R., Jusino C., Hollander E., Klein D.F. 1993. Fluoxetine for hypochondriacal patients without major depression. *Journal of Clinical Psychopharmacology* 13: 438–441.

Fallon B.A., Schneier F.R., Marshall R., Campeas R., Vermes D., Goetz D., Liebowitz M.R. 1996. The pharmacotherapy of hypochondriasis. *Psychopharmacology Bulletin* 32: 607–611.

First M.B., Spitzer R.L., Gibbon M., Williams J.B.W. 1997a. *User's Guide for the Structured Clinical Interview for DSM-IV Axis I Disorders (SCID-I)—Clinician Version.* Washington, DC: American Psychiatric Press.

First M.B., Gibbon M., Spitzer R.L., Williams J.B.W., Benjamin L.S. 1997b. *User's Guide for the Structured Clinical Interview for DSM-IV Axis II Personality Disorders (SCID-II).* Washington, DC: American Psychiatric Press.

Fishbain D.A., Goldberg M. 1991. Fluoxetine for obsessive fear of loss of control of malodorous flatulence. *Psychosomatics* 32: 105–107.

Fishbain D.A., Barsky S., Goldberg M. 1992. Monosymptomatic hypochondriacal psychosis: belief of contracting rabies. *International Journal of Psychiatry in Medicine* 22: 3–9.

Freed E. 1983. AIDophobia. *Medical Journal of Australia* 2: 479.

Goldenberg D.L., Mayskiy M., Mossey C.J., Ruthazer R., Schmid C. 1996. A randomized, double-blind crossover trial of fluoxetine and amitriptyline in the treatment of fibromyalgia. *Arthritis and Rheumatism* 39: 1852–1859.

Goodman W.K., Rasmussen S.A., Price L.H., Mazure C., Heninger G., Charney D.S. 1989. *The Yale–Brown Obsessive-Compulsive Scale (Y-BOCS).* New Haven, CT: Clinical Neuroscience Research Unit, Connecticut Mental Health Center.

Greene R.L. 1991. *The MMPI-2/MMPI: An Interpretive Manual.* Boston: Allyn & Bacon.

Gruber A.J., Hudson J.I., Pope H.G. 1996. The management of treatment-resistant depression in disorders on the interface of psychiatry and medicine. *Psychiatric Clinics of North America* 19: 351–369.

Guy W. 1976. *Early Clinical Drug Evaluation (ECDEU) Assessment Manual for Psychopharmacology. Publication No. 76-338.* Rockville, MD: National Institute of Mental Health.

Hamilton M. 1959. The assessment of anxiety states by rating. *British Journal of Medical Psychology* 32: 50–55.

Hamilton M. 1960. A rating scale for depression. *Journal of Neurology, Neurosurgery and Psychiatry* 23: 56–62.

Ichise M., Salit I.E., Abbey S.E., Chung D.G., Gray B., Kirsh J.C., Freedman M. 1992. Assessment of regional cerebral blood perfusion by 99Tcm-HMPAO SPECT in chronic fatigue syndrome. *Nuclear Medicine Communications* 13: 767–772.

Jenike M.A., Pato C. 1986. Disabling fear of AIDS responsive to imipramine. *Psychosomatics* 27: 143–144.

Jenike M.A., Vitagliano H.L., Rabinowitz J., Goff D.C., Baer L. 1987. Bowel obsessions responsive to tricyclic antidepressants in four patients. *American Journal of Psychiatry* 144: 1347–1348.

Kamlana S.H., Gray P. 1988. Fear of AIDS (letter). *British Journal of Psychiatry* 15: 1291.

Kellner R., Abbott P., Pathak D., Winslow W.W., Umland B.E. 1983–84. Hypochondriacal beliefs and attitudes in family practice and psychiatric patients. *International Journal of Psychiatry in Medicine* 13: 127–139.

Kellner R., Fava G.A., Lisansky J., Perini G.I., Zielezny M. 1986. Hypochondriacal fears and beliefs in DSM-III melancholia: changes with amitriptyline. *Journal of Affective Disorders* 10: 21–26.

Komaroff A., Goldenberg D. 1989. The chronic fatigue syndrome: definition, current studies and lessons for fibromyalgia research. *Journal of Rheumatology* 16 (Suppl. 19): S23–S27.

Kosek E., Ekholm J., Hansson P. 1995. Increased pressure pain sensibility in fibromyalgia patients is located deep in the skin but not restricted to muscle tissue. *Pain* 63: 335–339.

Kosek E., Ekholm J., Hansson P. 1996. Modulation of pressure pain thresholds during and following isometric contraction in patients with fibromyalgia and in healthy controls. *Pain* 64: 415–423.

Krishnan K.R.R. 1995. Monoamine oxidase inhibitors. In *Textbook of Psychopharmacology* (eds. Schatzberg A.F., Nemeroff C.B.), Washington DC: American Psychiatric Press.

Lesse S. 1967. Hypochondriasis and psychosomatic disorders masking depression. *American Journal of Psychotherapy* 21: 607–620.

Lipman R.S., Covi L., Shapiro A.K. 1979. The Hopkins Symptom Checklist (HSCL): factors derived from the HSCL-90. *Journal of Affective Disorders* 1: 9–24.

Lippert G.P. 1986. Excessive concern about AIDS in two bisexual men. *Canadian Journal of Psychiatry* 31: 63–65.

Max M.B., Lynch S.A., Muir J., Shoaf S.E., Smoller B., Dubner R. 1992. Effects of desipramine, amitriptyline, and fluoxetine on pain in diabetic neuropathy. *New England Journal of Medicine* 326: 1250–1256.

McDermid A.J., Rollman G.B., McCain G.A. 1996. Generalized hypervigilance in fibromyalgia: evidence of perceptual amplification. *Pain* 66: 133–144.

McNair D.M., Lorr M., Droppleman L.F. 1971. *Profile of Mood Sates.* San Diego: Educational and Industrial Testing Services.

Natelson B.H., Cheu J., Pareja J., Ellis S.P., Poliscastro T., Findley T.W. 1996. Randomized, double-blind, controlled placebo-phase in trial of low dose phenelzine in the chronic fatigue syndrome. *Psychopharmacology* 124: 226–230.

Norregaard J., Volkmann H., Danneskiold-Samsoe B. 1995. A randomized controlled trial of citalopram in the treatment of fibromyalgia. *Pain* 61: 445–449.

Noyes R., Reich J., Clancy J., O'Gorman T.W. 1986. Reduction in hypochondriasis with treatment of panic disorder. *British Journal of Psychiatry* 149: 631–635.

Noyes R., Kathol R.G., Fisher M.M., Phillips B.M., Suelzer M.T., Woodman C.L. 1994a. One-year follow-up of medical outpatients with hypochondriasis. *Psychosomatics* 35: 533–545.

Noyes R., Kathol R.G., Fisher M.M., Phillips B., Suelzer M.T., Woodman C.L. 1994b. Psychiatric comorbidity among patients with hypochondriasis. *General Hospital Psychiatry* 16: 78–87.

Noyes R., Happel R., Muller B., Holt C.S., Kathol R.G., Sieren L., Amos J. 1998. Fluvoxamine for somatoform disorders: an open trial. *General Hospital Psychiatry* 20: 339–344.

Onghena P., Van Houdenhove B. 1992. Antidepressant-induced analgesia in chronic nonmalignant pain: a meta-analysis of 39 placebo-controlled studies. *Pain* 49: 205–219.

Pilowsky I. 1967. Dimensions of hypochondriasis. *British Journal of Psychiatry* 113: 89–93.

Pilowsky I. 1968. The response to treatment in hypochondriacal disorders. *Australian and New Zealand Journal of Psychiatry* 2: 88–94.

Pilowsky I., Spence N.D. 1975. Patterns of illness behaviour in patients with intractable pain. *Journal of Psychosomatic Research* 19: 279–287.

Rowbotham M., Harden N., Stacey B., Bernstein P., Magnus-Miller L. 1998. Gabapentin for the treatment of postherpetic neuralgia: a randomized controlled trial. *Journal of the American Medical Association* 280: 1837–1842.

Russell I.J., Vaeroy H., Javors M., Nyberg F. 1992. Cerebrospinal fluid biogenic amine metabolites in fibromyalgia/fibrositis syndrome and rheumatoid arthritis. *Arthritis and Rheumatism* 35: 550–556.

Russell I.J., Orr M.D., Littman B., Vipraio G.A., Alboukrek D., Michalek J.E., Lopez Y., MacKillip F. 1994. Elevated cerebrospinal fluid levels of substance P in patients with the fibromyalgia syndrome. *Arthritis and Rheumatism* 37: 1593–1601

Scarone S., Gambini S. 1991. Delusional hypochondriasis: nosographic evaluation, clinical course and therapeutic outcome of 5 cases. *Psychopathology* 24: 179–184.

Schwartz R.B., Komaroff A.L., Garada B.M., Gleit M., Doolittle T.H., Bates D.W., Vasile R.G., Holman B.L. 1994. SPECT imaging of the brain: comparison of findings in patients with chronic fatigue syndrome, AIDS dementia complex, and major unipolar depression. *American Journal of Roentgenology* 162: 943–951.

Smith G.R., Monson R.A., Ray D.C. 1986. Psychiatric consultation in somatization disorder: a randomized controlled study. *New England Journal of Medicine* 314: 1407–1413.

Stone A.B. 1993. Treatment of hypochondriasis with clomipramine (letter). *Journal of Clinical Psychiatry* 54: 200–201.

Tollefson G.D. 1995. Selective serotonin reuptake inhibitors. In *Textbook of Psychopharmacology* (eds. Schatzberg A.F., Nemeroff C.B.), Washington DC: American Psychiatric Press.

Vercoulen J.H.M.M., Swainink C.M.A., Zitman F.G., Vreden S.G.S., Hoofs M.P.E., Fennis J.F.M., Galaga J.M.D., van der Meer J.W.M., Bleijenberg G. 1996. Randomized, double-blind, placebo-controlled study of fluoxetine in chronic fatigue syndrome. *Lancet* 347: 858–861.

Viswanathan R., Paradis C. 1991. Treatment of cancer phobia with fluoxetine. *American Journal of Psychiatry* 148: 1090.

Ware J.E., Sherbourne C.D. 1992. The MOS 36–Item Short-Form Health Survey (SF-36). *Medical Care* 30: 473–483.

Wesner R.B., Noyes R. 1991. Imipramine: an effective treatment for illness phobia. *Journal of Affective Disorders* 22: 43–48.

White K.P., Harth M. 1996. An analytical review of 24 controlled clinical trials for fibromyalgia syndrome (FMS). *Pain* 64: 211–219.

Wolfe F., Ross K., Anderson J., Russell I.J., Hebert L. 1995. The prevalence and characteristics of fibromyalgia in the general population. *Arthritis and Rheumatism* 38: 19–28.

Zitman F.G., Linssen A.C.G., Edelbroek P.M., Van Kempen G.M.J. 1991. Does addition of low-dose flupentixol enhance the analgesic effects of low-dose amitriptyline in somatoform pain disorder? *Pain* 47: 25–30.

# Epilogue

# Epilogue

DON R. LIPSITT
VLADAN STARCEVIC

This book comes to its close as the world celebrates its transition to a new millennium. Among a plethora of transitional images and cosmic questions, we associate the subject of the book—hypochondriasis—to a well-known painting by Paul Gauguin, searchingly titled "Whence do we come? What are we? Whither are we going?" In this final chapter, we approach our subject with a similar philosophic "longitudinal" view as we offer a summary and a conceptual synthesis not unlike the narrative sweep portrayed in Gaugin's painting.

We will consider lessons from the two-millennium history of hypochondriasis, its present status, and some perspectives on the future study of this disorder. Gaugin's paintings often conveyed melancholy, but almost always—even as he approached death—conveyed serenity and hope. We can only hope that, through our probing, the ancient malady of hypochondriasis, though as yet incompletely understood and imperfectly treated, will yield greater clarity and reduced suffering as we enter the new millennium.

## History Lessons

The opening chapter on the history of hypochondriasis reminds us that today hypochondriasis is no less a "challenge to medicine" than it was in previous centuries. Many views on hypochondriasis, now considered obsolete, have been abandoned. Yet, remarkably, certain "ancient" concepts and attitudes have withstood the test of time, and some have paved the way for models of hypochondriasis that now are considered products of "modern" times.

The observation made more than a hundred years ago that hypochondriasis had "a very wide meaning" (Savage, 1892) seems still to hold true today. More than three centuries ago, two important writers of the time, Molière and Cervantes, posited descriptive and explanatory models of hypochondriasis: One model portrays a "neurotic" and personality-associated form of the disorder, while the other describes a psychotic, delusional illness with hypochondriacal features. These models do not appear obsolete today, with the former corresponding to the concept of primary hypochondriasis, and the latter to delusional disorder, somatic type. The common difficulty acknowledged today in distinguishing between the two had been recognized as long ago as the early eighteenth century. And more than two centuries ago, a patient with hypochondriasis was described as "an object of derision and contempt," with symptoms regarded by others as "imaginary" (Blackmore, 1725), a bias that sadly persists today, readily reported by contemporary authors.

We see a striking consistency in the "antiquated" descriptions of hypochondriasis from Sydenham and Willis in the seventeenth century to the more "modern" notions of nineteenth-century writers like Guislain, Rush, and others. Many physicians had observed the essence of hypochondriasis to be worry over affection with an "imaginary" disease (Guislain, 1852; Rush, 1812; Willis, 1685), even while the suffering of hypochondriacal patients could be viewed as "real and unfeigned" (Blackmore, 1725). In some "archaic" writings, we can detect the "precursors" of some contemporary etiological models of hypochondriasis. Thus, it was speculated that the symptoms of hypochondriasis were the result of "wrong thinking" (Blackmore, 1725), excessive attention to body and bodily sensations (Feuchtersleben, 1847; Griesinger, 1861), amplification of bodily symptoms (Cotard, 1888), and misinterpretation of bodily sensations (Krafft-Ebing, 1893).

With such continuity in the conceptualization of hypochondriasis and the attendant, remarkable similarities, what, we may ask, has *really* changed in our understanding of hypochondriasis and what is *really* new in our approach to this disorder? We will consider these questions in the next section.

## The Present Status of Hypochondriasis

That hypochondriasis is an abnormal condition, very few would question today. Although usually regarded as a mental disorder, its conceptual status is uncertain. Disagreements prevail mainly in the realm of the utility and validity of current definitions and diagnostic concepts of primary hypochondriasis (i.e., hypochondriasis that is not considered a part of another disorder). Thus, the question of whether primary hypochondriasis is a valid and independent diagnostic category remains unanswered, although there is more evidence in support of an affirmative answer to this question. Likewise, although much has evolved to enhance the psychotherapeutic approach to the treatment of hypochondriasis, disagreements persist about preferred treatment techniques and goals. Let us consider current issues in the status of hypochondriasis.

## Diagnostic Matters and Classification of Hypochondriasis

Current conceptualizations of hypochondriasis rely on the diagnostic criteria in the classifications of mental disorders (*DSM-IV* [American Psychiatric Association, 1994] and ICD-10 [World Health Organization, 1992; 1993]). Essentially, there are two components of the disorder, one of which is *affective*, the other *cognitive*. The former pertains to the fear of a disease believed already to exist, but yet undetected, and the latter to a suspicion of the presence of such a disease. In contemporary language, the affective component is referred to by the sometimes overlapping terms "health anxiety," "disease fear," "disease phobia," and "illness worry," whereas the cognitive component is often referred to as "disease belief" and "disease conviction." It remains uncertain whether a predominance of one or another of these two components in the clinical picture of hypochondriasis defines two distinct subtypes of the disorder (Fallon, 1999; Kellner *et al.*, 1992). A behavioral component of hypochondriasis—in the form of obsessive-compulsive health-checking, repeated medical examinations, excessive preoccupation with bodily functioning and appearance, and with matters of health, illness, and the like—is a derivative of hypochondriacal disease fears and disease suspicions.

The refusal by many hypochondriacal patients to accept appropriate medical reassurance is often seen as an essential part of the current and specific definition of hypochondriasis, a diagnostic criterion that is a twentieth-century development. However, this recent addition has probably created the greatest controversy and has been criticized on several grounds. First, the patient's rejection of adequate and credible medical reassurance tends to blur the boundary between hypochondriasis and psychosis. In Chapters 2 and 13, it was noted that "appropriate" medical reassurance has been imprecisely defined, and it was proposed that a distinction be made between "routine" reassurance on the one hand, and complex, process-like, and explanation-oriented reassurance on the other, because hypochondriacal patients often do respond to the latter.

In Chapter 11, Pilowsky criticizes the "reassurance criterion" for a diagnosis of hypochondriasis on the grounds that this dimension of diagnosis implies that the diagnosis can be affirmed only "if there is a fundamental disagreement between the doctor and the patient." Pilowsky further argues that the ability to provide reassurance is "distorted" by imposed changes in the contemporary patient–physician relationship. Another view of the patient's rejection of medical reassurance as a diagnostic criterion for hypochondriasis comes from Gureje and associates (1997), who note that diagnostic adherence to this criterion *hampers* rather than *facilitates*, detection of hypochondriacal individuals in primary car

When this criterion was ignored, it was possible to estimate the prevalence of hypochondriasis more accurately, and the disorder was identified more than twice as often on the basis of its other, essential characteristics. Clearly, it is just such controversial points that call for reconsideration of the role of reassurance in the next revision of the diagnostic criteria for hypochondriasis.

Hypochondriasis is presently classified among the somatoform disorders, but many subscribe to the view that it may better be conceptualized as an anxiety or personality disorder and reclassified under those rubrics. This dissatisfaction with nosological "placement" of hypochondriasis stems from several sources: One is a general dissatisfaction with the broad group of somatoform disorders (Martin, 1999; Ono and Janca, 1999; Reid and Wessely, 1999) to which hypochondriasis "officially" belongs; the other is a view, espoused especially by cognitive therapists (e.g., Wells, 1997), that hypochondriasis is more strongly associated with anxiety, and that it is therefore a genuine anxiety disorder. The position that hypochondriasis should be reconceptualized as a personality disorder rests mainly on the longitudinal stability of the diagnosis of hypochondriasis and on certain trait-like characteristics of this condition (Tyrer et al., 1990).

Although retention of hypochondriasis among the somatoform disorders may be less than satisfactory, it does not seem that there is sufficient evidence presently to justify reclassification. Efforts to find a better nosological "solution" for hypochondriasis should go hand-in-hand with efforts to determine whether some of the proposed "subtypes" of hypochondriasis should be classified elsewhere (e.g., "disease phobia") among the anxiety disorders. The need to conceptualize the entire group of somatoform disorders in a more valid and meaningful way has already attracted robust attention (Bass and Murphy, 1990; Deary, 1999; Escobar and Gara, 1999; Martin, 1999; Wessely et al., 1999).

## Etiology and Pathogenesis of Hypochondriasis

Although still poorly understood, there is no shortage of theories about the etiology of hypochondriasis; the shortage would appear to prevail more in the dearth of carefully designed research studies that can test underlying assumptions and hypotheses.

Several etiologic and explanatory models of hypochondriasis dominate the field at the beginning of the twenty-first century. Briefly, these models are psychodynamic, behavioral, and cognitive. According to them, hypochondriasis may be conceived of as an enduring defensive style, an expression of an underlying conflict, a pattern of learned and reinforced maladaptive behavior, or a disorder of attention, perception, and/or thinking. These models do not necessarily exclude each other, and they may be integrated in a comprehensive explanatory model. The cognitive model, reviewed in Chapter 9 and centering on the notion of "catastrophic" misinterpretation of benign somatic sensations and misattribution of these sensations to a serious disease, has been particularly influential. Another model, elaborated and recently reviewed in Chapter 10, is that of somatosensory amplification. The psychodynamic model, discussed in Chapter 8, provides a basic foundation on which to build other therapeutic efforts. Psychodynamic and psychoanalytic treatment in and of themselves are not generally applicable to hypochondriacal patients whose orientation is most often one in search of physical (not psychological) explanation. However, the concepts of transference and countertransference help the physician immeasurably to understand and "get some distance" on the nuances of interpersonal interaction with hypochondriacal patients.

One of the main problems pertaining to etiology and pathogenesis of hypochondriasis is a difficulty in distinguishing among causes, consequences, and mere correlates or epiphenomena. For example, does misinterpretation of benign bodily sensations precede or follow the onset of hypochondriasis? Does low self-esteem play a role in causing hypochondriasis (so that hypochondriasis serves as a defense against low self-esteem) or is low self-esteem a consequence of hypochondriasis? Are any of the purported etiological factors merely correlates of hypochondriasis?

A related issue is the nature of primary disturbance. Is hypochondriasis primarily a disorder of amplification, altered perception, or overreporting of bodily sensations? This problem is perhaps best illustrated by the contradictory results of the studies of somatosensory amplification and accuracy of perception of somatic sensations, reviewed in Chapter 10. Although earlier studies (e.g., Tyrer *et al.*, 1980) supported the notion that hypochondriacal patients might be more sensitive to bodily sensations (i.e., that they perceived them more accurately), later it was discovered that hypochondriacal patients were less accurate perceivers of bodily sensations than were nonhypochondriacal individuals (Barsky *et al.*, 1995). Barsky notes that hypochondriasis is characterized by a "global proclivity to describe one's sensations as more uncomfortable," which may indicate that this disorder reflects a primary disturbance in the style of reporting somatic sensations. Barsky has also hypothesized that, in hypochondriasis, there may be a defect in somatic "stimulus barrier," as a result of which hypochondriacal patients are flooded with bodily sensations they cannot control.

Our current understanding of hypochondriasis is primarily that of the factors that maintain the disorder, not an understanding of the factors that initiate it. Thus, we know that heightened and selective attention to bodily events increases the likelihood of perceiving bodily sensations, and that one's mistrust in his or her own body makes "catastrophic" misinterpretations of innocuous bodily sensations more likely, thus reinforcing hypochondriacal concerns. However, the questions of why hypochondriacal individuals harbor more mistrust and why they are so "body-oriented" are usually answered with speculations that are left un-supported by objective data. Therefore, these fundamental questions about etiol-ogy remain essentially unanswered.

## Interpersonal and Social Aspects of Hypochondriasis

Patients with hypochondriasis continue to be disliked, avoided, and rejected. At-titudes toward them are less openly hostile than they were in the past, but this, unfortunately, does not appear to reflect greater compassion or higher tolerance for patients whose illness has a tendency to "get under the skin." Rather, it may now be more "vogueish" or a matter of "political correctness" to say that these are "difficult" patients (and not "crocks"), and that in most cases, their progno-sis is "poor" (and not that they are "incurable"). Thus, hypochondriacal patients continue to be stigmatized, and terms like "hypochondriasis" and "hypochon-driac" continue to carry derogatory connotations, as underscored by several con-tributors to this book.

To counteract the negative attitude toward hypochondriacal patients, some have proposed renaming hypochondriasis as "health anxiety disorder" (Rief and Hiller, 1998); Fallon and his associates use the term "heightened illness concern" in their work with hypochondriacal patients (see Chapter 15). But regardless of the name under which it appears, hypochondriasis is bound to "show its true face" when it emerges in the frustrating interactions of patients with their families, friends, and physicians. Although a laudable effort, any attempt to destigmatize patients with hypochondriasis by renaming their disorder is overridden by the negative connotations that have been entrenched for several centuries now.

Education of the general public and of physicians in particular may offer greater hope as a strategy for combating the stigma. In that process, special attention will need to be paid to the underlying, specific, and sometimes idiosyncratic causes of "sensitivity" to hypochondriacal patients usually predictive of discordant in-teractions with them. These causes can range from simple impatience to the un-dermining of the physician's self-image and identity caused by the patient's persistent and "unjustified" failure to get better. In most medical schools, the bias toward "difficult" patients may have its roots in the dualistic educational process that assigns greater valence to the biomedical than to the psychosocial aspects of human health and disease.

A more "modern" reason for harboring antagonistic feelings toward hypochon-driacal patients is related to health economics. Because these patients are exces-sive utilizers of more and more expensive health care services (which somehow must be paid for), they are not only "enemies to joy and hope" (Sydenham, 1850) of an earlier time, but they have more recently become "virtual enemies of the state" (Chapter 11). Health insurance companies and state insurance programs are not sanguine about covering the expenses of "unnecessary" medical examinations and of the "whimsical" illness behavior of hypochondriacal patients. These individuals are often alluded to dismissively as "the worried well" (rather than "the worried sick"). Managed care has focused to some extent on the problems of high cost of health care for hypochondriacal patients (or, indeed, for all somatizing illnesses) by attempting to contain patients within the system of primary care, with a single primary care physician "in charge" of each patient. Without involving an extensive educational process, there is evidence that an operational approach can reap economic benefits; a study by Smith and colleagues (1986) demonstrated very significant savings by having primary physicians follow a strict protocol in the form of a written "consultative letter" with somatizing patients.

## Treatment of Hypochondriasis

Although there is today little justification for regarding hypochondriacal patients as the physician's "hopeless cases" (Morel, 1860), therapeutic nihilism about hypochondriasis remains prevalent. This may be a consequence of the complexity of the treatment of primary hypochondriasis and its demands of time and commitment of both patient and physician. Today we are certainly equipped to help hypochondriacal patients; the main question is whether we wish to engage in a therapeutic process that often tests our patience, has an uncertain outcome, reminds us of our own vulnerabilities and limitations, frustrates our need to help, and undermines our sense of professional function.

Treatment principles in hypochondriasis have been outlined in Chapters 12 and 13, and other references to the salient treatment issues appear throughout this text. The therapeutic relationship between the patient and the physician is a cornerstone of the successful treatment of hypochondriasis. In our view, such a relationship is both a prerequisite for use of other treatment techniques and a treatment modality itself. The key elements in the therapeutic patient–physician relationship in hypochondriasis are the consistency of the interactions and the patient's development of a sense of firm interpersonal trust.

Psychotherapy is usually used as the main treatment modality in primary hypochondriasis that is uncomplicated by psychiatric comorbidity, although there is little controlled research into the efficacy of specific psychotherapies in hypochondriasis. A few controlled studies have demonstrated that cognitive therapy (Bouman and Visser, 1998; Clark *et al.*, 1998), cognitive-behavioral therapy (Warwick *et al.*, 1996), behavior therapy based on exposure *in vivo* and response prevention techniques (Bouman and Visser, 1998), and behavioral stress management (Clark *et al.*, 1998) are effective. Nonetheless, most hypochondriacal patients, especially those who seek help in primary care, are not likely to be treated by these highly elaborate procedures and techniques, which are offered in a relatively few specialized centers by appropriately trained therapists. Most patients with hypochondriasis in the real world of clinical practice are treated by other kinds of psychotherapy, usually of a supportive nature. While the value of these therapies remains unproven by controlled studies, clinical experience suggests that they may be useful, perhaps insofar as they pay attention to the subtleties of the patient–physician relationship and contribute to the establishment of a trusting therapeutic relationship.

Specific forms of psychotherapy are used when general indications for their use are present. Another important factor in the choice of psychotherapy is the postulation of treatment goals (Tables 1 and 2).

Treatment goals more specific or even unique to hypochondriasis (e.g., disappearance of the tendency to misinterpret somatic sensations and of related disease concerns; elimination of the excessive attention to bodily sensations and changes in the pattern of perception and attributional style so that patients learn to perceive their somatic sensations more accurately and to attribute them to innocuous causes) are particularly emphasized in cognitive therapy, cognitive-behavioral therapy, and cognitive-educational therapy. Treatment goals that are less associated with hypochondriasis *per se* (e.g., resolution of intrapsychic conflicts and acquisition of insight) characterize psychodynamically-oriented therapy and psychoanalysis, and these goals have been reported in detail in psychoanalytic case studies. Behavioral stress management and psychotherapy with systematic medical reassurance are concerned approximately equally with the specific and the more general treatment goals; thus, they emphasize both symptom relief and explanation of symptoms to hypochondriacal patients, as well

**Table 16.1.** Treatment considerations for hypochondriasis

I. Treatment setting

- Primary care (preferable)
- Psychiatric—more suitable for:
    1. Patients willing to undergo psychiatric treatment
    2. Patients with severe hypochondriasis and/or longer duration of illness
    3. Patients with numerous complications and greatly diminished quality of life
    4. Patients with psychiatric comorbidity and severe personality disturbance

II. There are no established "first-line" treatments for hypochondriasis, and the choice of treatment is determined by:

1. Treatment goals
2. Severity and duration of hypochondriasis
3. Presence of psychiatric comorbidity
4. Presence of personality disorders
5. Patient preferences (e.g., attitude toward medications, willingness to engage in long-term psychotherapy, etc.)

**Table 16.2.** Choice of treatment for hypochondriasis based on treatment goals

| If treatment goal is: | The choice of treatment is: |
| --- | --- |
| • Improved functioning and better quality of life | 1. All psychotherapies<br>2. Pharmacotherapy |
| • Alleviation of hypochondriacal fears and suspicions, freedom from excessive bodily preoccupation, and disappearance of repeated reassurance-seeking behavior | 1. All psychotherapies (more so in medical reassurance, cognitive-educational therapy, cognitive therapy* and behavioral stress management)<br>2. Pharmacotherapy |
| • Improved coping with symptoms (better control of symptoms) | 1. Medical reassurance<br>2. Cognitive-educational therapy<br>3. Behavioral stress management |
| • Assuring patients about benign nature of their symptoms | 1. Medical reassurance |
| • Better understanding of perception and reporting of physical symptoms | 1. Cognitive-educational therapy |
| • Better understanding of symptoms | 1. Medical reassurance<br>2. Cognitive-educational therapy<br>3. Cognitive therapy* |
| • Elimination of catastrophic misinterpretation of symptoms | 1. Cognitive therapy* |
| • Counteracting a sense of low self-esteem and excessive perception of personal vulnerability | 1. Medical reassurance<br>2. Psychodynamically oriented psychotherapy, psychoanalysis |
| • Better understanding of interpersonal and emotional difficulties and improvement in interpersonal functioning | 1. Medical reassurance<br>2. Behavioral stress management<br>3. Psychodynamically oriented psychotherapy, psychoanalysis |
| • Acquisition of insight into a relationship between hypochondriacal features and the underlying conflicts and deficits | 1. Psychodynamically oriented psychotherapy, psychoanalysis |

*Cognitive therapy also includes cognitive-behavioral therapy.

as shifting a focus of their attention from bodily events to their interpersonal problems, stressors, and emotions.

The use of pharmacotherapy alone is rare. Only one double-blind study shows that a medication (fluoxetine) is effective in hypochondriasis (Fallon *et al.*, 1996). However, there was a high placebo response in that study, suggesting the importance of nonspecific factors and the patient–physician relationship (Chapter 15).

Selective serotonin reuptake inhibitors may be particularly indicated for those forms of primary hypochondriasis that resemble obsessive-compulsive disorder. Insofar as one can be guided by analogy with results of the treatment studies of related disorders, psychotherapy of hypochondriasis may offer an advantage over pharmacotherapy in that its effects are likely to persist over longer periods of time. The practice of administering antipsychotic drugs to patients with hypochondriasis in the absence of clear-cut somatic (hypochondriacal) delusions is not justified and should be discouraged.

Pharmacotherapy (usually with antidepressants) and psychotherapy may be combined, either from the beginning of treatment or sequentially. Such a combination is usually used in patients with more severe and more chronic forms of hypochondriasis, and in those with comorbid psychiatric conditions, such as various anxiety and depressive disorders (Tables 3 and 4). Pharmacotherapy may be added to psychotherapy if there is no response or only a partial response to psychotherapy. However, it is not known how long a patient with hypochondriasis should be treated with psychotherapy before a medication is added.

Although there is no consensus among experts on the "first-line" treatments or "treatments of choice" for hypochondriasis, we have presented treatment recommendations and guidelines in Tables 1 through 4 on the basis of both con-

**Table 16.3.** Treatment choice for hypochondriasis based on severity and duration of condition and presence of psychiatric comorbidity and personality disorders

| Basis for making the choice | Choice of treatment |
| --- | --- |
| • Greater severity and longer duration of hypochondriasis | 1. Pharmacotherapy<br>2. Psychodynamically oriented psychotherapy, psychoanalysis<br>3. Combination of pharmacotherapy and psychotherapy (more so with medical reassurance) |
| • Presence of psychiatric comorbidity | 1. Pharmacotherapy<br>2. Combination of pharmacotherapy and psychotherapy (more so with medical reassurance) |
| • Presence of personality disorders | 1. Long-term psychotherapy*<br>2. Combination of psychotherapy and pharmacotherapy† |

*The type of psychotherapy used depends on general indications for its use and on the specific personality disorder. For example, *psychodynamically oriented psychotherapy and psychoanalysis* are more often used and appear more suitable in the treatment of obsessive-compulsive, histrionic and narcissistic personality disorders. *Medical reassurance* should not be used at all, or should be used very cautiously in the later stages of treatment of patients with paranoid, schizoid, and borderline personality disorders.

†Medications may be used as an adjunct to psychotherapy in some patients with specific personality disorders (see Table 4).

**Table 16.4.** General guidelines for pharmacotherapy in hypochondriasis

I. Medications of choice in the absence of psychiatric comorbidity

1st: SSRIs: fluoxetine, fluvoxamine
   a) Usually in higher doses
   b) Longer treatment preferable
2nd: TCAs:
   a) If associated with chronic pain: imipramine, amitriptyline (lower doses?)
   b) Clomipramine (lower or higher doses?)
   c) Imipramine preferable for "illness phobia" ("hypochondriasis with good insight")?

II. Medications of choice in the presence of psychiatric comorbidity

- Major depressive disorder, dysthymia:
   SSRIs (1st), TCAs (2nd), other (newer) antidepressants (3rd)
- Panic disorder:
   SSRIs (1st), clomipramine or imipramine (2nd), HPBDZ (3rd)
- Generalized anxiety disorder:
   SSRIs (1st), venlafaxine (2nd), TCAs (3rd), BDZ or buspirone (4th)
- Obsessive-compulsive disorder:
   SSRIs (1st), clomipramine (2nd)

III. Medications to be used as an adjunct to psychotherapy in the presence of specific personality disorders

- Borderline personality disorder:
   Antidepressants, carbamazepine, low-dose antipsychotic drugs
- Schizotypal personality disorder:
   Low-dose antipsychotic drugs
- Schizoid personality disorder:
   Low-dose antipsychotic drugs, BDZ, antidepressants
- Avoidant personality disorder:
   Antidepressants, BDZ, buspirone

SSRIs = selective serotonin reuptake inhibitors;
TCAs = tricyclic antidepressants;
HPBDZ = high-potency benzodiazepines (alprazolam, clonazepam);
BDZ = benzodiazepines.

trolled and uncontrolled studies, and also on the basis of clinical experience, case reports, and accounts of particular treatment modalities.

## Directions for the Future Study of Hypochondriasis

Despite advances in diagnosis and better treatment options, our knowledge of hypochondriasis remains comparatively meager, and we cannot be satisfied with our means of helping the patients. Fortunately, exciting prospects for the future study of hypochondriasis are emerging. This pertains particularly to the fact that we now have several reliable and valid instruments for the assessment of hypochondriasis (reviewed in Chapter 3) that are suitable for use in clinical and epidemiological research. Also, we are now able to test the criteria for various concepts and entities associated with hypochondriasis or that overlap with it. This would help us distinguish between hypochondriacal and nonhypochondriacal somatization, between hypochondriasis with "high insight" and hypochondriasis with "low insight" (Fallon, 1999), and between hypochondriasis as a mental state disorder and "hypochondriacal personality disorder" (Tyrer *et al.*, 1990). It would also clarify terms such as "health anxiety," "disease phobia," "thanatophobia" (all of them defined in Chapter 4), and "illness phobia" (Wesner and Noyes, 1991), as well as their relationship to hypochondriasis. As a result, the definitional boundary of the concept of hypochondriasis would be established more firmly.

Another "boundary issue" is the excessive internal heterogeneity of hypochondriasis. Future studies should address this problem by examining whether subtypes of hypochondriasis could be defined more clearly and then subjected to a process of diagnostic validation. Another approach to reducing the heterogeneity of hypochondriasis is to use the spectrum model, acknowledging that there is a wide range of hypochondriacal manifestations—from behaviors and attitudes that hardly depart from normality to a psychotic illness. As a first step, this approach calls for a careful delineation of entities that lie along the proposed spectrum of hypochondriacal manifestations.

The complex nature of the cognitive changes elucidated thus far in hypochondriasis suggests that studies of the etiology and pathogenesis of hypochondriasis would benefit from research paradigms that simultaneously take into account attention and perception, patterns of interpretation, attribution process, and reporting style. Research into the validity of psychodynamic concepts of hypochondriasis has been quite neglected, and it should receive appropriate attention in the future. Prospective, follow-up studies of individuals who may be at greater risk for developing hypochondriasis (e.g., those who were inordinately ill or abused in childhood or whose parents suffered from chronic and severe diseases) would help distinguish between causal factors in hypochondriasis and consequences of hypochondriasis.

A better understanding of the psychopathology of hypochondriasis is likely to contribute to more specific and more effective treatment. Future studies should aim to disentangle effects of nonspecific treatment factors from effects of specific components of the patient–physician relationship and of specific treatment techniques. Treatment studies should be conducted in the more homogeneous populations of hypochondriacal patients. These progressive steps would help bring us closer to the ideal situation of being able to match type of treatment to subtype of hypochondriasis (or to a particular "entity" in the hypochondriacal spectrum), knowing how to use such treatment, when, and for how long.

Finally, attempts to unravel the "mysteries" of hypochondriasis may tread on shifting ground. To the extent that comprehension of hypochondriasis will depend on appreciation of complex mind–body interactions, we must guard against those economic, political, technological, and social forces that erect barriers against the integration of *psyche* and *soma* (Lipsitt, 1997).

## References

American Psychiatric Association. 1994. *Diagnostic and Statistical Manual of Mental Disorders, Fourth Edition (DSM-IV)*. Washington, DC: American Psychiatric Association.

Barsky A.J., Brener J., Coeytaux R.R., Cleary P.D. 1995. Accurate awareness of heartbeat in hypochondriacal and nonhypochondriacal patients. *Journal of Psychosomatic Research* 39: 489–497.

Bass C.M., Murphy M.R. 1990. Somatization disorder: critique of the concept and suggestions for further research. In *Somatization: Physical Symptoms and Psychological Illness* (eds. Bass C.M., Cawley R.H.), Oxford: Blackwell Scientific.

Blackmore R. 1725. *A Treatise of the Spleen and Vapours: or, Hypochondriacal and Hysterical Affections with Three Discourses on the Nature and Cure of Cholick, Melancholy, and Palsies*. London: Pemberton.

Bouman T.K., Visser S. 1998. Cognitive and behavioural treatment of hypochondriasis. *Psychotherapy and Psychosomatics* 67: 214–221.

Clark D.M., Salkovskis P.M., Hackmann A., Wells A., Fennell M., Ludgate J., Ahmad S., Richards H.C., Gelder M. 1998. Two psychological treatments for hypochondriasis: a randomised controlled trial. *British Journal of Psychiatry* 173: 218–225.

Cotard J. 1888. Hypocondrie. In *Dictionnaire Encyclopédique des Sciences Médicales, Vol. 51* (eds. Dechambre A., Lereboullet A.), Paris: Masson.

Deary I. 1999. A taxonomy of medically unexplained symptoms. Journal of *Psychosomatic Research* 47: 51–59.

Escobar J.L., Gara M.A. 1999. DSM-IV Somatoform disorders: do we need a new classification? *General Hospital Psychiatry* 21: 154–156.

Fallon B. 1999. Hypochondriasis vs. anxiety disorders: why should we care? *General Hospital Psychiatry* 21: 5–7.

Fallon B.A., Schneier F.R., Marshall R., Campeas R., Vermes D., Goetz D., Liebowitz M.R. 1996. The pharmacotherapy of hypochondriasis. *Psychopharmacology Bulletin* 32: 607–611.

Feuchtersleben Baron E. von. 1847. *The Principles of Medical Psychology* (translated by H.E. Evand and B.G. Babington). London: The Sydenham Society.

Griesinger W. 1861. *Die Pathologie und Therapie der psychischen Krankheiten, Second Edition*. Stuttgart: Krabbe.

Guislain J. 1852. *Leçons orales sur les phrénopathies, ou traité théorique et pratique des maladies mentales*, 3 vols. Gand: L. Hebbelynck.

Gureje O., Üstün T.B., Simon G.E. 1997. The syndrome of hypochondriasis: a cross-national study in primary care. *Psychological Medicine* 27: 1001–1010.

Kellner R., Hernandez J., Pathak D. 1992. Hypochondriacal fears and beliefs, anxiety, and somatization. British Journal of Psychiatry 160: 525–532.

Krafft-Ebing R. v 1893. Lehrbuch der Psychiatrie, Fifth Edition. Stuttgart: Enke.

Lipsitt D.R. 1997. From fragmentation to integration: a history of comprehensive patient care. In Primary Care Meets Mental Health: Tools for the 21st Century (eds. Haber J.D., Mitchell G.E.), Tiburon, California: CentraLink Publications.

Martin R.D. 1999. The somatoform conundrum: a question of nosological values. General Hospital Psychiatry 21: 177–186.

Morel B.A. 1860. Traité des Maladies Mentales. Paris: Masson.

Ono Y., Janca A. 1999. Rethinking somatoform disorders. Journal of Psychosomatic Research 46: 537–539.

Reid S., Wessely S. 1999. Somatoform disorders. Current Opinion in Psychiatry 12: 163–168.

Rief W., Hiller W. 1998. Somatization—future perspectives on a common phenomenon. Journal of Psychosomatic Research 44: 529–536.

Rush B. 1812. Medical Inquiries and Observations upon the Diseases of the Mind. New York: Hafner, 1962.

Savage G. 1892. Hypochondriasis and insanity. In A Dictionary of Psychological Medicine, Vol. 1 (ed. Tuke D.H.), London: J & A Churchill.

Smith G.R. Jr., Monson R.A., Ray D.C. 1986. Psychiatric consultation in somatization disorder: a randomized, controlled study. New England Journal of Medicine 314: 1407–1413.

Sydenham T. 1850. The Works of Thomas Sydenham M.D. (transl. by G. Latham), 2 vols. London: The Sydenham Society.

Tyrer P., Lee I., Alexander J. 1980. Awareness of cardiac function in anxious, phobic and hypochondriacal patients. Psychological Medicine 10: 171–174.

Tyrer P., Fowler-Dixon R., Ferguson B., Kelemen A. 1990. A plea for the diagnosis of hypochondriacal personality disorder. Journal of Psychosomatic Research 34: 637–642.

Warwick H.M.C., Clark D.M., Cobb A.M., Salkovskis P.M. 1996. A controlled trial of cognitive-behavioural treatment of hypochondriasis. British Journal of Psychiatry 169: 189–195.

Wells A. 1997. Cognitive Therapy of Anxiety Disorders: A Practice Manual and Conceptual Guide. Chichester: John Wiley.

Wesner R.B., Noyes R. 1991. Imipramine: an effective treatment for illness phobia. Journal of Affective Disorders 22: 43–48.

Wessely S., Nimnuan C., Sharpe M. 1999. Functional somatic syndromes: one or many? Lancet 354: 936–939.

Willis Th. 1685. The London Practice of Physick. London: Thomas Basset.

World Health Organization. 1992. The ICD-10 Classification of Mental and Behavioural Disorders: Clinical Descriptions and Diagnostic Guidelines. Geneva: World Health Organization.

World Health Organization. 1993. The ICD-10 Classification of Mental and Behavioural Disorders: Diagnostic Criteria for Research. Geneva: World Health Organization.

# Coda

In closing, we are pleased that the idea to produce an international resource on hypochondriasis, born in Spain at the time of the World Congress of Psychiatry in 1996, has completed a journey over the high seas of enthusiasm and inspiration and through the arid lands of doubts and obstacles. We acknowledge the mutual satisfaction of a transoceanic editorship that has weathered both national and personal crises and has been a heartwarming testimony to international colleagueship and collaboration. We have not only edited each other but also educated each other, especially with the aid of our dedicated contributors. We hope that the original idea, now represented in this book, will continue its exploratory and exciting journey in the minds of our readers.

We wish also to express our appreciation to Fiona Stevens and Jeff House of Oxford University Press for their encouragement and support from beginning to end of this project. We are grateful for their patience at times when we needed it most.

And in bringing closure to this extraordinary journey, we wish to thank Susan Hannan of Oxford University Press for her thoughtful guidance with final editing, and Sydney Wolfe Cohen for his indexing expertise in constructing the ultimate guide to the book's contents.

*Vladan Starcevic*
*Don R. Lipsitt*

# Appendices

# Appendix 1

## The Structured Diagnostic Interview for Hypochondriasis (modified from Barsky et al., 1992)*

*PROBE QUESTIONS:*
1) Do you have a lot of medical problems?          Yes   No
2) Do you have symptoms that bother you a lot?     Yes   No

- **Persistent Symptoms and Inadequate Physical Explanation**

1) What kinds of symptoms have you been having in the last six months?

**Interviewer note:** List each of the patient's symptoms. Probe each one using the techniques and probe flow chart from the DIS-3R. If patient gets a "5", code them as having somatic symptoms without a medical explanation.

| | | | | | |
|---|---|---|---|---|---|
| Symptom #1 _____ | 1 | 2 | 3 | 4 | 5 |
| Symptom #2 _____ | 1 | 2 | 3 | 4 | 5 |
| Symptom #3 _____ | 1 | 2 | 3 | 4 | 5 |
| Symptom #4 _____ | 1 | 2 | 3 | 4 | 5 |
| Symptom #5 _____ | 1 | 2 | 3 | 4 | 5 |

| **Somatic Symptoms** | **No Somatic Symptoms** | **Adequate Physical Explanation** | **No Adequate Physical Explanation** |
|---|---|---|---|

*Reprinted with permission from Dr. Arthur Barsky

Barsky A.J., Cleary P.D., Wyshak G., Spitzer R.L., Williams J.B.W., Klerman G.L. 1992. A structured diagnostic interview for hypochondriasis: a proposed criterion standard. *Journal of Nervous and Mental Disease* 180: 20–27.

- **Not Reassurable**
1) Has the doctor tried to reassure you about these symptoms (ask about symptoms which got a "5")?                                                    Yes     No
2) Did the reassurance make you feel better?                                   Yes     No
3) Do you feel that your doctor(s) examined and handled your illness well or were you dissatisfied with the way it was examined or handled?

                                                        Handled Well      Dissatisfied
4) Did you often think your doctors were mistaken about the cause or diagnosis, or what should be done about it?                No     Sometimes    Yes
**Reassurable        Not Reassurable**

- **Disease Fear or Conviction**
1) Is your health on your mind a lot?                                          Yes     No
2) Are you concerned about your health?                                        Yes     No
3) Do you worry about getting sick or being sick?                              Yes     No
4) Are you concerned that you might have a serious illness that has not been detected yet?                                                             Yes     No
5) In the past twelve months have you had a period of 6 months or more when you worried about having a serious physical illness most of the time?

                                                                              Yes     No

**Diagnosis of DSM-IV Hypochondriasis**
**Interviewer note:** Based on the patient's answers to the above questions, code whether or not they meet each of the following criteria. All criteria must be met to receive the diagnosis.

*Criterion A)*
    Preoccupation with the fear of having, or the belief that one has, a serious disease, based on the person's interpretation of the physical signs or sensations as evidence of physical illness.
**1** = Criterion A met
**0** = Criterion A not met

*Criterion B)*
    Appropriate physical evaluation does not support the diagnosis of any physical disorder that can account for the physical signs or sensations or the person's unwarranted interpretation of them, and the symptoms in A are not just symptoms of panic attacks.
1 = Criterion B met
0 = Criterion B not met

*Criterion C)*
    The fear of having, or belief that one has, a disease persists despite medical reassurance.

**1** = Criterion C met
**0** = Criterion C not met

DSM-IV hypochondriasis
**1** = Diagnosis of hypochondriasis
**0** = No diagnosis of hypochondriasis

**History of Hypochondriasis**
*PROBE QUESTIONS:*
1) When did concerns and worries about your health start bothering you like this?
2) Since your concerns began bothering you, has your health worried you all of the time, or have you had any periods of time when you weren't worried a lot (more days than not) about your health?
   **Worried all the time about health     Periods not worried about health**
3) What is the longest period of time you remember when concerns about your health did not bother you a lot?
   _____months (**Interviewer note:** a period of *6 months or more* required for course to be episodic)
4) For what percentage of time, since the start of your concerns, has your health worried you or been on your mind a lot? _____ %

*Interviewer note:* Based on the patient's answers to the above questions, code the following information for history of the diagnosis.
- Age onset _____
- Course: 0 = Chronic; 1 = Episodic
- If Episodic, estimation of percentage of time spent worried _____ % (since the onset of concerns)

# Appendix 2

## The Whiteley Index (Pilowsky, 1967)*

In response to each of the following questions, please circle Yes or No.

1. Do you often worry about the possibility that you have a serious illness?      Yes    No
2. Are you bothered by many pains and aches?      Yes    No
3. Do you find that you are often aware of various things happening in your body?      Yes    No
4. Do you worry a lot about your health?      Yes    No
5. Do you often have the symptoms of a very serious illness?      Yes    No
6. If a disease is brought to your attention (through the radio, television, newspapers, or someone you know) do you worry about getting it yourself?      Yes    No
7. If you feel ill and someone tells you that you are looking better, do you become annoyed?      Yes    No
8. Do you find that you are bothered by many different symptoms?      Yes    No
9. Is it hard for you to forget about yourself and think about all sorts of other things?      Yes    No
10. Is it hard for you to believe the doctor when he tells you there is nothing to worry about?      Yes    No
11. Do you get the feeling that people are not taking your illness seriously?      Yes    No
12. Do you think that you worry about your health more than most people?      Yes    No
13. Do you think there is something seriously wrong with your body?      Yes    No
14. Are you afraid of illness?      Yes    No

*Reprinted with permission from Dr. Issy Pilowsky.

Pilowsky I. 1967. Dimensions of hypochondriasis. *British Journal of Psychiatry* 113: 89–93.

# Appendix 3

# The Illness Behaviour Questionnaire (Pilowsky et al., 1984)*

1. Do you worry a lot about your health?     Yes    No
2. Do you think there is something seriously wrong with your body?     Yes    No
3. Does your illness interfere with your life a great deal?     Yes    No
4. Are you easy to get on with when you are ill?     Yes    No
5. Does your family have a history of illness?     Yes    No
6. Do you think you are more liable to illness than other people?     Yes    No
7. If the doctor told you that he could find nothing wrong with you would you believe him?     Yes    No
8. Is it easy for you to forget about yourself and think about all sorts of other things?     Yes    No
9. If you feel ill and someone else tells you that you are looking better, do you become annoyed?     Yes    No
10. Do you find that you are often aware of various things happening in your body?     Yes    No
11. Do you ever think of your illness as a punishment for something you have done wrong in the past?     Yes    No
12. Do you have trouble with your nerves?     Yes    No
13. If you feel ill or worried, can you be easily cheered up by the doctor?     Yes    No

*Reprinted with permission from Dr. Issy Pilowsky.

Pilowsky I., Spence N., Cobb J., Katsikitis M. 1984. The Illness Behavior Questionnaire as an aid to clinical assessment. *General Hospital Psychiatry* 6: 123–130.

14. Do you think that other people realize what it's like to be sick?            Yes    No

15. Does it upset you to talk to the doctor about your illness?     Yes    No

16. Are you bothered by many pains and aches?                 Yes    No

17. Does your illness affect the way you get on with your family or friends a great deal?                        Yes    No

18. Do you find that you get anxious easily?                   Yes    No

19. Do you know anybody who has the same illness as you?      Yes    No

20. Are you more sensitive to pain than other people?        Yes    No

21. Are you afraid of illness?                               Yes    No

22. Can you express your personal feelings easily to other people?   Yes    No

23. Do people feel sorry for you when you are ill?           Yes    No

24. Do you think that you worry about your health more than most people?                               Yes    No

25. Do you find that your illness affects your sexual relations?    Yes    No

26. Do you experience a lot of pain with your illness?       Yes    No

27. Except for your illness, do you have any problems in your life?                                   Yes    No

28. Do you care whether or not people realize you are sick?     Yes    No

29. Do you find that you get jealous of other people's good health?                                Yes    No

30. Do you ever have silly thoughts about your health which you can't get out of your mind, no matter how hard you try?   Yes    No

31. Do you have any financial problems?                   Yes    No

32. Are you upset by the way people take your illness?       Yes    No

33. Is it hard for you to believe the doctor when he tells you there is nothing for you to worry about?               Yes    No

34. Do you often worry about the possibility that you have got a serious illness?                              Yes    No

35. Are you sleeping well?                                 Yes    No

36. When you are angry, do you tend to bottle up your feelings?   Yes    No

37. Do you often think that you might suddenly fall ill?      Yes    No

38. If a disease is brought to your attention (through the radio, television, newspapers, or someone you know) do you worry about getting it yourself?                            Yes    No

39. Do you get the feeling that people are not taking your illness seriously enough?                             Yes    No

40. Are you upset by the appearance of your face or body?     Yes    No

41. Do you find that you are bothered by many different symptoms?                                Yes    No

| | | | |
|---|---|---|---|
| 42. | Do you frequently try to explain to others how you are feeling? | Yes | No |
| 43. | Do you have any family problems? | Yes | No |
| 44. | Do you think there is something the matter with your mind? | Yes | No |
| 45. | Are you eating well? | Yes | No |
| 46. | Is your bad health the biggest difficulty of your life? | Yes | No |
| 47. | Do you find that you get sad easily? | Yes | No |
| 48. | Do you worry or fuss over small details that seem unimportant to others? | Yes | No |
| 49. | Are you always a co-operative patient? | Yes | No |
| 50. | Do you often have the symptoms of a very serious disease? | Yes | No |
| 51. | Do you find that you get angry easily? | Yes | No |
| 52. | Do you have any work problems? | Yes | No |
| 53. | Do you prefer to keep your feelings to yourself? | Yes | No |
| 54. | Do you often find that you get depressed? | Yes | No |
| 55. | Would all your worries be over if you were physically healthy? | Yes | No |
| 56. | Are you more irritable toward other people? | Yes | No |
| 57. | Do you think that your symptoms may be caused by worry? | Yes | No |
| 58. | Is it easy for you to let people know when you are cross with them? | Yes | No |
| 59. | Is it hard for you to relax? | Yes | No |
| 60. | Do you have personal worries which are not caused by physical illness? | Yes | No |
| 61. | Do you often find that you lose patience with other people? | Yes | No |
| 62. | Is it hard for you to show people your personal feelings? | Yes | No |

# Appendix 4

## Illness Attitude Scales (modified from Kellner et al., 1983–84)*

Please describe how you feel *now* or how you have felt *recently*, not how you generally feel. Circle your answer. Please answer the other few questions with a few words or sentences.

0 = No ("Not at all" for question 15b)
1 = Rarely
2 = Sometimes
3 = Often
4 = Most of the time

| | |
|---|---|
| 1. Do you worry about your health? | 0  1  2  3  4 |
| 2. Are you worried that you may get a serious illness in the future? | 0  1  2  3  4 |
| 3. Does the thought of a serious illness scare you? | 0  1  2  3  4 |
| 4. If you have a pain, do you worry that it may be caused by a serious illness? | 0  1  2  3  4 |
| 5. If a pain lasts for a week or more, do you see a physician? | 0  1  2  3  4 |
| 6. If a pain lasts a week or more, do you believe that you have a serious illness? | 0  1  2  3  4 |
| 7. Do you avoid habits that may be harmful to you such as smoking? | 0  1  2  3  4 |

*Reprinted with permission of The University of New Mexico from Kellner R., Abbott P., Pathak D., Winslow W.W., Umland B.E. 1983–84. Hypochondriacal beliefs and attitudes in family practice and psychiatric patients. *International Journal of Psychiatry* in Medicine 13: 127–139.

8. Do you avoid foods that may not be healthy?     0   1   2   3   4

9. Do you examine your body to find whether there is
   something wrong?     0   1   2   3   4

10. Do you believe that you have a physical disease but
    the doctors have not diagnosed it correctly?     0   1   2   3   4

11. When your doctor tells you that you have no
    physical disease to account for your symptoms,
    do you refuse to believe him?     0   1   2   3   4

12. When you have been told by a doctor what he found,
    do you soon begin to believe that you may have
    developed a new illness?     0   1   2   3   4

13. Are you afraid of news that reminds you of death
    (such as funerals, obituary notices)?     0   1   2   3   4

14. Does the thought of death scare you?     0   1   2   3   4

15. Are you afraid that you may die soon?     0   1   2   3   4

15a. Has your doctor told you that you have an illness now?     Yes     No
    If yes, what illness? _____

15b. How often do you worry about this illness?     0   1   2   3   4

16. Are you afraid that you may have cancer?     0   1   2   3   4

17. Are you afraid that you may have heart disease?     0   1   2   3   4

18. Are you afraid that you may have another serious illness?     0   1   2   3   4
    Which illness? _____

19. When you read or hear about an illness, do you
    get symptoms similar to those of the illness?     0   1   2   3   4

20. When you notice a sensation in your body, do you
    find it difficult to think of something else?     0   1   2   3   4

21. When you feel a sensation in your body, do you
    worry about it?     0   1   2   3   4

22. How often do you see a doctor?     0 = Almost never
        1 = Only very rarely
        2 = About 4 times a year
        3 = About once a month
        4 = About once a week

23. How many different doctors, chiropractors or other healers have you seen
    in the past year?     0 = None
        1 = 1
        2 = 2 or 3
        3 = 4 or 5
        4 = 6 or more

24. How often have you been treated during the past year? (For example, drugs, change of drugs, surgery, etc.)     0 = Not at all
                                                              1 = Once
                                                              2 = 2 or 3 times
                                                              3 = 4 or 5 times
                                                              4 = 6 or more times

If you have been treated,
what were the treatments? _____

_____

The next three questions concern your bodily symptoms (for example, pain, aches, pressure in your body, breathing difficulties, tiredness, etc.).

25. Do your bodily symptoms stop you from working?          0  1  2  3  4
26. Do your bodily symptoms stop you from concentrat-
    ing on what you are doing?                              0  1  2  3  4
27. Do your bodily symptoms stop you from enjoying
    yourself?                                               0  1  2  3  4

# Appendix 5

## The Somatosensory Amplification Scale (modified from Barsky et al., 1990)*

Please indicate the degree to which each of the following statements are true of you in general. Circle your answer.

1 = Not at all true
2 = A little bit true
3 = Moderately true
4 = Quite a bit true
5 = Extremely true

| | |
|---|---|
| 1. I can't stand smoke, smog, or pollutants in the air. | 1 2 3 4 5 |
| 2. I am often aware of various things happening within my body. | 1 2 3 4 5 |
| 3. When I bruise myself, it stays noticeable for a long time. | 1 2 3 4 5 |
| 4. I sometimes can feel the blood flowing in my body. | 1 2 3 4 5 |
| 5. Sudden loud noises really bother me. | 1 2 3 4 5 |
| 6. I can sometimes hear my pulse or my heartbeat throbbing in my ear. | 1 2 3 4 5 |
| 7. I hate to be too hot or too cold. | 1 2 3 4 5 |
| 8. I am quick to sense the hunger contractions in my stomach. | 1 2 3 4 5 |
| 9. Even something minor, like an insect bite or a splinter, really bothers me. | 1 2 3 4 5 |
| 10. I can't stand pain. | 1 2 3 4 5 |

*Reprinted with permission from Dr. Arthur Barsky.

Barsky A.J., Wyshak G., Klerman G.L. 1990. The Somatosensory Amplification Scale and its relationship to hypochondriasis. *Journal of Psychiatric Research* 24: 323–334.

# Index